Veterinary Physiology and Applied Anatomy:

A textbook for veterinary nurses and technicians

Commissioning editor: Mary Seager
Development editor: Caroline Savage
Production controller: Anthony Read
Desk editor: Jackie Holding
Cover designer: Gregory Harris

Veterinary Physiology and Applied Anatomy:

A textbook for veterinary nurses and technicians

Louise Tartaglia BSc(Hons) MSc
with
Anne Waugh BSc(Hons) MSc cert ed SRN RNT ILTM

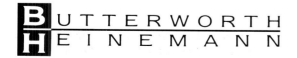

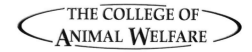

OXFORD   AUCKLAND   BOSTON   JOHANNESBURG
MELBOURNE   NEW DELHI

BUTTERWORTH-HEINEMANN
An imprint of Elsevier Science

First published 2002

British Library Cataloguing in Publication Data
Tartaglia, Louise
  Veterinary physiology and applied anatomy of small snimals:
  a textbook for veterinary nurses and technicians
  1. Veterinary anatomy   2. Veterinary physiology   3. Pet medicine
  I. Title   II. Waugh, Anne   III. College of Animal Welfare
  636'.089'2

ISBN 0 7506 4802 3

Composition by Genesis Typesetting, Laser Quay, Rochester, Kent
Printed and bound in Italy by Printer Trento S.r.l.

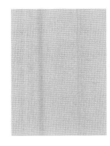

Contents

Preface   vii

Acknowledgements   ix

1 Basic principles of living matter   1
  1.1 Basic biochemistry   1
      Introduction   1
      The chemistry of life   1
      The atom   1
      Chemical bonding   3
      Solutes and solvents   5
      Acids, alkalis and pH   6
      SI units in practice   7
  1.2 Cells, tissue and organs   10
      Introduction   10
      Cellular structure and function   10
      Cell division   14
      Tissues   17
      Organs and body systems   23
  1.3 The mammalian body   23
      Introduction   23
      Anatomical terminology   24
      Basic anatomy of the dog and cat   24
      Body cavities   24
      Homeostasis and body fluids   28
  Review questions   31

2 Co-ordination and control   34
  2.1 Nervous tissue   34
      Introduction   34
      Neurones and neuroglia   34
      Classification of neurones   36
      Nerve fibres   38
      Neurophysiology   39
      The transmembrane potential   39
      The action potential   40
      The nervous impulse   41
  2.2 The nervous system   45
      Introduction   45

      The central nervous system   46
      The brain   46
      The spinal cord   48
      The peripheral nervous system   48
      The autonomic nervous system   53
  2.3 Special senses   55
      Introduction   55
      Vision   56
      Optic chambers   58
      The lens   58
      Rods and cones   59
      Protection of the eye   60
      Audition   60
      Gustation   64
      Olfaction   64
  2.4 The endocrine system   64
      Introduction   64
      Hormone   65
      The hypothalamus   66
      The pituitary gland   66
      The pineal gland   69
      The parathyroid glands   69
      The thyroid gland   69
      The thymus   69
      The heart   70
      The digestive tract   70
      The kidneys   70
      The adrenal glands   70
      The pancreas   71
      The gonads   72
  Review questions   73

3 Support and movement   77
  3.1 The skeletal system   77
      Introduction   77
      The skeleton   77
      The formation and structure of bone   77
      Classification of bones   81
      Features of the surfaces of bone   82

3.2 The muscular system   83
    Introduction   83
    Muscle tissue   83
    Striated (voluntary) muscle   83
    Muscle contraction   83
    Aerobic and anaerobic respiration   85
    Smooth (involuntary) muscle   86
    Cardiac muscle   86
    Skeletal muscles   86
3.3 Joints   88
    Introduction   88
    Joint classification   88
    Movement of a synovial joint   89
    Ligaments   90
    Tendons   91
Review questions   91

4 Transport   93
4.1 Blood   93
    Introduction   93
    Blood   93
        Plasma   93
        Blood corpuscles (cells)   94
    Haemopoiesis   96
    Haemostasis   97
    Fibrinolysis   99
4.2 The cardiovascular system   99
    Introduction   99
    Anatomy of the heart   99
    Cardiac muscle   100
    Heart valves   101
    Heartbeat and conduction   102
    The vascular system   104
    Heart rate and cardiac output   108
    Blood pressure   108
    Shock   110
Review questions   111

**5 Attainment of nutrients and disposal
of waste**   113
5.1 The digestive system   113
    Introduction   113
    The digestive process   113
    The digestive or alimentary tract   114
    Digestive secretions   118
    The exocrine function of the pancreas 119
    Bile   120
    Absorption of the products of digestion 120
    Defecation   122
    Vomiting or emesis   122
5.2 The liver   122
    Introduction   122

    Metabolism of the products of
        digestion   122
    The composition of blood   123
5.3 The urinary system   123
    Introduction   123
    Structure of the urinary system   123
    Structure and function of the kidney 124
    The ureters, urinary bladder and urethra 128
    Neural control of urination   128
    Composition of urine   128
5.4 The respiratory system   129
    Introduction   129
    Basic principles of respiration   129
    Composition of inspired and expired
        air   130
    Structure of the respiratory system   130
    The mechanism of respiration   132
    Control of respiration   134
Review questions   136

6 Survival, development and defence   139
6.1 The integument   139
    Introduction   139
    Structure of the integument/skin   139
    Specialization of the integument   141
    Hair   143
    Specialized glands   144
6.2 The defence function   144
    Introduction   144
    Non-specific defences   144
    Specific defence: immunity   145
6.3 The lymphatic system   147
    Introduction   147
    Circulation of tissue fluid   147
    Structure of the lymphatic system   148
    Lymphatic tissue   149
6.4 Reproduction   149
    Introduction   149
    The male reproductive system   150
    The female reproductive system   152
    Mating and pregnancy   154
    Parturition   162
    Lactation   163
Review questions   164

References   167

Further Reading   168

Answers   169

Glossary   183

Index   205

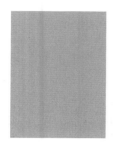

Preface

Before we can start to consider the complex structure and function of the mammalian body we should consider some general terminology.

The word around which the content of this book is focused is 'physiology'. This is derived from Greek and means 'the science of the processes of life in plants and animals' or, to be more specific to veterinary studies, 'the study of how animals perform their vital functions'.

Another closely related word, without which physiology would have difficulty existing, is 'anatomy'. This is 'the science of the structure of the body' or, more specifically, 'the study of the structure of the internal and external body structures'.

As the structure of an object is always related to its function (there would be little point in trying to use a spoon to cut a steak or a knife to eat a bowl of soup), it is difficult, if not impossible, to study the physiology of any living organism without considering its anatomy. Consequently, although this text will focus primarily upon the physiology of the mammalian body, reference will also be needed to basic anatomy.

Louise Tartaglia
Anne Waugh

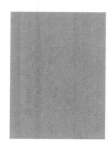

Acknowledgements

I would like to thank the College of Animal Welfare, in particular Barbara Cooper for the opportunity to write this text and for her support, advice and guidance. I would also like to thank my husband Andy for his Veterinary advice and Anne for her constructive comments during its completion. Finally, I would like to thank my students past, present and future for the continuing challenge in helping each of them reach an understanding of what to many, is a complex subject. I hope that this text goes some way in helping them and encouraging them to keep asking 'How?' and 'Why?'

Louise Tartaglia

1
Basic principles of living matter

1.1 Basic biochemistry

> The chemistry of life
> The atom
> Chemical bonding
> Solutes and solvents
> Acids, alkalis and pH
> SI units in practice

Introduction

To examine the complex working systems of the mammalian body, we need to have an understanding of the basic chemical principles and theories that determine the biochemical reactions involved in living processes. These will, in turn, help us to understand the more complex processes occurring at a cellular level and ultimately within the tissues, organs, and systems that form the body as a whole.

The chemistry of life

The study of the chemistry of living systems is termed biochemistry. It examines the molecular reactions that occur during living processes and consequently requires an understanding of both chemistry and biology.

Perhaps the best place to start is at the beginning, with the smallest, indivisible (until recently) part of everything, the atom.

The atom

Before we think about the atom, we need to consider some other chemical terminology.

An **element** is a pure substance that cannot be split up by a chemical reaction. There are 92 naturally occurring elements and some 13 more man-made. The majority are solid or metallic but some are liquid or gases at room temperature and atmospheric pressure.

Examples of solids include: carbon, calcium, iron, zinc
Examples of liquids include: mercury, bromine
Examples of gases include: hydrogen, oxygen, nitrogen

Each element has its own chemical symbol that is used as a form of shorthand. The symbols for some of the more common elements found in the mammalian body are shown in Table 1.1.

A **compound** is the combination of two or more elements to form a chemical substance. Certain mixtures or elements react together (usually when heated) to form compounds. Energy is usually released when mixtures/elements combine to form compounds. The compounds formed have very different properties from their constituent elements. Splitting a compound is not usually an easy process.

An example of a compound is water, which is formed from hydrogen and oxygen

- The chemical symbol for the element hydrogen is H
- The chemical symbol for the element oxygen is O
- As gases, hydrogen and oxygen atoms always exist in pairs, therefore the symbol for oxygen gas is O_2 and for hydrogen gas, H_2.
- When forming the compound water, two hydrogen atoms always combine with one atom of

Table 1.1 Common elements found in the mammalian body

Element	Atomic symbol	Approximate percentage by weight
Oxygen[a]	O	65
Carbon[a]	C	18
Hydrogen[a]	H	10
Nitrogen[a]	N	3
Calcium[a]	Ca	2
Phosphorus[a]	P	1
Potassium[b]	K	0.35
Sulphur[b]	S	0.25
Sodium[b]	Na	0.15
Chlorine[b]	Cl	0.15
Magnesium[c]	Mg	*
Iron[c]	Fe	*
Zinc[c]	Zn	*
Copper[c]	Cu	*
Iodine[c]	I	*
Manganese[c]	Mn	*
Chromium[c]	Cr	*
Molybdenum[c]	Mo	*
Cobalt[c]	Co	*
Selenium[c]	Se	*

[a] 99% approximate weight;
[b] 0.9% approximate weight;
[c] 0.1% approximate weight.
* denotes 'trace'.

Table 1.2 Properties of sub-atomic particles

Particle	Relative mass	Relative charge	Location
Neutron	1	0	nucleus
Proton	1	+1	nucleus
Electron	5.4×10^{-4}	−1	orbital shells

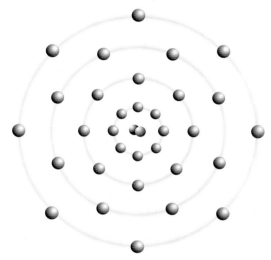

Figure 1.1 Diagrammatic representation of the structure of an atom. Electrons travel around the nucleus at certain energy levels and protons and neutrons pack together in the nucleus

oxygen gas, therefore the reaction can be represented as:

$$2H_2 \text{ (g)} + O_2 \text{ (g)} \rightarrow 2H_2O \text{ (l)},$$

or as

$$\text{Hydrogen}_{\text{(gas)}} + \text{Oxygen}_{\text{(gas)}} \rightarrow \text{Water}_{\text{(liquid)}}$$

The **atom** can be defined as the smallest part of an element that can exist whilst retaining the physical and chemical properties of that element. Each element has its own particular atom which is different from all other atoms, however they are all made up of three basic subatomic particles:

1. Protons (p)
2. Neutrons (n)
3. Electrons (e⁻)

Table 1.2 shows the mass and charge of the different sub-atomic particles. A diagrammatic representation of their location within the atom is shown in Figure 1.1.

Protons and neutrons are located in the nucleus and have the same relative mass. The much smaller electrons (with negligible mass) are located in orbital shells around the nucleus. Each shell can only accommodate a certain number of electrons and those further away from the nucleus contain electrons with a higher energy level than those in the inner orbitals.

In an atom, the number of negatively charged electrons always equals the number of positively charged protons and consequently, the atom has no charge (is neutral). The **atomic number** of an atom is equal to the number of electrons or protons and is different for each element. The **mass number** of an element is the sum of the neutrons and protons in the atom (those sub-atomic particles that have a significant mass). For example:

● Hydrogen has an atomic number of 1, because it has 1 proton and 1 electron. Its mass number is also 1, as it has 1 proton but no neutrons.

- The atom hydrogen can be written as ^1_1H. The lower number is the atomic number and is equal to the number of protons or electrons. The upper number is the mass number and represents the number of protons and neutrons.
- Sodium has an atomic number of 11 and a mass number of 23. It therefore has 11 protons, 11 electrons, and 12 neutrons and can be written as $^{23}_{11}Na$.

The mass number determines the relative atomic mass of the element and can be referred to as its atomic weight.

Some elements have more than one type of atom, the difference being in the number of neutrons within the nucleus. These different atoms are called **isotopes** of a particular element.

For example, the oxygen atom exists in three forms (isotopes):

- Oxygen-16, which has 8 protons, 8 electrons, and 8 neutrons
- Oxygen-17, which has 8 protons, 8 electrons, and 9 neutrons
- Oxygen-18, which has 8 protons, 8 electrons, and 10 neutrons

These three isotopes are all oxygen elements as they have the same number of protons and electrons. The difference in neutrons means that they have similar chemical properties but slightly different physical properties.

Some isotopes of certain elements have unstable nuclei due to the presence of extra neutrons in the nucleus. They have a tendency to change into other more stable structures whilst emitting energy and some sub-atomic particles. Such isotopes can be described as radioactive isotopes and break down into their more stable form over time (a process known as radioactive decay). For example:

- The radioactive form of carbon, carbon-14 (^{14}C), exists in all living tissue in a fixed ratio to the more stable ^{12}C that is not radioactive. After death, the ^{14}C starts to decay slowly at a fixed rate. Therefore, measurement of the levels of ^{14}C in organic materials can allow an accurate determination of the age of the material. This process, called radio-carbon dating, is used extensively in archaeology to date materials of organic origin.
- Radioactive forms of Iodine can be used in the medical field to study the activity of the thyroid gland.

Chemical bonding

Most elements in living systems exist as compounds. When two elements react to produce a compound, the atoms of the elements join together through the sharing or transfer of electrons in their outer orbitals. Each atom has a number of electrons that it can share, donate or receive. This number is termed the **valency** of the atom. An atom with a valency of 1 can share, donate, or receive 1 electron; hydrogen is an atom with a valency of 1. Oxygen has a valency of 2 and therefore uses two of its electrons in the formation of a chemical bond with another element or elements.

Covalent bonding

When electrons are shared between atoms during chemical bonding, the resultant **molecule** can be described as having **covalent bonds** between each atom.

An oxygen atom has an electron arrangement of 2, 6. This shows that the atom has 2 electrons in the inner orbital and 6 in the outer orbital. When forming an oxygen molecule, two oxygen atoms each donate two electrons and these four electrons are shared between the two atoms, to form the oxygen molecule, O_2, as shown in Figure 1.2.

This is known as a double covalent bond as two pairs of electrons are shared between the atoms. The electron arrangement within the molecule is more stable than in the single atom.

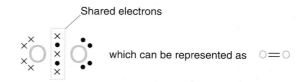

Figure 1.2 Formation of an oxygen molecule. **X** Represents electrons in the outer orbital of the first oxygen atom; • represents electrons in the outer orbital of the second oxygen atom

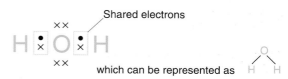

Figure 1.3 Formation of a water molecule. **X** Represents electrons in the outer orbital of the oxygen atom; • represents the single electron of each of the hydrogen atoms

An example of single covalent bonds can be seen in the formation of a water molecule. Two hydrogen atoms combine with an oxygen atom, each sharing an electron with the oxygen in a single covalent bond, as illustrated in Figure 1.3.

Ionic bonding

Sometimes, instead of sharing electrons as in covalent bonding, electrons are transferred from one atom to another, to form an **ionic** or **electrovalent** bond. The number of electrons transferred is determined by the valency of the atom (as with covalent bonding). An **ion** is formed when an atom gains or loses an electron. When an atom loses an electron it becomes a positively charged ion called a **cation**. If an atom gains an electron, it becomes a negatively charged ion called an **anion**. The cations are attracted to the anions within the compound and are held together by the electrical attraction of the opposite charges. For example, consider the formation of sodium chloride:

- Sodium (Na) has a valency of 1. It has an electron arrangement of 2,8,1. The single outer electron is unstable.
- Chlorine (Cl) also has a valency of 1. It has an electron arrangement of 2,8,7. The seven outer electrons are unstable, as 8 is the ideal number of electrons in the third orbit conferring a stable structure.

Consequently, when sodium chloride is formed, the sodium atom donates its single electron to the chlorine atom to form a stable ionic bond. The sodium atom loses an electron and becomes a sodium ion (Na^+) and the chlorine atom gains an electron, becoming a chloride ion (Cl^-). The compound formed is sodium chloride, or common salt (NaCl).

We can express this in the following equations:

$$Na \rightarrow Na^+ + e^- \text{ and } e^- + Cl \rightarrow Cl^-$$

Therefore, overall $Na + Cl \rightarrow Na^+ Cl^-$

The term 'salt' can be applied generically to any compound which exists in an ionic form. When dissolved in water, salts dissociate (or break up) into their anions and cations in solution. A substance that dissociates into ions in solution is called an **electrolyte.** These are important components of body fluids and are particularly important when considering rehydration therapy in practice.

Whilst other types of bonding can occur between atoms during chemical reactions, covalent and ionic bonds are the main types of bonding found in biochemical molecules and compounds. There is one final type of bonding, **hydrogen bonding**, that also plays an important role.

Hydrogen bonding

Hydrogen bonding differs from covalent and ionic bonding in that it does not involve the strong bonds formed between atoms during chemical reactions. Instead it describes the weaker bonds whereby molecules are attracted to other molecules. These are often called **intermolecular** bonds meaning 'between molecules'. One important type of intermolecular bonding that affects biological systems is the weak bonds that exist between the hydrogen atoms of different water molecules.

As discussed previously, a molecule of water is formed by single covalent bonds between hydrogen and oxygen, as represented in Figure 1.3. Two hydrogen atoms each share a single electron with one of the six electrons in the outer orbital of the oxygen atom. Consequently, the oxygen atom gains a stable structure of eight electrons and the hydrogen atoms a stable structure of 2 electrons (note that the inner orbital can only contain 2 electrons). However, there are 4 electrons of the oxygen atom that are unpaired and these give the oxygen part of the water molecule a slight negative charge. In addition, as the electrons of the hydrogen atoms have been drawn into the orbital of the oxygen atom, the hydrogen parts of the water molecule have a slight positive charge. This is illustrated in Figure 1.4.

Consequently, the slightly negatively charged oxygen component of one water molecule is

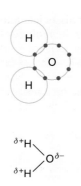

Figure 1.4 Polarity of the water molecule

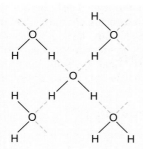

Figure 1.5 Hydrogen bonding in water

attracted to the slightly positively charged hydrogen component of another water molecule, to form weak intermolecular hydrogen bonds. These are represented in Figure 1.5.

Hydrogen bonding results in water being a liquid at room temperature and atmospheric pressure instead of a gas. This is critical to all life processes, which depend ultimately upon water and its properties as a liquid.

Solutes and solvents

Salts dissolve in water to form a solution of ions, as discussed previously. Any substance that dissolves to form a liquid (solution) can also be called a **solute**. The liquid in which it dissolves is called the **solvent.** Sodium chloride is a particular type of solute which dissociates into ions in solution and can be called an **electrolyte**. An electrolyte can be defined as a substance that dissolves in water to give a solution of ions. Sugar molecules, which are formed by covalent bonds rather than ionic bonds, like sodium chloride, also dissolve in water, due to the weak hydrogen bonds that form between the sugar and water molecules. Sugar can therefore still be described as a solute, although it is not an electrolyte as it does not dissociate into ions in solution.

Most reactions in biological systems occur in solutions in water (aqueous solutions). Therefore, the ability of a substance to dissolve in water and the way it behaves in solution is of great significance. A substance that dissolves in water can be termed **hydrophilic** ('water loving'). One that does not dissolve in water, for example lipid (fat), is termed **hydrophobic** ('water hating').

Diffusion and osmosis

Diffusion is the movement of molecules of a substance (usually gases) from an area of high concentration to an area of low concentration, until the concentration of the substance is uniform in both areas. For example, the smell of a stink bomb set off at the front of a classroom will gradually diffuse from the front of the classroom to the back, until all areas of the classroom smell the same.

Diffusion is the process whereby oxygen and nutrients move from blood vessels (where there is a high concentration of oxygen and nutrients) to the tissues (lower concentrations) where they are needed for cells to function.

Osmosis is the movement of a solvent (in biological systems, usually water) through a **semi-permeable membrane** in order to equalize the solute concentrations on both sides of the membrane. This is illustrated in Figure 1.6.

As the solute molecules cannot pass across the membrane (due to its partial permeability), the solvent molecules (water) move from a high water concentration (weak solution) to a low water concentration (strong solution) until the concentrations of the solvent are equal on both sides of the semi-permeable membrane. The **osmotic pressure** is the pressure that would need to be applied to prevent the movement of solvent (water) molecules from high to low concentration.

Osmosis is important in many biological processes. When a cell is surrounded by fluid that has a higher osmotic pressure than the fluid inside, then water moves out of the cell into the fluid surrounding it, in an effort to equalize the osmotic pressure within and outside the cell. Ultimately, if the osmotic pressure is very different, the cell shrinks and shrivels up. This is termed **crenation**. When the cell is surrounded by fluid with a lower osmotic pressure, then water moves into the cell, ultimately causing it to burst. This is termed **haemolysis**. Crenation and haemolysis can be demonstrated by placing blood cells into a strong salt solution or water, as illustrated in Figure 1.7.

The term **tonicity** is used to describe the **osmotic concentration** of a solution in relation to body fluids. A **hypertonic** (or **hyperosmotic**) solution is more concentrated than normal body fluids and will result in the situation illustrated in Figure 1.7(c). Conversely, a **hypotonic** (or **hypo-osmotic**) solution is less concentrated than body fluids and will result in the situation illustrated in Figure 1.7(b). An **isotonic** (or **iso-osmotic**) solution has the same concentration as body fluids and cells placed in such a solution will neither lose nor gain water. Normal saline (a 0.9% solution of sodium chloride) is isotonic with blood plasma.

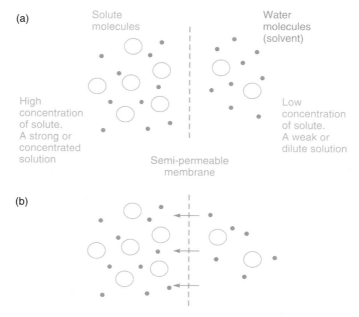

Figure 1.6 Diagrammatic illustration of the principle of osmosis

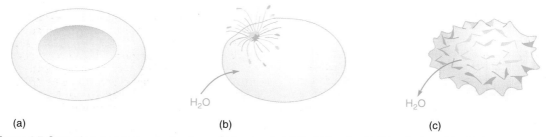

Figure 1.7 Crenation and haemolysis of a red blood cell. (a) Red blood cell; (b) cell placed in distilled water which causes it to swell and burst; (c) cell placed in a concentrated salt solution which causes it to shrink and shrivel

Acids, alkalis and pH

An acid is a molecule that, when dissolved in water, dissociates to release a hydrogen ion (H^+) or proton. For example:

$$HA \leftrightarrows H^+ + A^-$$

HA is an acid

The strength of the acid depends on how many protons are released. Strong acids (e.g. sulphuric acid) release a large number of protons and weak acids (e.g. acetic acid) release a small number of protons.

An alkali is a molecule that accepts protons (H^+), usually by dissolving in water to release hydroxide ions. For example:

$$H^+ + A^- \leftrightarrows HA$$

A^- is an alkali

The strength of an alkali depends upon the readiness with which it accepts protons. Sodium

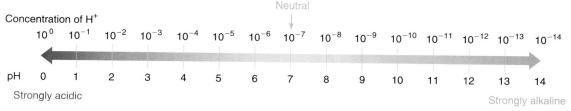

Figure 1.8 The pH scale of acids and bases

hydroxide is an example of a strong alkali. Weak alkalis are also called **bases** (e.g. ammonia).

The strength of an acid or alkali can be measured by assessing the concentration of hydrogen ions (protons) in solution. A logarithmic scale, where an increase in one unit represents a ten-fold increase in hydrogen ion concentration, is used to express the concentration of hydrogen ions in solution. This is known as the **pH scale**. The pH of a solution is always expressed relative to pH = 7 (or neutral) for pure water (neutrality is always taken as pH = 7, the pH of pure water). The pH scale goes from 1 to 14, 1 being strongly acidic and 14 strongly alkaline. Figure 1.8 shows the relation between pH and hydrogen ion concentration.

SI units in practice

Mathematical notation

Before considering the units of measurement we use in practice, it is useful to appreciate the correct mathematical approach to writing both the large and the small numbers that are involved with biological measurement.

The current system of measurement (the metric system) uses numbers that are based upon 10 (decimal numbers). For example, there are 10 millimetres in 1 centimetre and 100 (10 × 10) centimetres in 1 metre. When we consider larger numbers there is a mathematical short hand that allows us to abbreviate the number of decimal places in a number and to express that number to the power of 10. For example, 100 can be written as 10^2 because $100 = 1 \times 10 \times 10 = 1 \times 10^2$ (or 10^2, ten to the power of two, or ten squared).

Similarly:

$1000 = 1 \times 10^3 \ (10^3)$

$100 \times 100 = 10\,000 = 1 \times 10^4 \ (10^4)$, etc.

An alternative way to express the final example would be:

$10^2 \times 10^2 = 10^4$

Should the number contain numbers other than 1, e.g. 5000, then the number has to be expressed before the power ten, for example:

$5000 = 5 \times 10^3$

$5\,000\,000 = 5 \times 10^6$

If the number is not a whole number (i.e. contains a fraction or decimal place), then the number is expressed as a decimal with only one number to the left of the decimal point, for example:

Five and a half million = 5.5×10^6

Two and a quarter thousand = 2.25×10^3

(where $0.5 = \frac{1}{2}$, $0.25 = \frac{1}{4}$ and $0.75 = \frac{3}{4}$).

Living cells must maintain a constant pH in order for cellular enzymes and proteins to function correctly. If the environment within the cell becomes too hostile (e.g. too acidic or too alkaline) then the enzymes and proteins will be **denatured**, losing their structural shape and ability to function correctly. The normal pH range for living tissue is 7.0 to 7.8. That of canine arterial blood is 7.3–7.43 and for the cat is 7.27–7.4. When considering pH we need to consider the particular tissue or fluid in question. The pH of gastric acid would be far lower than either of the ranges previously mentioned. The maintenance of pH within the ideal range is achieved through **buffering**. A buffer is a substance which in solution, resists changes in pH by either 'mopping up' excess protons if the environment becomes too acidic, or by releasing protons if the environment become too alkaline. Examples of buffers in biological systems are some proteins and amino acids in the blood plasma (e.g. albumin, globulin and fibrinogen) and ammonia (and ammonium ions) excreted by the kidney to help stabilize the pH of urine.

Table 1.3 Common prefixes indicating the power of ten

Prefix	Symbol	Value	Factor by which the unit is multiplied
tera	T	1000 000 000 000	10^{12}
giga	G	1000 000 000	10^{9}
mega	M	1000 000	10^{6}
kilo*	k	1000	10^{3}
hecto	h	100	10^{2}
deca	da	10	10^{1}
deci	d	0.1	10^{-1}
centi*	c	0.01	10^{-2}
milli*	m	0.001	10^{-3}
micro*	μ†	0.000 001	10^{-6}
nano	n	0.000 000 001	10^{-9}
pico	p	0.000 000 000 001	10^{-12}
femto	f	0.000 000 000 000 001	10^{-15}
atto	a	0.000 000 000 000 000 001	10^{-18}

*Prefixes in common clinical use; †Greek 'mu' read as 'micro'.

When considering small numbers, the number is still expressed as a power of ten but a minus sign is used to indicate that the number is being divided by ten rather than multiplied by it, for example:

$$0.001 = 1 \times 10^{-3}$$

As a rule of thumb, the power 10 equals the number of decimal places that the decimal point has to move to express the number with one digit in front of the decimal place. If the movement is to the left, then the power 10 is positive and if the movement is to the right, the power 10 is negative. For example:

$$0.0045 = 4.5 \times 10^{-3}$$

$$0.000273 = 2.73 \times 10^{-4}$$

Prefixes can be used to indicate the power 10, as illustrated in Table 1.3.

SI units

Also, although 's' is added to the imperial measurements when plural, this is NOT the case with metric units.

Conversion from imperial units

In some cases it may be necessary to convert from imperial to metric units. The most common imperial units that were used in veterinary practice before the introduction of the metric system were stones (sts), pounds (lbs) and ounces (ozs) for weight and degrees Fahrenheit (F) for temperature.

Weight

For weight, 1 st = 14 lbs, 1 lb = 16 ozs, 1 kg = 2.2 lbs. Consequently, to convert pounds into kilograms, we divide by 2.2, for example:

$$26 \text{ lbs} = 26 \div 2.2 = 11.82 \text{ kg (to 2 decimal places)}$$

Note that although 's' is added to the imperial measures when plural, this is not the case with metric units.

Standard units based upon metric measurements are used in science and it is important to have an understanding of the basic units that may be encountered in practice. These standard units are called SI units (from the French, 'Systeme Internationale d'Unites') and they provide a standardized format for measurement in science.

There are seven basic SI units, shown in Table 1.4. These are used in combination with the prefixes in Table 1.3 to express units of measurement (N.B. although the SI unit for temperature is the Kelvin, K, this is not used in veterinary practice. For this type of work the Celsius scale is internationally recognized. For conversion, 0K = −273°C and 37°C = 273 + 37 = 310 K. Note that K is not preceded by a degree (°) symbol).

Table 1.4 Basic SI units

Physical quantity	Symbol of SI unit	Name of SI base unit
Length	m	metre
Mass	kg	kilogram
Time	s	second*
Temperature	K	Kelvin
Amount of substance	mol	mole
Electrical current	A	ampere
Luminous intensity	Cd	candela

*Although the second is the basic unit of time, the minute (min), hour (h) and day (d) may also be used.

9 sts = 9 × 14 = 126 lbs

126 lbs = 126 ÷ 2.2 = 57.27 kg (to 2 decimal places)

Temperature

For temperature, the conversion from Fahrenheit to Celsius is a little more complex and can be represented by the following equation:

$$\frac{(F-32) \times 5}{9} = °C$$

Therefore, to convert 98°F into °C:

Step 1. 98–32 = 66

Step 2. 66 × 5 = 330

Step 3. 330 ÷ 9 = 36.67°C (to 2 decimal places)

To convert °C into °F, the above steps should be reversed (i.e. multiply by 9, divide by 5 and add 32).

Concentrations

In chemical terminology the quantity of a substance is measured in moles (mol). One mole of a substance is the weight of one molecule of that substance in grams (g). For example:

> The molecular mass of Carbon is 12. Therefore one mole of Carbon atoms weigh 12 g

You should think of a mole as a fixed quantity rather like a dozen (12) eggs or a ream of paper (480 sheets). A mole of a substance is always equal to 6.023×10^{23} molecules. This is rather a large number, as molecules are very, very, small.

The concentration of a substance (i.e. the amount of a substance present in a given volume) is usually expressed using moles and litres (l). For example:

> The plasma glucose concentration of a healthy dog is 4 to 5.5 mmol/l (millimoles per litre)

Note that mmol/l may also be expressed as $mmol/l^{-1}$. The use of −1 as a superscript indicates that the unit directly preceding it should be understood to be 'per'. This notation system is more common in the USA.

More complex substances such as proteins are usually measured in grams per litre (g/l or $g\,l^{-1}$)

and enzymes are measured in international units (IU) per litre (IU/l or $IU\,l^{-1}$). For example:

> The total plasma protein concentration in the dog is approximately 50 g/l
> Plasma concentration of the enzyme lipase may be over 500 IU/l in a dog with pancreatitis

The only exception to the above is seen in the measurement of the haemoglobin concentration of blood and this is always measured in grams per decilitre (g/dl or $g\,dl^{-1}$). As 1 decilitre = 0.1 of a litre, then one decilitre is equivalent to 100 ml. Therefore haemoglobin is expressed as g per 100 ml (g/100 ml). For example:

> The mean corpuscular haemoglobin concentration (MCHC) is normally about 35 g/100 ml, irrespective of species

Concentrations may also be expressed as milli-equivalents per litre (mEq/l). It is now more usual to use the millimole, although a working knowledge of both is useful. The number of equivalents (Eq) can be calculated as follows:

$$\text{No. of equivalents} = \frac{\text{Weight in grams} \times \text{Valency}}{\text{Molecular weight}}$$

and the number of moles (mol) can be calculated using a similar equation without using the valency of the atom/ion:

$$\text{Number of moles (mol)} = \frac{\text{Weight in grams}}{\text{Molecular weight}}$$

When the valency of the ions concerned is 1 (e.g. Na^+, K^+) then the values from the above equations are the same. For example:

> A solution of potassium with a concentration of 100 mEq/l also has a concentration of 100 mmol/l

If the solution contains ions with a valency other than 1 (e.g. Mg^{2+}, Ca^{2+}), then the old units (mEq/l) should be divided by the valency. For example:

> A solution of calcium with a concentration of 100 mEq/l has a concentration of 50 mmol/l

Pressure

Although not used routinely in veterinary practice, it can be useful to measure blood pressure whilst monitoring anaesthesia or in the diagnosis of hypertension and some cardiac conditions. Whilst the standard unit of pressure is the Pascal (Pa) those more routinely used in the measurement of blood pressure include centimetres of water (cmH_2O) or millimetres of mercury (mmHg).

1.2 Cells, tissue and organs

Cellular structure and function
Cell division
Tissues
Organs and body systems

Introduction

The cell is the basic structural and functional unit of all living organisms. This section examines aspects of cellular structure and function, and looks at the structures of some specialized cells and tissues and their role within the mammalian body. The concept of specialization is expanded further to examine the generalized role of organs and body systems.

Cellular structure and function

Life evolved based upon a cellular structure, allowing the cell to become a system, isolated from the external environment, yet able to exchange chemical raw materials and waste products necessary for its function and for the maintenance of **homoeostasis**. Homoeostasis is the ability to maintain within acceptable limits, a constant cellular composition (pH, temperature, state of hydration, concentration of electrolytes, etc.) to permit normal cellular metabolism. The barrier between the cellular environment and that outside is the cell membrane (or **plasma membrane**) which controls the substances entering and leaving the cell. Two distinct regions of the cell can be identified, the **nucleus** and the **cytoplasm**. The nucleus contains the genetic material of the cell in the form of thin threads of **chromatin** and a dense area called the **nucleolus.** It is surrounded by the **nuclear membrane.** The cytoplasm is a semi-fluid, aqueous, substance and contains the nucleus, **cell organelles**, glucose, protein and salts.

Cells have specialized characteristics dependent upon their function within the animal. They may differ in their shape and content. For example, all cells contain a nucleus except mature red blood cells. The absence of a nucleus means that the red blood cell is lacking genetic material and consequently cannot directly reproduce itself. However, as a cell specialized to carry oxygen in the form of haemoglobin to other cells, the absence of a nucleus confers more advantages than it does disadvantages. The red blood cell has more available volume for the oxygen-carrying pigment, haemoglobin, and also has a greater degree of flexibility, allowing it to pass through the narrowest of capillaries in tissues. Consequently, although we will examine the structure of a generalized mammalian cell, we should remember that the structure of a cell may differ, depending upon its location and function.

Generalized structure of a mammalian cell

A diagrammatic representation of the structure of a typical mammalian cell is illustrated in Figure 1.9. Those structures within the cell (the nucleus and organelles) are visible under an electron microscope. This type of microscope is extremely powerful and allows the minute detail of cellular structure to be examined. Those structures that would be visible under a normal light microscope would be the nucleus and cell membrane only. In the next section we shall consider the structure and function of each part of the cell.

The cell membrane

The cell membrane or **plasma membrane** is composed of **phospholipid** molecules that have a hydrophilic ('water loving') phosphate head and a hydrophobic ('water hating') lipid tail (see Figure 1.10). These molecules are arranged in a **bilayer**, with the hydrophilic phosphate heads in contact with the aqueous environment inside and outside the cell. Integrated throughout the lipid bilayer are protein molecules that act as transport mechanisms for molecules that are unable to pass across the cell membrane by simple diffusion. Other membrane proteins act as **enzymes**, **receptor molecules** or **electron transporters**. Enzymes act to speed up

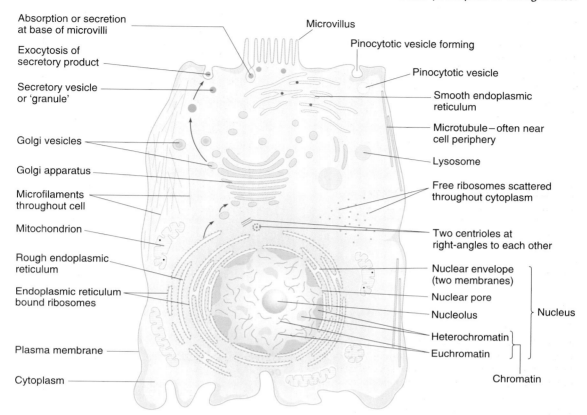

Figure 1.9 Generalized structure of a mammalian cell

chemical reactions whereas receptor molecules act as sites for the recognition of specific substances, the arrival of which may change the permeability of the cell membrane for example. Electron transporters carry electrons across the membrane.

Glycoproteins are proteins linked covalently to a carbohydrate, and are an important constituent of the cell membrane. The branching carbohydrate portions on the outer surface of the membrane are thought to assist in the recognition and adhesion of adjacent cells in the formation of tissues during cell differentiation. The glycoproteins also act as antigens in the immune response (see Chapter 6). Current theory proposes that the protein complexes and phospholipid molecules are mobile within the membrane, giving the membrane fluid-like characteristics. Figure 1.10 illustrates the fluid mosaic model of cell membrane structure.

Transport across the cell membrane

There are four basic methods of transport of substances across the cell membrane: **diffusion**, **osmosis**, **active transport**, and **endocytosis** or **exocytosis**.

Diffusion has been discussed earlier and is the movement of a substance from an area of high concentration to an area of low concentration. It is a passive process, i.e. does not require the input of energy. Substances that can dissolve in the lipid or protein part of the cell membrane can pass into the cell by diffusion. Similarly, those substances that are at a higher concentration inside the cell may dissolve in the lipid or protein part of the membrane and diffuse out of the cell. Not all substances can move across the membrane by simple diffusion. Examples of substances that can are the respiratory gases (oxygen and carbon dioxide) in solution and most ions.

Facilitated diffusion is a method of transport that relies on the principles of diffusion but utilizes a carrier molecule that is specific for the substance being transported (i.e. can carry no other substance). Transport still occurs when there is a concentration gradient, from high to

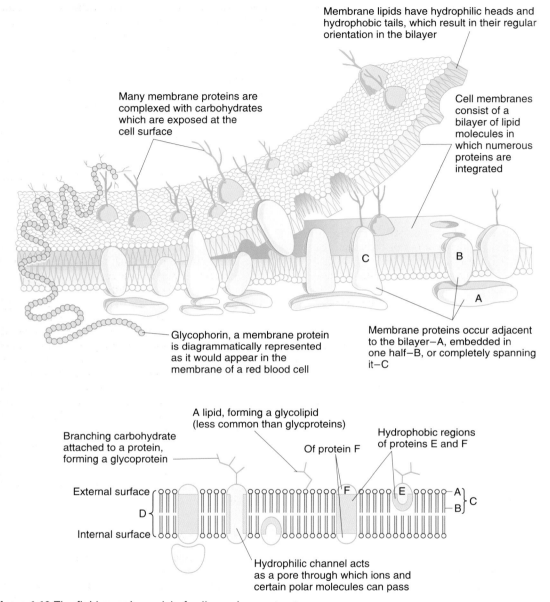

Membrane lipids have hydrophilic heads and hydrophobic tails, which result in their regular orientation in the bilayer

Many membrane proteins are complexed with carbohydrates which are exposed at the cell surface

Cell membranes consist of a bilayer of lipid molecules in which numerous proteins are integrated

C

B

A

Glycophorin, a membrane protein is diagrammatically represented as it would appear in the membrane of a red blood cell

Membrane proteins occur adjacent to the bilayer–A, embedded in one half–B, or completely spanning it–C

A lipid, forming a glycolipid (less common than glycproteins)

Branching carbohydrate attached to a protein, forming a glycoprotein

Of protein F

Hydrophobic regions of proteins E and F

External surface

F   E   A

B

C

D

Internal surface

Hydrophilic channel acts as a pore through which ions and certain polar molecules can pass

Figure 1.10 The fluid mosaic model of cell membrane structure

low concentration but the use of a carrier molecule results in a much quicker transport process. An example of facilitated diffusion is the transport of glucose into red blood cells and cells of the liver.

The principles of **osmosis** have also been discussed in the section on Solutes and Solvents. It is the movement of water molecules across a semipermeable membrane, from a dilute to a strong solution, until the osmotic pressures of the fluids on both side of the membrane are equal. The cell membrane acts as a semi-permeable membrane, as if it had small 'holes' or 'channels' that would let very small molecules (such as ions and water), pass through.

Active transport requires the use of energy to transport molecules or ions across the cell membrane against a **concentration gradient**. Energy is necessary as the substance needs to be moved against a tendency for it to move in the opposite direction (with the concentration gradient, i.e. from high concentration of solute to low concentration of solute). This can be compared with trying to push a car up a steep hill. Sodium, potassium, calcium, and chloride ions are transported across cell membranes by active transport which requires the release of energy from adenosine triphosphate (ATP, a molecule which can be said to 'carry' chemical energy). Active transport is carried out by all cells but is particularly associated with the epithelial cells of the lining of the intestine and kidney tubules during the process of active secretion and absorption.

Endocytosis and **exocytosis** involve the transport of materials through the cell membrane, either into cells (endocytosis) or out of cells (exocytosis). Endocytosis involves an in-folding of the cell membrane forming a vesicle or vacuole. A vacuole can be defined as a fluid-filled, membrane-bound sac, while a vesicle is a small vacuole. Endocytosis can be of two types:

1. **Phagocytosis** or 'cell eating', when the material taken into the cell is of solid form. Cells that specialize in this function are called **phagocytes**, e.g. some white blood cells. The sac formed during uptake is a **phagocytic vacuole**.
2. **Pinocytosis** or 'cell drinking' is when material taken into the cell is of liquid form (e.g. a solution or fine suspension). This process is particularly associated with leucocytes, liver cells and cells of the kidney involved with fluid exchange.

Each vesicle or vacuole fuses with a lysosome that contains digestive enzymes. The contents of the vacuole/vesicle are digested and, following a change in permeability of the vacuole/vesicle membrane, pass into the cytoplasm for use by the cell.

Exocytosis is the reverse of endocytosis and is a process that removes materials from the cell. It is associated particularly with the **Golgi apparatus** of the cell, glandular cells, and nerve cells.

The nucleus (pl = nuclei)

Every mammalian cell except red blood cells contains a nucleus. The nucleus is the largest constituent of the cell and is visible with a light microscope. The nucleus is surrounded by a double-layered **nuclear membrane** that contains nuclear pores through which certain substances can pass into and out of the nucleus. It contains the genetic material of the cell, deoxyribonucleic acid (DNA), in the form of **chromatin**. During cell division the chromatin coils and condenses to form **chromosomes.**

A dense round structure, the **nucleolus**, is visible within the nucleus when viewed under the electron microscope. This contains ribonucleic acid (RNA) as well as some DNA. The function of the nucleolus is the manufacture of ribosomal RNA which forms the RNA of the ribosomes in the cytoplasm.

The endoplasmic reticulum

The endoplasmic reticulum is a network of membranes that runs through the cytoplasm of the cell and can only be seen under an electron microscope. Some of the endoplasmic reticulum is covered with ribosomes and is called **rough endoplasmic reticulum** due to its granular appearance. That without ribosomes is termed **smooth endoplasmic reticulum**. Both types are associated with the synthesis and transport of substances within the cell. Rough endoplasmic reticulum transports and modifies proteins made by the ribosomes on its surface. They are taken to the Golgi apparatus for further modification and secretion. Smooth endoplasmic reticulum is responsible for lipid synthesis and secretion of some steroid hormones. It is often associated with the Golgi apparatus. In the liver, both rough and smooth endoplasmic reticulum are associated with detoxification.

The ribosome

Ribosomes are small organelles only visible with an electron microscope. They are the site of protein synthesis within the cell. Each ribosome consists of a large and small subunit that together contain the ribosomal RNA of the cell plus some protein. At the ribosomes, amino acids are joined together in a specific sequence to form a polypeptide chain. Some ribosomes exist as free organelles within the cell whilst others are bound to the endoplasmic reticulum, as discussed previously. The proteins synthesized by the ribosomes on the rough endoplasmic reticulum are usually secreted by the cell. An example of a protein made by free ribosomes is haemoglobin in the immature red blood cell.

The mitochondrion (pl = mitochondria)

The mitochondrion is frequently described as the 'power house' of the cell. It is the site of aerobic cell respiration, where energy is produced from the breakdown of nutrients and stored in the high-energy bonds of ATP molecules. It has a double membrane structure, the inner membrane being folded to form a larger surface area on which the chemical reactions can occur. The number of mitochondria within a cell is related to the level of its metabolic activity.

The Golgi apparatus

The Golgi apparatus consists of a system of membrane-bound sacs and associated vesicles that have connections with the endoplasmic reticulum. It is larger in those cells associated with secretion. The function of the Golgi apparatus is to transport and modify the materials within. Proteins are passed from the endoplasmic reticulum to the Golgi apparatus where they are chemically modified by the addition of carbohydrate chains, forming glycoproteins. The products may then be secreted by exocytosis. The Golgi apparatus also has a role in the production of lysosomes and may be involved with the transport of lipid in the cell.

Lysosomes

Lysosomes are found in all cells but are particularly abundant in cells with phagocytic activity. They are formed from a single membrane and contain digestive enzymes. Their function is to digest the contents of phagocytic and pinocytic vesicles. They may also release their contents out of the cell (exocytosis) and are involved in the removal of damaged parts of cells, or dead cells (a process known as **autolysis**).

Microbodies

Microbodies (also called peroxisomes) are spherical organelles, bound by a single membrane. They contain the enzyme catalase which facilitates the decomposition of hydrogen peroxide, a toxic by-product of many cellular reactions, into oxygen and water. They are particularly abundant in liver cells.

Microtubules and microfilaments

Microtubules and microfilaments are complex networks of fibrous structures that exist within the cytoplasm of the cell. Microtubules are very fine tubes that form **cilia** (motile processes that arise from the surfaces of cells) as well as giving form and structure to cells in general. They also form the spindle during cell division. Microfilaments are involved with cell division, cell motility, endocytosis and exocytosis. They are also predominant in striated muscle tissue where they are composed of the proteins **actin** and **myosin** and are called **myofibrils** (refer to Chapter 3).

Cell division

Prior to cell division, each adult cell contains two pairs of chromosomes, one from the mother (often referred to as the maternal chromosome) and the other from the father (the paternal chromosome). This cell is diploid, $2n$, where n is the number of chromosome pairs.

Mitosis

Mitosis is the process whereby a cell nucleus divides to produce two daughter nuclei containing identical sets of **chromosomes** to the parent cell. The cytoplasm also divides and the cell membrane reforms, forming two separate daughter cells which are each an exact duplicate of the parent cell, and contain the same genetic material. Mitotic cell division results in an increase of cell numbers and is the method by which an animal grows and repairs or replaces existing cells. The stages of mitosis are prophase, metaphase, anaphase and telophase with a resting stage known as interphase both before and after the cell division sequence. These are illustrated in Figure 1.11.

Cellular division is necessary for every animal to maintain their structure and function, to grow and reproduce. Most cells have the ability to produce new cells that are genetically identical to themselves. This process is called **mitosis**. Some cells have the ability to produce cells that are involved in sexual reproduction, i.e. the creation of another animal. These cells are termed **gametes**. In the female they are known as **ova** (sing = **ovum**) and in the male they are called **spermatozoa** (sing = **spermatozoon**). These cells divide during development so that they contain half the amount of the genetic material of their parent cell. This process is known as **meiosis**.

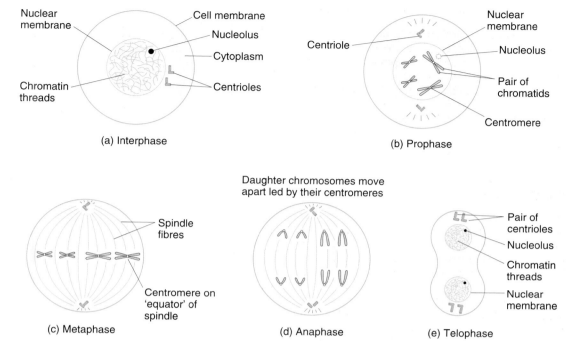

Figure 1.11 Summary of the stages of mitosis

Meiosis

Meiosis is the process whereby the cell nucleus divides to produce **four daughter nuclei**, each with half the number of chromosomes of the **parent cell**. It can also be referred to as reduction division, as it reduces the number of chromosomes from diploid (2n, two sets of each chromosome) to haploid (n, one set of each chromosome). Meiosis is necessary as it enables the chromosome number to remain constant in any sexually reproductive species. Each gamete contains the haploid number of chromosomes (n) and consequently the fertilized zygote produced by the male and female gametes has the same number of chromosomes as either of its parents (diploid, 2n), one half being from its mother and the other from its father. Meiosis is similar to mitosis, but it has two stages of cellular division rather than one. The changes occurring in meiosis are represented in Figure 1.12.

Thus, meiosis produces four daughter cells, each with half the number of chromosomes of the parent cell. This allows the chromosome number of the next generation to remain constant, as the gametes combine to restore the diploid number (2n) of chromosomes. Meiosis also provides the opportunity for genetic variation to occur. Each gamete only contains one copy of each chromosome which has undergone a process or random assortment (the separation of the randomly positioned chromosomes during anaphase I and II as illustrated in Figure 1.12). This is in addition to the genetic exchange of material, with the formation of chiasmata during prophase I (see Figure 1.12), creating new genetic sequences on each chromosome. Consequently, each gamete may

> The study of tissues is known as histology. A tissue is defined as a collection of similar cells (and their component parts) that perform specialized homeostatic functions. Within the tissues, cells develop specialized functions dependent upon their role within the body. For example, muscle tissue cells are specialized to carry out movement and skeletal tissue cells are specialized to support the body. Some cells, once specialized, lose their ability to carry out other functions, for example, a mature red blood cell is concerned with transport and exchange of respiratory gases but loses its ability to reproduce itself.

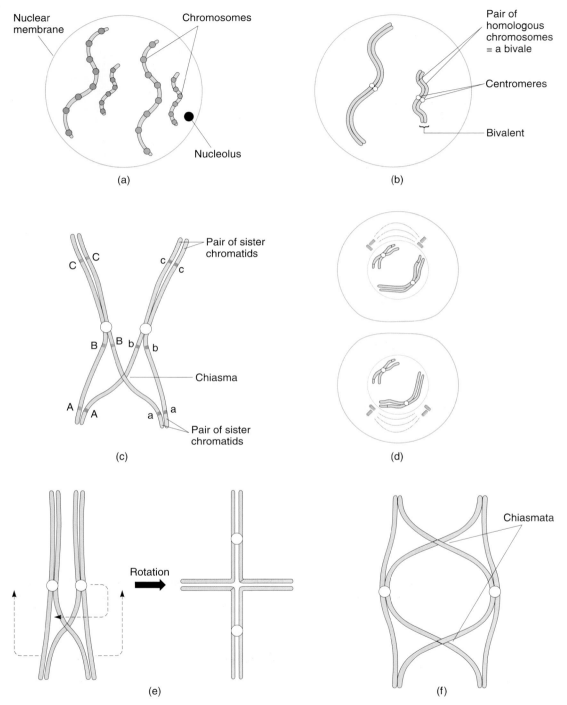

Figure 1.12(a–f) Summary of the stages of meiosis. (a) Early prophase I; (b) prophase I; (c) crossing-over during prophase I; (d) prophase II; (e) bivalent with a single chiasma; (f) bivalent with a double chiasmata;

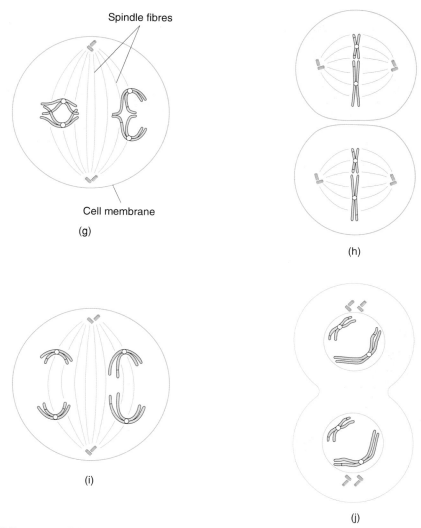

Figure 1.12(g–j) Summary of the stages of meiosis. (g) late metaphase I; (h) metaphase II; (i) anaphase I; (j) telophase

contain genetic sequences that differ from those expressed by the parent. This concept is expanded in Chapter 6 on reproduction.

Tissues

There are four main types of tissue that can be identified in the mammalian body:

● epithelial tissue
● connective tissue
● nervous tissue
● muscular tissue

Epithelial and connective tissues will be discussed in detail below. Nervous and muscular tissues will be discussed in Chapters 2 and 3, respectively.

Epithelial tissue

The functions of epithelial tissue can be summarized as follows:

● protection: epithelial tissue covers all surfaces of the body, for example, the skin and the lining of body cavities and hollow organs.

- transport: epithelial tissue is located where there is the rapid transport of substances, e.g. in the alveoli of the respiratory tract (see Chapter 2).
- lining: epithelial tissue lines the internal cavities and tubes of the body, for example, the respiratory and digestive tracts. The functions of protection and lining are closely interlinked.
- secretion: epithelial tissue produces a variety of substances with specific homeostatic functions, for example, sweat and tears.

It is important to note that not all types of epithelial tissue possess all the properties mentioned above. The function of a particular type of epithelial tissue depends very much upon its structure and location.

There are three different types of epithelial tissue:

1. **Simple epithelium**
   This type of epithelial tissue consists of flat sheets of cells and is associated with covering and lining surfaces of the body. It comprises a single layer of cells held together by a basement membrane. It is located in areas of the body where diffusion, absorption, secretion, or filtration occur, for example, the respiratory surfaces of the lungs, internal surfaces of blood and lymph vessels, and linings of major body cavities.

   Simple epithelia may be squamous (pavement or flattened), cuboidal or columnar (elongated). Figure 1.13 illustrates these different types of simple epithelia, with an example of their location within the body.

   Ciliated epithelium: Some simple epithelial tissue consists of cells that secrete **mucus**, a thick proteinaceous fluid secreted by specialized epithelial cells, known as goblet cells. Its function is to protect the underlying tissue. Mucous membranes (mucus is the noun and mucous the adjective) usually possess small hair-like projections on their surface, known as cilia. These are constantly moving and 'waft'

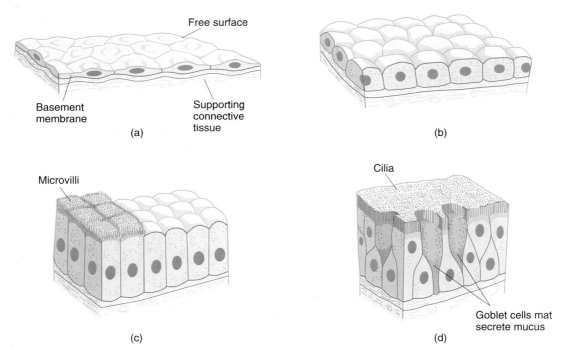

Figure 1.13 Diagrammatic illustration of the different types of simple epithelia. (a) Simple squamous epithelium, found lining body cavities, blood and lymphatic vessels and respiratory surfaces of lungs; (b) Simple cuboidal epithelium, found lining the nephron of the kidney and ducts of the reproductive tract; (c) Simple columnar epithelium, found lining the gastrointestinal tract. The free surface may be covered with finger-like projections that increase the surface area of the cell for secretion and/or absorption; (d) Ciliated mucous epithelium, found lining the ducts of the reproductive and respiratory tracts. Although this tissue appears to consist of more than one layer of cells, it is, in fact, one layer of simple columnar cells bunched together; each cell is attached to the basement membrane. This can also be called pseudostratified columnar epithelium, the prefix 'pseudo' meaning 'false'

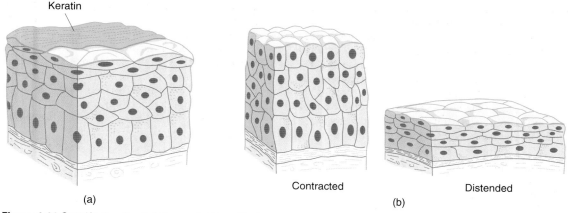

Figure 1.14 Stratified epithelial tissue. (a) Stratified squamous epithelium, found in the epidermis of the skin, where it is keratinized, and also lining the oral cavity, pharynx, oesophagus, vagina and anus; (b) Transitional epithelium found lining the bladder. This tissue is capable of great distension

the mucus along the surface. This type of tissue lines the ducts of the reproductive and respiratory tracts, and is illustrated in Figure 1.13.

2. **Compound or stratified epithelium**

   This type of epithelial tissue consists of more than one layer of cells. The tissue is resistant to wear and tear as the surface cells are replaced by those underneath, consequently this tissue type is located in areas that are subject to some degree of friction. Examples of stratified epithelial tissue can be seen in Figure 1.14.

   Stratified squamous epithelial tissue lines the skin, oral cavity, oesophagus, vagina and anus. The basal cells are columnar and germinal (i.e., they produce new cells by **mitosis**). The cells

change shape as they age and are squamous in shape at the surface. Squamous epithelial tissue of the skin also contains a tough, waterproof protein known as keratin and consequently the tissue is sometimes referred to as **cornified** or **keratinized stratified squamous epithelium**.

Transitional epithelial tissue lines the bladder and urinary tract. It is capable of great extension due to its elastic properties.

3. **Glandular epithelium**

   This type of epithelial tissue is comprised of glandular cells that produce and secrete (release a substance) or excrete (separate or discharge a substance) materials such as milk, sweat, sebum, cerumen, hormones, or enzymes. It

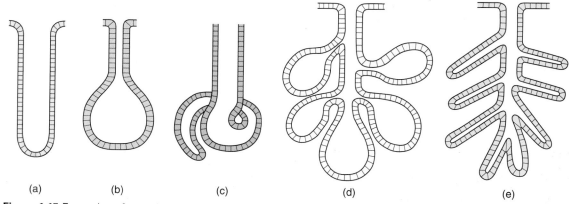

Figure 1.15 Examples of exocrine glands. Simple glands: (a) tubular glands found in the wall of the stomach and small intestine; (b) saccular gland, e.g. the sebaceous glands in the skin. Also termed 'alveolar' glands; (c) coiled gland, e.g. the sweat glands in the nose and foot pads. Compound glands: (d) alveolar glands, e.g. salivary glands; (e) tubular glands, e.g. duodenal glands

contains specialized contractile epithelial cells called **myoepithelial cells** that assist with the secretion of the glandular products.

Exocrine glands such as sweat glands, sebaceous glands, glands of the pancreas, and mammary glands, secrete their glandular products onto the surface of a cavity or skin. They are formed from pockets of epithelial tissue with a duct to the surface. Exocrine glands can be one of many shapes, examples of which are illustrated in Figure 1.15.

Endocrine glands develop from epithelial tissue but lose their connections to the surface during development. They secrete their products into the blood supply for distribution to target organs. Examples of endocrine glands include the adrenal glands, thyroid gland, ovary and testis (refer to Chapter 2).

Connective tissue

There are five different types of connective tissue: loose or areolar connective tissue, dense connective tissue, bone, blood and cartilage. The

> The function of connective tissue includes:
>
> - to surround and protect delicate organs
> - to provide a structural framework for the body
> - to support and bind other interconnecting tissues with organs
> - to transport substances from one part of the body to another, e.g. blood
> - to provide an internal defence mechanism against pathogens
> - to store energy reserves as fat/adipose tissue

development and structure of bone will be discussed in Chapter 3 and blood in Chapter 4. The following section describes loose and dense connective tissue, as well as cartilage.

1. **Loose or areolar connective tissue**
   Loose or *areolar* connective tissue consists of many cells in a loose, irregular network of

Elastic fibres
Capillary
Collagen fibres
Fibroblast
Matrix
Fat cell

(a)

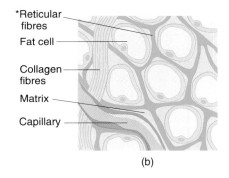

*Reticular fibres
Fat cell
Collagen fibres
Matrix
Capillary

(b)

Fibroblast
Collagen fibres
Matrix
Capillary

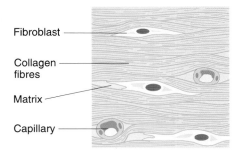

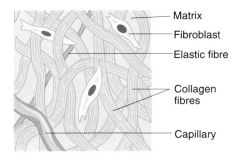

Matrix
Fibroblast
Elastic fibre
Collagen fibres
Capillary

(c)

Figure 1.16 Loose and dense connective tissue. (a) Loose/areolar connective tissue; (b) adipose connective tissue; (c) dense regular connective tissue; (d) dense irregular connective tissue. *Reticular fibres are a smaller form of collagen, forming supporting networks around cell groups

fibres. The fibres are both **collagen fibres** (a structural protein) and **elastic fibres** (formed from the protein elastin). **Fibroblast cells** (those that produce collagen fibres) are also present, along with a few fat cells (for lipid storage). The tissue also has a blood supply via the capillaries. Loose connective tissue forms the subcutaneous tissue of the skin (the hypodermis) and is located between the organs of the body. A diagrammatic representation of the structure of loose connective tissue is shown in Figure 1.16.

    Adipose or **fatty tissue** has a similar structure to loose connective tissue except that it contains a greater number of fat cells. This type of tissue acts as a food reserve, storing energy as well as fat-soluble vitamins, and provides a layer of insulation. It also provides mechanical protection for organs such as the kidneys and eye. A diagrammatic representation of the structure of adipose tissue is shown in Figure 1.16.

2. **Dense or fibrous connective tissue**
   Dense or fibrous connective tissue exists in two forms, regular and irregular. The names refer to the arrangement of the collagen and elastic fibres within the tissue. Dense regular connective tissue forms ligaments and tendons. The parallel arrangement of the fibres means that it is resistant to tension whilst allowing some stretching. Irregular connective tissue forms joint capsules and sheaths of **fascia** that surround muscle tissue. It also covers certain organs, including the liver and spleen, and forms the dermis of the skin. Fibres in this tissue are irregularly arranged, making the tissue impact-resistant, bearing stress in all directions. Both irregular and regular dense connective tissue have minimal vascularization. A diagrammatic representation of the structure of dense connective tissue is shown in Figure 1.16.

3. **Cartilage**
   Cartilage is considered as a supporting connective tissue along with bone. It consists of cartilage-producing cells called **chondrocytes** which are located in small cavities called lacunae, surrounded by a hard and flexible matrix containing fine collagen fibres. Cartilage does not have a blood supply; it is **avascular**, receiving all its nutrition from the surrounding membrane known as the **perichondrium**. There are three types of cartilage: hyaline, elastic, and fibrocartilage. These are illustrated in Figure 1.17.

   ● **Hyaline cartilage**. Hyaline cartilage is flexible and compressible. It consists of chondrocytes within a hyaline matrix with fine collagen fibres. Its major function within the mammalian body is covering bone ends at synovial joints, where it is called **articular** cartilage. Here it provides a smooth, durable

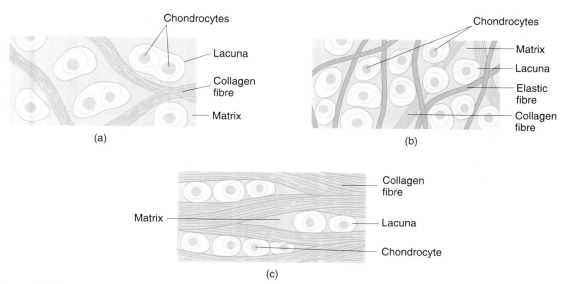

Figure 1.17 Structure of the different types of cartilage. (a) Hyaline cartilage; (b) elastic cartilage; (c) fibrocartilage

surface facilitating movement of the joint whilst acting to absorb some of the forces within the joint.

- **Elastic cartilage**. Elastic cartilage also has a hyaline matrix and chondrocytes. However, it also contains elastic fibres and a slightly different type of collagen, both of which give the tissue a great degree of flexibility. Elastic cartilage forms the pinna of the external ear and the epiglottis of the larynx.

- **Fibrocartilage**. Fibrocartilage is the strongest of the cartilage tissues, containing more collagen fibres and showing increased tensile strength. It is located within the intervertebral discs of the vertebral column, the sacroiliac joint, the pubic symphysis, and in the acetabulum of the pelvis and glenoid fossa of the scapula. It also forms the intra-articular **menisci** of the stifle (see Chapter 3). Fibrocartilage is resistant to tension and impaction.

Table 1.5 Major organ systems of the mammalian body

Organ system		Major function
Cardiovascular system		Internal transport of cells and dissolved materials, including nutrients, wastes, and gases
Digestive system		Processing of food and absorption of nutrients, minerals, vitamins and water
Endocrine system		Directing long-term changes in the activities of other organ systems
Integumentary system		Protection from environmental hazards; temperature control
Lymphatic system		Defence against infection and disease
Muscular system		Locomotion; support; heat production
Nervous system		Directing immediate response to stimuli, generally by co-ordinating the activities of other organ systems
Reproductive system		Production of sex cells and hormones
Respiratory system		Delivery of air to sites where gas exchange can occur between the air and circulating blood
Skeletal system		Support; protection of soft tissues; mineral storage; blood formation
Urinary system		Elimination of excess water, salts and waste products

Organs and body systems

Several different types of tissue are arranged to form organs, which exist as functional units within the body. Organs are described as **tubular (hollow)** or **parenchymal (compact)**.

Tubular organs have three basic layers:

- an inner layer of epithelial tissue
- a middle layer of smooth/involuntary muscle and connective tissue
- an outer layer of connective and epithelial tissue

Examples of tubular organs include the heart, lungs and stomach.

Compact organs have a solid form and vary in shape and size. They are enclosed by a capsule of connective tissue and may be covered with serous membrane. They have an extensive network of connective tissue and are sometimes divided into sections called **lobules**. The functional tissue of the organ is called **parenchyma** and this may be divided into an outer **medulla** and an inner **cortex**. Examples of compact organs include the liver and the ovaries.

Organs are arranged in groups within the body and work together to perform specific bodily functions. A summary of the major organ systems is shown in Table 1.5.

1.3 The mammalian body

Anatomical terminology
Basic anatomy of the dog and cat
Body cavities
Homeostasis and body fluids

Introduction

All living organisms share a number of basic biological characteristics. These include:

Responsiveness:
The ability to respond to changes in the environment. These responses can be short-term, for example, a cat hunting a mouse as potential prey, or more long-term, for example, a dog developing a thicker coat in the autumn in preparation for the winter months.

Movement:
The ability to produce movement. This can be movement of the animal within its surroundings, as well as movement of materials inside the body, e.g. movement of food along the digestive tract.

Growth:
The ability to grow larger over time through an increase in **cellular** size and number. Complex organisms such as mammals demonstrate cellular differentiation. Groups of cells develop specialist functions within the body, e.g. red blood cells are specially adapted to transport oxygen and carbon dioxide. Once cells specialize, they lose their ability to perform certain functions at the expense of their specialization, e.g. a red blood cell would not be able to function as a hepatocyte (liver cell) and vice versa.

Reproduction:
The ability to create a generation of similar offspring and ensure survival of the species.

Metabolism:
The ability to utilize materials to provide energy for all the above processes. Nutrients are taken in from the surrounding external environment and are used in complex chemical processes to provide energy and products for growth and maintenance. Most animals require oxygen from the atmosphere for metabolism to occur and this process of oxygen acquisition by cells is called **aerobic respiration**. As well as producing useful substances, metabolism also produces by-products that are not required and may be potentially harmful. These by-products are excreted from the animal. An example is given by exhalation of carbon dioxide, a by-product of cellular respiration.

The more complex the organism, the more complex the above processes. For example, in the case of a very small, simple organism consisting of one cell, the nutrients for metabolism can be absorbed through the cell membrane. Complex organisms, such as the dog and cat, have to digest their food, using a specially adapted area of the body (the digestive tract) before it can be utilized. Specialized systems are also required for excretion and respiration and, as all these areas are located in different parts of the body, a transport system is required to allow each area to transfer substances. This is the cardiovascular system.

So you can begin to see that, although we can define the basic functions of living things, complex organisms have developed specialized areas to conduct specific processes which have allowed them to develop a more advanced and complex existence. In the rest of this book we will examine the entire process of existence from a basic cellular level through to that of complex systems, which will allow a greater understanding of the ways in which the mammalian body develops, exists and functions.

Anatomical terminology

When considering the physiology and anatomy of any organism it becomes necessary to refer to direction and position, to allow structures to be correctly located and identified. This is termed **anatomical terminology**. The basic anatomical directions relating to the dog are shown in Figure 1.18 and a description and example is given in Table 1.6.

We might also need to refer to **planes** of the body, as if we were taking a slice through the animal. Planes in relation to the dog are shown in Figure 1.18.

Basic anatomy of the dog and cat

For a deeper understanding of further chapters, it is necessary to be familiar with the basic skeletal structure of the dog and cat, as illustrated in Figures 1.19 and 1.20, respectively. This will allow us to apply the theoretical principles of physiology and associated anatomy, to the living animal.

Body cavities

The body cavities of the dog and cat are the chambers within the body that contain the internal organs or **viscera**. The function of the body cavities is to provide protection for the delicate organs, e.g. the brain, by allowing a cushioning effect in response to jarring. They also allow for changes in shape and size of the internal organs

Table 1.6 Anatomical terms

Term	Region	To note
Ventral	Towards or relatively near the belly and corresponding surface head, neck, thorax and tail	Never used for limbs
Dorsal	Towards or relatively near the back and corresponding surface of head, neck, thorax and tail	On limbs, applies to upper or front surface of carpus, tarsus and digits
Cranial/anterior	Towards or relatively near the head. When relating to the head it is replaced by rostral	On limbs, applies proximal to carpus and tarsus
Caudal/posterior	Towards or relatively near the tail. Also used in reference to the head	On limbs, applies proximal to carpus and tarsus
Rostral	Towards or relatively near the nose	Applies to head only
Lateral	Away from or relatively farther from the medial plane	
Medial	Towards or relatively near the medial plane	
Proximal	Relatively near main mass or origin	In limbs and tail, the attached end
Distal	Away from main mass or origin	In limbs and tail, the free end
Palmar	Aspect of fore paw on which pads are located	Opposite surface known as dorsal
Plantar	Aspect of hind paw on which pads are located	Opposite surface known as dorsal
Superficial	Relatively near the surface of the body or an organ	
Deep	Relatively near the centre of the body or an organ	

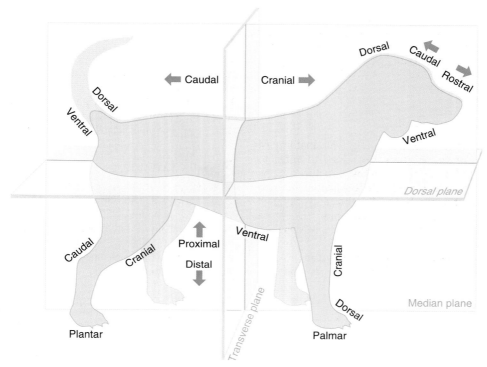

Figure 1.18 Anatomical directions and anatomical planes of the dog

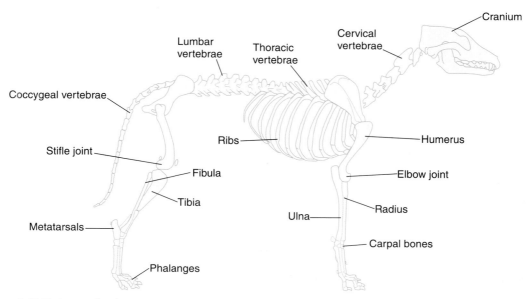

Figure 1.19 Skeleton of a dog

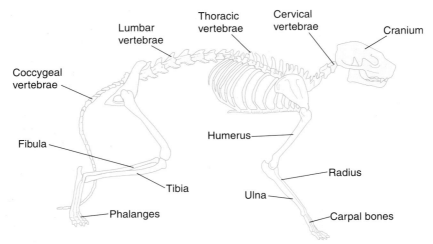

Figure 1.20 Skeleton of a cat

without disrupting other tissues and organs, e.g. the lungs can expand during respiration and the stomach can distend after eating a meal.

The body cavities of the dog can be distinguished as follows:

Dorsal body cavity
This is bounded by the bones of the skull and vertebral column and contains the brain and spinal cord. It is subdivided into the cranial cavity containing the brain and the **spinal cavity** containing the **spinal cord**

Ventral body cavity
This is divided by the diaphragm into the thoracic cavity and the abdominal cavity (see below)

Thorax or thoracic cavity
This is bound on the anterior aspect by the thorax, on the dorsal aspect by the thoracic vertebrae and

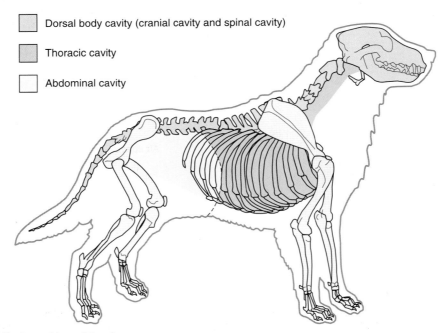

Figure 1.21 Body cavities of the dog

All body cavities are lined with **serous endothelial cells**. These specialized endothelial cells form a smooth, shiny membrane (the serous membrane) and secrete a watery fluid that acts as a lubricant between surfaces. The serous membrane that lines the thoracic cavity is called the pleura and consists of the visceral and parietal pleural membranes (see Figure 1.23). That lining the abdominal cavity is called the peritoneum.

hypaxial muscles (those below the spinal column), ventrally by the sternum, laterally by the ribs and intercostal muscles, and posteriorly by the diaphragm

Abdomen or abdominal cavity
This is bound on the anterior aspect by the diaphragm, dorsally by the hypaxial muscles of the lumbar region, ventrally by the abdominal muscles and floor of the pelvis, on the lateral aspect by the abdominal muscles and the wall of the pelvis, and posteriorly by the posterior part of the pelvis (pelvic diaphragm). The abdomen is sometimes divided into the abdominal and pelvic cavities, although there is no actual physical barrier between them.

Figure 1.21 illustrates the body cavities of the dog.

Thoracic cavity

The thoracic cavity consists of three internal chambers, the **pericardial cavity**, containing the

heart, and the left and right **pleural cavities**, containing the left and right lungs, respectively.

Figure 1.22 demonstrates the relationship between the heart and the pericardial cavity. The serous membrane surrounding the heart is the **pericardium**. The **visceral** (or **serous**) **pericardium** covers the heart whilst the **parietal** (or **fibrous**) **pericardium** lies opposite. Both the visceral and parietal pericardium form one continuous membrane. They are separated by a small amount of fluid which enables the two layers to slide across each other easily and without friction.

The space between the two pleural cavities is called the **mediastinum**. This part of the thoracic cavity contains the heart and pericardial cavity, the thymus, trachea, oesophagus, large arteries and veins. Each pleural cavity is lined by serous membranes called **pleura**. The pleural layer lining the lungs is called the **visceral pleura** and that lining the pleura cavity is called the parietal pleura. Figure 1.23 demonstrates the relationship between the pericardial cavity, mediastinum and pleural cavities.

Abdominal cavity

The abdominal cavity (sometimes referred to as the abdominopelvic cavity) contains the liver, stomach, spleen, small intestine and some of the large intestine. The lining of serous membrane is called the **peritoneum**. The **parietal peritoneum** lines the inner body wall whilst the **visceral peritoneum** lines the surface of the organs within the cavity. The kidneys and pancreas lie outside the peritoneum, between the parietal peritoneum and

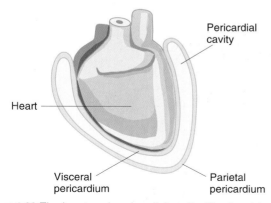
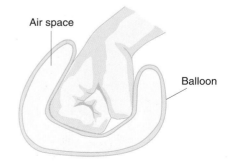

Figure 1.22 The heart and pericardial cavity. The heart is suspended within the pericardial cavity like a fist pushed into a balloon. The attachment site, corresponding to the wrist of the hand in the model, lies at the connection between the heart and major blood vessels

Veterinary Physiology and Applied Anatomy

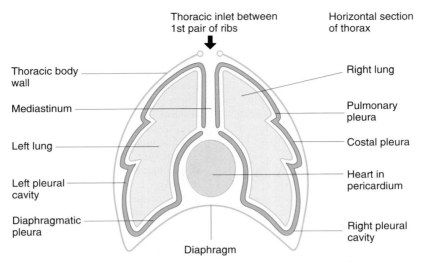

Figure 1.23 Relationship between the pericardial cavity, mediastinum and pleural cavities

the muscle of the body wall. The ventral portion of the abdominal cavity, sometimes referred to as the **pelvic cavity**, lies within the pelvic bones. It contains the bladder, the final section of the large intestine, and the reproductive organs of the female (ovaries, fallopian tubes and uterus) or the prostate gland and seminal vesicles of the male. The pelvic organs are located outside of the peritoneum, although some are covered by it as mentioned earlier.

The pelvic diaphragm is located towards the posterior part of the ventral abdominal cavity and is a collection of muscles forming a 'sheet' enclosing the posterior region of the pelvis, sometimes referred to as the pelvic cavity. It allows passage of the urethra, vagina and anus, each of which is surrounded by a muscular sphincter.

Homeostasis and body fluids

Cellularity

Animal cells can only function if their internal and external environments can be kept within acceptable limits. If either of these environments becomes too hostile, e.g. the temperature becomes too high, the cell contents become too acidic, or the cell becomes dehydrated, then the functioning of the cellular proteins and enzymes will be disrupted or deactivated. Cells are therefore in a state of constant flux. They use nutrients and produce waste products as part of their metabolic processes. In order to prevent a shortage of one and an excess

of the other, they need to be able to exchange substances with their external environment. The cell must also be able to protect itself against fluctuations in the external environment, e.g. temperature.

For a multicellular species such as the dog and cat, cellular exchange requires some form of transport mechanism in order that the exchange of substances can be conducted efficiently. Consider a cell of the intestine, deep within the body of an animal. It is not in direct contact with the atmosphere and consequently cannot obtain the oxygen necessary for cellular respiration by simple exchange across its membrane, as would a simple organism consisting of one or two cells. Thus, in order to obtain oxygen, a specialized transport system is required which not only provides all the essential cellular requirements but also removes by-products for excretion. If these by-products were allowed to build up within the cell they would prevent the cell from functioning normally, ultimately destroying it completely. So the complex organism has evolved specialized systems to obtain nutrients (e.g. the respiratory system to obtain oxygen and the gastrointestinal system to obtain glucose and other nutrients) and excrete waste products (e.g. the respiratory system to eliminate carbon dioxide and the urinary system to eliminate nitrogen-containing compounds). A transport system has also evolved to connect these systems with others and with the external environment. This is the blood, which is part of the cardiovascular system.

The total amount of fluid within the body of an animal constitutes between 50% and 70% of its total body weight. This amount varies and depends upon the amount of fat (adipose tissue). The amount of adipose tissue is dependent upon the age, sex, and nutritional status of the animal. As adipose tissue contains relatively less water than other tissues, the percentage of body water is lower in females, and in obese and older animals (as these all have proportionately more body fat) and greater in males and young animals. The average amount of body water in the 'normal' adult animal is approximately 65% (range 60–70%).

Body water and compartments

From an understanding of these basic principles, it becomes apparent that, in multicellular, complex organisms, the majority of cells exist within an **internal environment** consisting of the fluid surrounding them and the adjacent cells. The small amount of fluid surrounding each cell is called **interstitial fluid** (or **tissue fluid**). Fluid that exists inside cells is called **intracellular fluid** and that existing outside cells is termed extracellular fluid. Consequently, **interstitial fluid** is part of the extracellular fluid of an animal.

The total body fluid of an animal is distributed between the intracellular and extracellular fluid compartments. In the healthy animal, approximately 60% exists as intracellular fluid with the remaining 40% being extracellular fluid mainly in the plasma and as interstitial fluid.

Extracellular fluid

The extracellular fluid compartment of an animal can be broken down into three components:

- interstitial fluid: the fluid surrounding the cells (also called tissue fluid). It allows the exchange of substances between the cells and the external environment
- plasma: fluid in the vascular compartment of the body, i.e. blood vessels and lymphatic vessels
- transcellular fluid: specialized fluids are separated from the blood by capillary endothelium and epithelium. These fluids are usually formed by active secretion of specialized cells, e.g. gastrointestinal secretions, synovial fluid, and cerebrospinal fluid. The proportion of these fluids secreted accounts for less than 1% of total extracellular fluid.

Fluid composition

Each fluid compartment has a specific chemical composition. Plasma and interstitial fluid are quite similar in composition while there is a great difference between these and intracellular fluid. The difference is primarily due to the variation in the concentrations of different electrolytes, and is illustrated in Table 1.7.

The major cations of intracellular fluid are potassium (K^+) and magnesium (Mg^{2+}) and the major anions are phosphate (PO_4^{3-}) and **proteins**

Table 1.7 Electrolyte composition of body fluid compartments. Concentrations of main ionic constituents of intracellular and extracellular fluids

	Extracellular fluid (mmol/l)		Intracellular fluid
	Plasma	*Interstitial fluid*	
Cations			
Sodium Na^+	138	130	10
Potassium K^+	4	4	110
Calcium Ca^{2+}	2	2	4
Magnesium Mg^{2+}	2	2	15
Anions			
Chloride Cl^-	102	110	4
Bicarbonate HCO_3^-	24	27	12
Phosphate PO_4^{2-}	2	2	40
Neutral or slightly –ve			
Proteins	70	approx 0	25

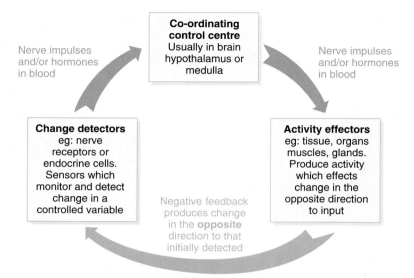

Figure 1.24 A simple homeostatic negative feedback loop

with a slight negative charge. This is in direct contrast to the composition of extracellular fluid where the major cation is sodium (Na^+) and the major anions, chloride (Cl^-) and bicarbonate (HCO_3^-). Note that the composition of plasma is very similar to interstitial fluid except that plasma also includes a high concentration of **negatively charged protein**. The selective permeability of the capillary endothelial cells allows the diffusion of simple electrolytes and other small substances between the two compartments. However, the large plasma proteins are too big to cross the membrane due to their size, and consequently they remain in the plasma fluid compartment, along with a slightly increased concentration of cations (Na^+) to counteract their negative charge.

The difference in the fluid composition of the intracellular and extracellular fluid compartments is due to the presence of a sodium/potassium ion pump within the cell membrane that can pump sodium ions out of the cell in exchange for potassium ions maintaining the physiological concentrations of these inside and outside cells.

The interstitial fluid forms the true cellular environment as it bathes the cells throughout the body. Consequently its composition is crucial, ensuring a stable environment for cellular function. The process by which the internal environment is maintained within an optimum range is called **homeostasis** and this will be examined in the following section.

Homeostasis

Maintaining the internal environment within an optimum range requires the co-ordination of a large number of physiological processes. These are termed **homeostatic mechanisms**, and they contribute to the maintenance of **homeostasis** within the animal.

A change in a property of the extracellular fluid triggers the homeostatic mechanisms that will return it to within its optimal range. This may involve the communication systems of the body (the nervous and endocrine systems) as well as those systems that are in contact with the external environment (the respiratory, digestive and urinary systems). The homeostatic mechanism triggered may be simple or complex, depending upon the type of change that has occurred within the extracellular fluid. It usually involves some form of negative feedback, where a change in the opposite direction returns the properties of the extracellular fluid to its optimal range. Examples of homeostatic mechanisms include the regulation of body temperature, respiratory rate, blood pH, heart rate, blood pressure, levels of blood glucose and body water and electrolyte concentrations. An example of a simple homeostatic mechanism is illustrated in Figure 1.24.

For example, when a dog has acute diarrhoea, fluid is lost from the body and the osmolarity (concentration) of plasma increases. This is detected by receptors that respond to changes in plasma osmolarity (or osmostic) osmoreceptors in the hypothalamus of the brain that stimulate a control centre, again within the hypothalamus. This centre regulates the synthesis and release of antidiuretic hormone (ADH) from the anterior pituitary gland. ADH secretion is increased and levels of this hormone within the blood increase. This stimulates the kidneys of the animal to secrete less water in urine and consequently the concentration of urine increases as the water is retained in the body. Providing that the bout of diarrhoea is not prolonged, the conservation of water by the kidneys should cause the osmolarity of plasma to fall back towards its normal value. This is further assisted by the activation of 'thirst' centres within the brain, which stimulate the dog to drink water. In prolonged cases, intravenous fluid therapy may be necessary to assist the restoration of plasma osmolarity.

Review questions

1. What is the name given to the sub-atomic particles that orbit the nucleus of the atom?
   (a) protons
   (b) neutrons
   (c) electrons
   (d) electrovalents
2. Which type of bonding occurs during the formation of salt (sodium chloride)?
   (a) ionic
   (b) covalent
   (c) hydrogen
   (d) shared
3. Which of the following best describes the process of dissolving salt in water?
   (a) Water is the solute, salt the solvent, and an ionic solution is formed
   (b) Water is the solute, salt the solvent, and a covalent solution is formed
   (c) Salt is the solute, water the solvent, and a cationic solution is formed
   (d) Salt is the solute, water the solvent, and an ionic solution is formed
4. 0.9% Saline is
   (a) hypertonic
   (b) hypotinic
   (c) hyperosmotic
   (d) iso-osmotic
5. If a red blood cell is placed into a hypotonic solution which of the following will occur?
   (a) Water molecules will move out of the red blood cell, causing the cell to become crenated
   (b) Water molecules will move into the red blood cell, causing the cell to haemolyse
   (c) Solute molecules will move into the red blood cell, causing the cell to haemolyse
   (d) The concentration of fluid inside the cell is the same as outside the cell, therefore there will be no net movement of fluid
6. Which of the following represents the pH of a strong acid?
   (a) 1
   (b) 5
   (c) 7
   (d) 12
7. 10 000 can also be written as
   (a) 1×10^4
   (b) 1×10^3
   (c) 1×10^2
   (d) 1×10^{-4}
8. Which sub-atomic particles are equal in number in the atom?
   (a) protons and neutrons
   (b) protons and electrons
   (c) neutrons and electrons
   (d) they are all equal
9. Which of the following statements is most accurate?
   (a) Diffusion is the movement of water through a semi-permeable membrane from a strong to a weaker solution
   (b) Diffusion is the movement of water through a semi-permeable membrane from a weak to a stronger solution
   (c) Osmosis is the movement of water through a semi-permeable membrane from a strong to a weaker solution
   (d) Osmosis is the movement of water through a semi-permeable membrane from a weak to a stronger solution
10. Which of the following is liquid at room temperature?
    (a) mercury
    (b) carbon
    (c) calcium
    (d) zinc
11. Describe the structure of an atom.
12. Define the term isotope.
13. Explain the formation of a water molecule.
14. Briefly describe the effects of osmosis.
15. What is buffering?
16. Explain the pH scale for acids and alkalis.
17. What is 25 000 expressed as a number to the power of 10?

18. Convert 30 lb to kg.
19. Convert 101°F into Centigrade.
20. Convert 40°C into Fahrenheit.
21. Energy to run the various activities of cells is the result of cell respiration which occurs in the:
    (a) endoplasmic reticulum
    (b) Golgi body
    (c) ribosomes
    (d) mitochondria
22. State which of the following organelles is responsible for the packaging and secretion of secretory products such as enzymes:
    (a) endoplasmic reticulum
    (b) Golgi body
    (c) ribosomes
    (d) mitochondria
23. Name the structure that controls the activities of the cell and contains genetic information:
    (a) nucleolus
    (b) nucleus
    (c) nucleosome
    (d) centrosome
24. The cell membrane is best described as:
    (a) a phospholipid monolayer
    (b) a phospholipid bilayer
    (c) a lipid membrane
    (d) a lipid bilayer
25. Identify which sub-atomic particles are equal in number in the atom:
    (a) protons and neutrons
    (b) protons and electrons
    (c) neutrons and electrons
    (d) they are all equal
26. State which of the following is the largest structure within a cell:
    (a) nucleus
    (b) mitochondrion
    (c) ribosome
    (d) Golgi body
27. Identify which of the following describes the mechanism whereby solid particles are ingested by the cell:
    (a) phagocytosis
    (b) pinocytosis
    (c) phagosytosis
    (d) pinosytosis
28. Body fluid comprises what percent of total body weight in a healthy adult animal?
    (a) 40%
    (b) 50%
    (c) 65%
    (d) 70%

29. The substance that gives connective tissue its strength is
    (a) collagen
    (b) collogen
    (c) fibrogen
    (d) protein
30. Hyaline cartilage is found in:
    (a) cartilaginous joints
    (b) intervertebral discs
    (c) synovial joints
    (d) the mandibular symphysis
31. List the four types of tissue in the body.
32. List three types of epithelial tissue and draw a diagram to represent the structure of each.
33. For each type of epithelial tissue above identify where in the body they are found.
34. State what type of tissue is skin.
35. State what type of tissue lines the bladder.
36. Name the two different types of glands and give an example of each.
37. Give an example of a simple coiled gland.
38. Give an example of a compound alveolar/acinar gland.
39. Explain the events which occur during mitosis.
40. In what way is meiosis different from mitosis?
41. Which one of the following body fluids contains the highest concentration of proteins?
    (a) interstitial fluid
    (b) intracellular fluid
    (c) plasma
    (d) cerebrospinal fluid
42. Which one of the following body cavities contains the heart?
    (a) pleural
    (b) cardium
    (c) pericardial
    (d) peritoneum
43. In anatomical terminology, to which one of the following directions does dorsal refer?
    (a) Towards or on the back of an animal
    (b) Towards or on the belly of an animal
    (c) Towards the head of an animal
    (d) Towards the tail of an animal
44. In the mammalian body, the main extracellular anion is:
    (a) bicarbonate
    (b) chloride
    (c) potassium
    (d) sodium

45. In the mammalian body, the main extracellular cation is:
    (a) bicarbonate
    (b) chloride
    (c) potassium
    (d) sodium
46. In the mammalian body, the main intracellular cation is:
    (a) bicarbonate
    (b) chloride
    (c) potassium
    (d) sodium
47. The thoracic cavity is lined with a serous membrane called the:
    (a) mediastinum
    (b) perineum
    (c) peritoneum
    (d) pleura
48. The mediastinum is located in the:
    (a) head
    (b) thorax
    (c) abdomen
    (d) pelvis
49. Cerebrospinal fluid is an example of:
    (a) interstitial fluid
    (b) plasma fluid
    (c) tissue fluid
    (d) transcellular fluid
50. What percentage of total body water does intracellular fluid comprise?
    (a) 30%
    (b) 40%
    (c) 50%
    (d) 60%
51. Give details of what a serous membrane is.
52. Describe the difference between the visceral and parietal pleura membranes.
53. Explain what is meant by the term homeostasis.
54. Detail the difference between interstitial fluid and intracellular fluid.
55. Would you expect the percentage body water of a puppy to be less than or greater than that of an adult dog?
56. What are the three types of extracellular fluid?
57. Describe what is meant by the anatomical term 'distal'.
58. What is the correct anatomical term to describe 'towards the middle of'?
59. What is the opposite term to the answer to question 58?
60. Explain what the term 'superficial' means.

Co-ordination and control

2.1 Nervous tissue

Neurones and neuroglia
Classification of neurones
Nerve fibres
Neurophysiology
The transmembrane potential
The action potential
The nervous impulse

Introduction

The nervous system controls the co-ordination of the body's organ systems, in close cooperation with the endocrine system. In this chapter we will examine the role of each in providing a rapid means of communication that allows the animal to adjust to the ever-changing environment in which it has to survive. The nervous system is probably the most complex system in the mammalian body, transmitting electrical signals at very high velocity along specialized nerve fibres. It provides a means of communication between the various parts of the body that is essential for the animal's survival. It is the means by which sensations from both the external environment (outside the animal) and internal environment (inside the animal) are received and interpreted, whilst it enables appropriate action to be initiated by sending electrical impulses to other parts of the body.

Broadly speaking the nervous system can be considered to consist of two parts, the central nervous system (CNS) and the peripheral nervous system (PNS). The CNS comprises the brain and spinal cord that together, control and co-ordinate the PNS. The PNS comprises all of the neural tissue that is outside the CNS. These concepts will be discussed later in this chapter, however we shall start at the very beginning by considering the structure and function of nervous tissue.

Neurones and neuroglia

Neurones have the same structural components as any other animal cell, however, their shape is adapted for their function. As they are involved in the transmission of impulses over long distances they are long, thin cells with branching processes at the ends, where they 'connect' with other neurones. The structure of a typical neurone is illustrated in Figure 2.1.

The neurone can be seen to consist of three main sections:

1. The **cell body** (or soma) is large and contains the nucleus of the cell. It also contains the majority of the cell organelles that synthesize the materials needed by the neurone, particularly energy (synthesized by the mitochondria) and **neurotransmitters** (synthesized by the ribosomes and rough endoplasmic reticulum [Rough ER]). Some of the areas containing large amounts of Rough ER and ribosomes stain

Nervous tissue consists of cells, as does any other kind of tissue. Two types of cells can be identified in nervous tissue, **neurones**, which are the cells that are involved in the transmission of the electrical nervous impulse, and **neuroglia** (or satellite cells), the cells that provide support and protection.

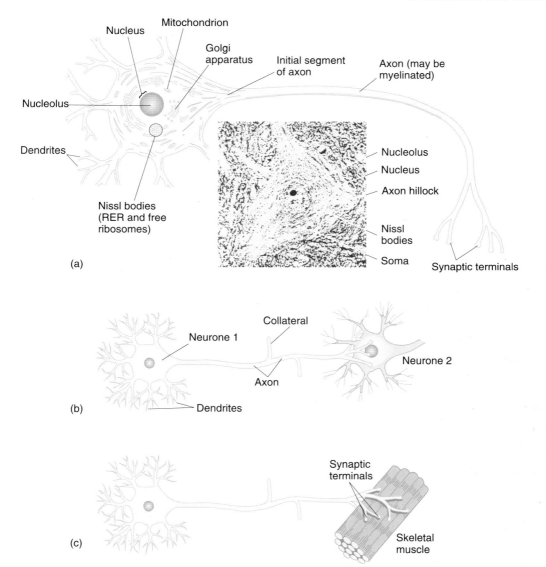

Figure 2.1 (a) The structure of a typical neurone; (b) synapses with another neurone; (c) neuromuscular junctions

darkly and these areas may be referred to as **Nissl bodies**. These give the grey colouration to areas of the spinal cord that contain the cell bodies of the neurones, the so-called **grey matter**.

2. The **dendrites** are short, branching processes extending out from the cell body. They increase the surface area of the cell and provide a means for nervous impulses from other neurones to enter the cell. The dendrites may themselves have small fine processes called **dendritic spines**.

3. The **axon** is a single nerve fibre through which the nervous impulses leave the neurone. It conducts the nervous impulse away from the cell body, down its length to its synaptic terminals. In some cases the axon may branch along its length producing **collaterals** that allow the nervous impulse to be transmitted to more than one other cell. Some axons have closely associated **neuroglial cells**. In the CNS these are **astrocytes**, **oligodendrocytes**, **microglia** and **ependymal cells**, whereas in the PNS they are **satellite cells** and **Schwann cells**.

Astrocytes have a variety of functions. They are thought to be responsible for the blood–brain barrier, a concept based on the observations that certain substances, although present in the bloodstream, are excluded from the CNS. The purpose of this is one of protection, protecting the delicate CNS from substances that may be toxic or that may alter the functioning of the nervous tissue. The blood–brain barrier also serves to prevent substances leaving the CNS. The astrocytes are thought to secrete a substance that maintains the selective permeability of the endothelial cells lining the CNS. Astrocytes are also thought to have some structural function within the CNS, supporting neurones, as well as aiding the stabilization of damaged neural tissue to prevent further damage. They may also be able to change the composition of interstitial fluid, if necessary.

Oligodendrocytes are similar to **Schwann cells** (the latter being present in the PNS as opposed to the CNS). They line the cell membrane of the axon (the **axolemma**) and protect it from direct contact with the extracellular fluid. In some cases several cells form a pad that winds around the axon creating a sheath. The sheath consists primarily of phospholipid and protein and is called a **myelin sheath**. Those neurones with a myelin sheath are said to be **myelinated** and those without, **non-myelinated**. The presence of a myelin sheath increases the speed of transmission of the nervous impulse along the neurone. All axons have either oligodendrocytes or Schwann cells but in some cases a myelin sheath is not formed and the axon is non-myelinated. The outer surface of oligodendrocytes or Schwann cells is called the **neurilemma**. Where several oligodendrocytes or Schwann cells form a sheath, a small gap can be seen between the adjacent cells. This is called the **node of Ranvier** and is illustrated in Figure 2.2.

The function of **microglial cells** is to wander through the CNS and with their phagocytic activity, engulf and destroy cellular waste products, debris and pathogens.

Ependymal cells line the ventricles of the brain and spinal canal (see section on the Nervous System). They are responsible for the circulation of **cerebrospinal fluid** that surrounds and protects the brain and spinal cord. They may also aid in its production and the monitoring of its composition.

Satellite cells are located in the PNS (in addition to Schwann cells discussed previously). They surround the clusters of cell bodies known as **ganglia** (sing = **ganglion**), insulating them from their surroundings.

The function of each type of neuroglial cells is summarized in Table 2.1. A myelinated neurone is illustrated in Figure 2.2.

Classification of neurones

Neurones can be classified anatomically (i.e. based upon their structure) into one of four different types. These are illustrated in Figure 2.3.

The classification relates to the position of the cell body in relation to the axon. **Anaxonic** neurones (Figure 2.3a): there is no anatomical

Table 2.1 Neuroglial cells of the CNS and PNS

Cell type	Location	Function
Astrocyte	CNS	• Maintain the blood–brain barrier, isolating the CNS from the general circulation • Structural support • Support damaged neural tissue • Control the composition of interstitial fluid
Oligodendrocyte	CNS	• Form a sheath around every axon of the CNS • Responsible for myelination of some axons
Microglia	CNS	• Remove debris, waste and pathogens by phagocytosis
Ependymal cell	CNS	• Line the ventricles of the brain and spinal canal • Assist with the production, monitoring and circulation of cerebrospinal fluid
Satellite cell	PNS	• Surround cell bodies of neurones in ganglia
Schwann cell	PNS	• Form a sheath around every axon of the PNS • Responsible for myelination of some peripheral axons

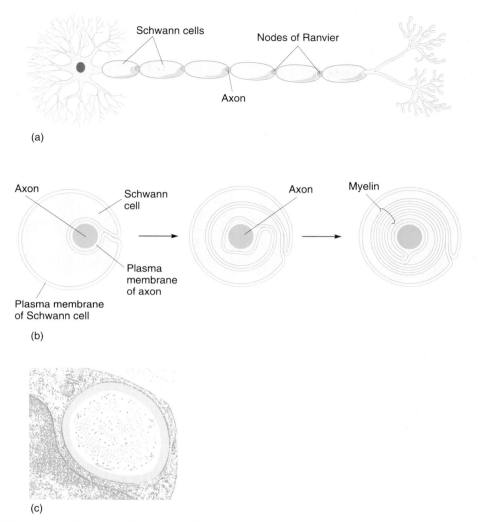

Figure 2.2 Schwann cells and myelination. (a) Schwann cells wrap around some axons, leaving them exposed only at nodes between the cells forming the sheath; (b) during development of a nerve a myelin sheath is formed by Schwann cells wrapping themselves around the axon; (c) part of the nucleus of the Schwann cell

method of differentiating between axons and dendrites. All cell processes appear similar. They are small and are usually located within the brain and special sense organs. **Bipolar** neurones (Figure 2.3b) have two processes arising from the cell body; the dendritic process and one axon, with the cell body in the middle. This type of neurone is rare but can be found in the eye, ear and nose. **Unipolar** neurones (Figure 2.3c) appear to have a continuous dendritic and axonal process with the cell body lying off to one side. These neurones usually have very long axons and are usually located in the PNS. **Multipolar** neurones (Figure

2.3d) have one axon running from the cell body with several dendrites coming in. These are the most common type of neurone found in the CNS.

In addition to anatomical classification, neurones can also be classified on the basis of their function. **Sensory** neurones of the PNS are **afferent**, that is, they carry impulses from sensory receptors towards or into the CNS. **Somatic** sensory neurones carry information from the external environment to the CNS, while **visceral** sensory neurones carry information from within the animal (its organs and other systems). Sensory

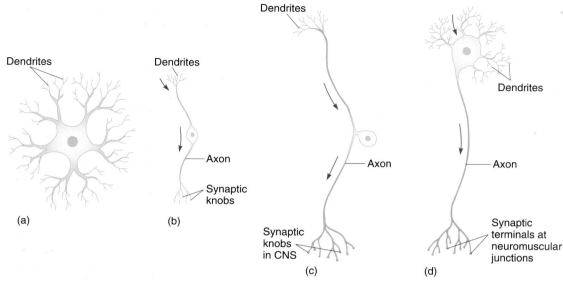

Figure 2.3 Anatomical classification of neurons: (a) anaxonic; (b) bipolar; (c) unipolar; (d) multipolar (somatic motor neuron)

neurones terminate at a **sensory receptor**, either located on a specialized cell or on the process of the neurone itself.

Motor neurones are **efferent**, that is, they carry impulses from the CNS to peripheral tissues, organs or organ systems. Somatic motor neurones carry impulses to the muscles of the body under voluntary control, i.e. the skeletal muscles of the animal. Visceral motor neurones carry impulses to the muscle in the body that are not under conscious control, e.g. the smooth muscle of the intestine and cardiac muscle of the heart. **Interneurones** are those situated between sensory and motor neurones and are found only in the CNS. They distribute sensory information and co-ordinate motor responses.

Nerve fibres

Nerve fibres contain many nerve axons and associated structures and vary in length and diameter. A mixed nerve contains both afferent and efferent fibres and may innervate several different organs, muscles or glands. The structure of a nerve fibre is shown in Figure 2.4.

It can be seen from Figure 2.4 that each axon is surrounded by a fibrous connective tissue called the **endoneurium** (endo = on the inside) and that groups of these axons are held in bundles by connective tissue known as the **perineurium** (peri = on the outside). These are further held together

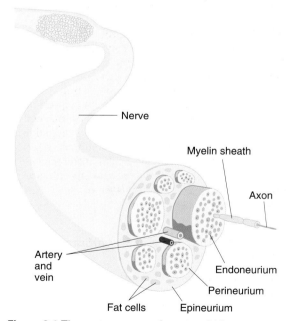

Figure 2.4 The arrangement of axons within a nerve fibre

by an outer fibrous sheath called the **epineurium** which also encloses a blood supply and fat deposits. This arrangement of connective tissues ensures that a protective framework exists for the nerve axons.

Neurophysiology

Neurophysiology is the study of the functioning of nervous tissue, i.e. how the neurones and glial cells transmit and process information. We have already mentioned that neurones can transmit nervous impulses along their length. This impulse is in the form of an electrical stimulus caused by changing the concentration of certain ions (Na^+ and K^+) on the inside and outside of the membrane of the neurone. In the following sections we will examine exactly how this occurs.

The transmembrane potential

In Chapter 1 we discussed the difference in electrolyte composition of extracellular (ECF) and intracellular fluid (ICF). ECF has a high concentration of sodium ions (Na^+) and chloride ions (Cl^-) whereas ICF has a high concentration of potassium ions (K^+) and negatively charged proteins. This difference in ionic concentration exists due to the semipermeability of the cell membrane that will not allow the ions to move across to equalize their distribution. Some ions can pass through more easily than others, for example, proteins carrying a negative charge inside the cell cannot move to the outside whereas K^+ can move out of the cell through a specialized channel more easily than Na^+ can enter through its specialized channel. This leads to a difference in the distribution of positive and negative charges on either side of the cell membrane. There is an overall excess of negative charge on the inner surface of the membrane when compared to the outer surface. This difference in electrical charge is called the **transmembrane potential** or **resting potential** of the cell membrane.

Factors affecting the transmembrane potential

There are several factors that affect the transmembrane potential of a cell, and it is necessary to understand these before we can consider the passage of a nervous impulse in nervous tissue.

Chemical gradients exists across the cell membrane, i.e. there is a difference in concentration of certain electrolytes on either side of the membrane, as discussed previously. The concentration of K^+ is relatively high inside the cell and these ions tend to diffuse along their concentration gradient out of the cell through open potassium channels in the cell membrane. These channels will only allow K^+

through and the movement is with the chemical gradient, i.e. from high to low concentration. The transport of K^+ therefore does not require any input of energy and can be described as **passive** transport.

Electrical gradients also exist across the cell membrane. K^+ can move more easily out of the cell than Na^+ can enter. Consequently, there is a loss of positive charge from the inside of the cell, leaving the inside of the cell with a negative charge relative to the outside. This difference in electrical charge is measured in millivolts (mV). For a resting neurone, the transmembrane potential is 0.07 V or -70 mV (the negative sign indicating that the inner surface is negatively charged when compared to the outside of the cell).

When both the chemical and electrical gradients are considered together, we call this the **electro-chemical gradient**. Let us consider the movement of Na^+; as it is at a higher concentration outside the cell than inside, the chemical gradient that exists results in movement into the cell. There is also an electrical attraction of the positively charged ions towards the negatively charged interior of the cell. Consequently, both the chemical and electrical forces combine to result in movement of the ions into the cell. If we apply this theory to the movement of K^+, then the chemical gradient results in movement out of the cell. However, the electrical gradient means that this movement is resisted by the pull of the negative charge inside the cell and the repulsion of the positive charge outside the cell. The electrochemical gradient that exists across the cell membrane acts as a store of energy. Anything that causes a change in the permeability of the membrane to a particular ion for which an electrochemical gradient exists would cause a sudden movement of that ion across the membrane. The larger the gradient, the more dramatic the movement of ions.

In neurones, K^+ and Na^+ are the two major ions that play a role in transmission of the nervous impulse.

The sodium/potassium pump

We have discussed the concentration of K^+ and Na^+ in relation to the cell in the previous section. If the cell is to maintain homeostasis then it must be able to retrieve some of the lost K^+ from outside the cell and get rid of excess Na^+ from inside the cell. This presents a problem, as both these activities will involve moving the ions against their electrochemical gradients. In order to do this, energy is used to activate a mechanism known as the sodium/potassium pump. This mechanism permits the exchange of intracellular Na^+ for extracellular K^+, using a carrier protein molecule located in the cell membrane, called sodium/potassium ATPase, (Na^+,K^+-ATPase). This mechanism uses energy derived from the conversion of adenosine triphosphate (ATP) to adenosine diphosphate (ADP) to move the ions against their electrochemical gradients, a process known as **active transport**. In a resting neurone, three Na^+ ions diffuse into the cell for every two K^+ ions that diffuse out. The sodium/potassium pump counteracts this by moving, three Na^+ ions out for every two K^+ ions that it moves in. As a result, the transmembrane potential of the cell remains stable.

Now that we have an appreciation of the electrochemical activity of a resting cell, we can apply these theories to the transmission of a nervous impulse along a neurone. This will be considered in the following section.

The action potential

In the previous section we learnt that the transmembrane potential across the cell membrane is approximately $-70\,mV$ in a resting neurone. This may also be referred to as the **resting potential** and the cell membrane can be said to be **polarized**.

Cells of nerve and muscle tissues have a special ability to alter their transmembrane potential and reverse it momentarily. This results in the inside of the cell becoming positively charged and the outside negatively charged, for a short period of time. This process is known as **depolarization** and the change in potential is called the **action potential**. The whole process lasts for approximately 1 millisecond and the resting potential is very quickly restored. Figure 2.5 is an illustration of the stages during an action potential.

We can see from Figure 2.5 that, following a suitable stimulus, sodium channels open in the cell membrane and Na^+ rapidly enters the cell, moving along its electrochemical gradient. This results in the inside of the cell membrane having a transient positive charge and the cell membrane being **depolarized**. Following depolarization, the sodium channels are closed and potassium channels are opened. This results in K^+ leaving the cell moving with its electrochemical gradient, and **repolarization** of the cell membrane commences. There is a slight fall below the resting potential (**hyperpolarization**) as the potassium channels start to

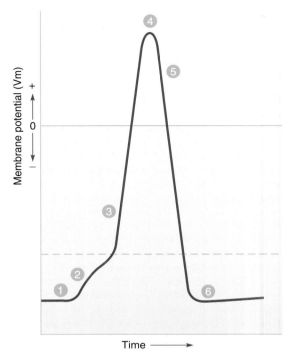

Figure 2.5 The action potential of a neurone. 1, Membrane at rest (no net charge movement); 2, depolarizing electronic potential; 3, Na^+ moving in rapidly; 4, no net charge movement; 5, K^+ moving out rapidly; 6, Na^+ channels recovering from refractoriness

close, however this is soon corrected and the transmembrane potential returns to its normal resting level of $-70\,mV$.

Generation of an action potential

As is indicated in Figure 2.5, there is a certain level of depolarization that is required before an action potential can be triggered. This is called the **threshold**. Once the stimulus (which may be light, heat, mechanical force, electrical or chemical energy) has caused the neurone to become depolarized above the threshold level, then an action potential is triggered. Generation of action potentials can be said to follow the **all-or-none law**. This means that they either occur or not, a graded response is not possible. A certain threshold exists, but once that threshold is exceeded, whether it is by a gradual or sudden stimulus, the magnitude and duration of the response is the same.

The frequency of the stimulus that is of a magnitude to exceed the threshold, also has some effect upon the generation of further action potentials within the same neurone. If a second stimulus acts upon a neurone in which an action potential is ongoing, then a second action potential will not be produced. The neurone at this stage is unresponsive and is said to be in a **refractory** stage. The time that it takes for the neurone to be able to generate a second action potential from the start of the first is called the **absolute refractory period**. It is possible to generate a second action potential in a neurone that has not completely returned to its resting potential; this is only possible in the very late stages of the action potential, however, and the stimulus needs to be stronger in order to overcome the increased threshold depolarization. The period between the end of the absolute refractory period (when it is impossible to initiate another action potential) and a return to the resting potential is known as the **relative refractory period**. This is the period during which a second action potential can be triggered, although, as stated above, this requires the stimulus to exceed the threshold depolarization. The sodium channels at this stage can be re-opened and the influx of Na^+ exceeds the movement of K^+ leaving the cell, triggering a second action potential. An action potential triggered during the relative refractory period may be distorted in both amplitude and duration.

The nervous impulse

In the previous section we discussed how an action potential is generated in nervous tissue. We now need to consider how action potentials are propagated along the axon of the neurone and between neurones, forming a nervous impulse within the body.

When a stimulus generates an action potential, the potential difference across the membrane is altered by the sudden movement of Na^+ out of the cell into the extracellular fluid. This only occurs at one point along the axon, however the efflux of Na^+ causes a local change in the electric potential of both the extracellular fluid and axoplasm. This local disturbance in the electric field generates a potential difference that causes an electrical current (a movement of positive charge) to flow to the next segment of the axon. This in turn causes a depolarization of this section of the axon, reaching the threshold and triggering an action potential. Consequently, action potentials are triggered successively along different regions of the axon as the nervous impulse travels away from the point of initial stimulation. This effect is illustrated in Figure 2.6.

Due to the fact that the axon becomes refractory for a period following the generation of an action potential, action potentials can only travel in one direction along the axon, away from the region of initial stimulation.

Myelination of the nerve fibres alters the electrical properties of the axon, as the myelin sheath causes an increase in resistance to the flow of electrical current. The nodes of Ranvier are the only point along myelinated axons at which the action potentials can be generated as they are the only places where K^+ can move out of the axoplasm into the extracellular fluid. Impulse transmission between the nodes is by local current within the axon. Action potentials are often said to 'jump' from one node of Ranvier to another in myelinated fibres and this is often referred to as **saltatory conduction** (from **saltare** – Latin – to leap). This type of nervous transmission occurs much more quickly than that in non-myelinated axons as the action potential can 'leap' across lengths of the myelinated axon from node to node.

Speed of impulse transmission is not only dependent on the myelination of the nerve fibre, but also on its diameter. Those of a larger diameter conduct action potentials at a greater speed than those with a smaller diameter.

The synapse

Nerve fibres have a finite length and consequently it is necessary for the nervous impulse to be transmitted from one neurone to another, or from a neurone to a muscle cell. The point at which this transmission occurs is called the **synapse** (between one neurone and the next) or **neuromuscular junction** (between a neurone and muscle fibre). At the synapse, the action potential from the axon of first nerve cell (the presynaptic neurone) is carried across the interstitial, known as the **synaptic cleft**, space to the dendrites of the next nerve cell (the postsynaptic neurone). This occurs in one of two ways.

1. **Electrical transmission**
    Electrical transmission occurs when the two cells are very close together, i.e. the synaptic gap or cleft was small. In some cases the membranes of the cells may even be fused. In cells that were close together, the action potential is automatically propagated into the adjacent cell by causing a membrane depolarization, just as the action potential is propagated along the axon itself.

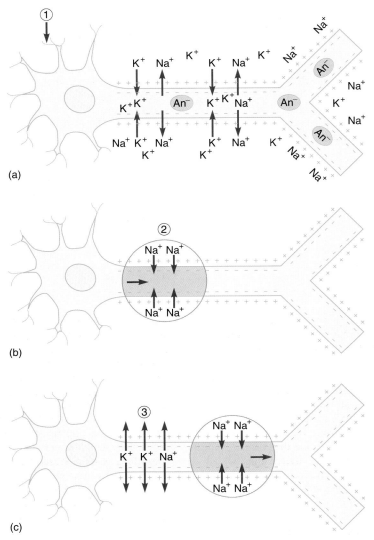

Figure 2.6 Impulse transmission along an axon. (a) At rest, and being stimulated sufficiently to depolarize the membrane; (b) and (c) the conduction of the wave of depolarization along the axon. An⁻=large anions. 1, Stimulus; 2, area of action potential travelling along neurone; 3, area of repolarization

2. **Chemical transmission**

When the synaptic gap is large, an impulse in the presynaptic neurone causes the release of a chemical into the gap. This chemical is known as a **neurotransmitter**. The neurotransmitter diffuses across the synaptic gap to the postsynaptic neurone and triggers a change in the membrane potential of the postsynaptic neurone. This depolarizes the postsynaptic neurones generating an action potential in the postsynaptic cell.

Transmission across the synapse occurs primarily by the second method, chemical transmission and this method forms the basis of synaptic transmission in the majority of mammalian neurones. We will examine the mechanism of chemical transmission in more detail.

Chemical transmission

Figure 2.7 illustrates the basic structure of the chemical synapse. Synaptic vesicles in the

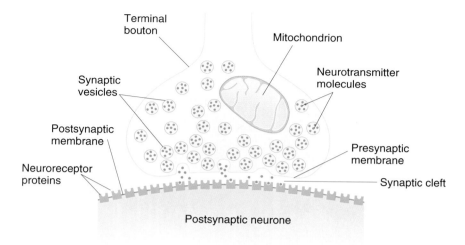

Figure 2.7 The synapse

terminal bouton (the swollen end of the presynaptic neurone) contain the neurotransmitter that is synthesized by the neurone. When an impulse reaches the terminal boutons, the synaptic vesicles migrate towards the presynaptic membrane, with which they fuse, and release their contents into the synaptic gap. The neurotransmitter diffuses across the gap until it reaches the membrane of the postsynaptic cell. It causes a change in the potential difference across the membrane that can either: (a) depolarize the cell, thereby increasing the likelihood of the generation of an action potential; or (b) hyperpolarize the cell, thereby reducing the chance of an action potential being generated.

This action occurs by one of two mechanisms. Firstly, the neurotransmitter can react with specific **receptor sites** in the postsynaptic membrane. This opens gates in the membrane that allows the movement of ions into the neurone, causing changes in the membrane potential and the generation of an action potential. The excitator neurotransmitter **acetylcholine** is released at synapses of the peripheral nervous system (see section on the Nervous System) and generates an action potential in this way). The neurotransmitter gamma-aminobutyric acid (GABA) causes hyperpolarization (i.e. is an inhibitory neurotransmitter) by a similar mechanism. The second mechanism is thought to be less direct and is not yet clearly understood.

Once the neurotransmitter has reacted with the receptors, the presynaptic neurone must prepare for the arrival of another nervous impulse. Con-

sequently, any neurotransmitter that remains in the synaptic gap must be broken down or removed before another impulse arrives. Some neurotransmitters are deactivated by the action of enzymes, for example, acetylcholine is broken down by the enzyme **acetylcholinesterase**, which is found in the membrane of the postsynaptic neurone. Some of the by-products of the breakdown are taken up by the presynaptic membrane and used to synthesize more neurotransmitter for future use. Other neurotransmitters, such as noradrenaline, are removed from the synaptic gap by active re-uptake into the presynaptic neurone using a biological 'pump', similar to that used to move ions across cell membranes, against a concentration gradient.

The neuromuscular junction

In addition to a nervous impulse travelling from one neurone to the next we should also consider the transmission of an impulse from a neurone to a muscle to stimulate contraction. The region where this occurs is called the neuromuscular junction and each muscle fibre is controlled by a single neurone. At the neuromuscular junction the axon forms a number of small branches within the perimysium of the muscle (see Chapter 3). Each branch ends in a swollen synaptic terminal that contains the neurotransmitter acetylcholine (ACh). The surface of the muscle surrounding the synaptic terminals contains membrane receptors that bind to

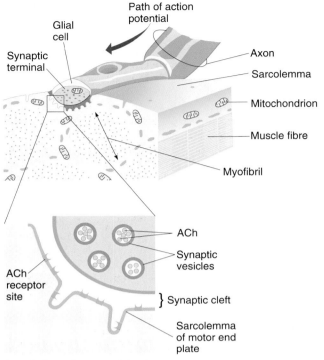

Step 1: An action potential arrives at the synaptic terminal.

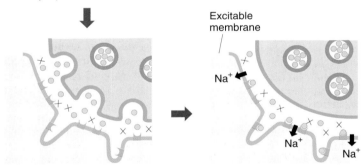

Step 2: Acetylcholine is released. Vesicles in the synaptic terminal fuse with the membrane of the neurone and release ACh into the synaptic cleft.

Step 3: ACh binds at the motor end plate. An action potential is generated causing muscle contraction.

Figure 2.8 The neuromuscular junction and mechanism of impulse transmission

the ACh. This region of the membrane is called the motor end plate. The release of ACh and binding at the motor end plates triggers changes within the muscle fibre that stimulates contraction of the muscle. The structure of a neuromuscular junction and the mechanism of impulse transmission is illustrated in Figure 2.8.

Postsynaptic receptors

The receptors on the postsynaptic membrane are specific to a particular type of neurotransmitter and a postsynaptic neurone may have several different kinds of receptors, meaning that it can respond to several neurotransmitters. For example, **nicotinic**

receptors respond to nicotine and acetylcholine whereas **muscarinic receptors** respond to muscarine and acetylcholine (but are insensitive to nicotine). Nicotinic receptors are usually located in skeletal muscle and ganglia of the autonomic nervous system (see the section on the Nervous System) and muscarinic receptors can be found in smooth muscle, cardiac muscle and exocrine glands.

Receptors that cause an excitatory response in the postsynaptic membrane act to increase its permeability to potassium and sodium ions, although the influx of sodium ions tends to predominate. This causes a depolarization of the membrane. An inhibitory response is caused by receptors that trigger the opening of the 'gates' that allow the movement of potassium and chloride ions. This acts to stabilize the resting potential of the cell and in some cases may cause hyperpolarization.

When one neurone has many synapses with other neurones, the activity within the cell is determined by the net effect of excitatory and inhibitory impulses at any one time. If excitatory impulses predominate, then a wave of depolarization spreads along the postsynaptic dendrites to the axon hillock where it produces an action potential that is propagated along the axon. If inhibitory impulses predominate, the threshold level at the axon hillock is not reached and an action potential is not generated. So it can be seen that the axon hillock acts as a type of 'collection point' where excitatory and inhibitory impulses are gathered and a 'total' of all synaptic activity is taken into account.

An understanding of the way that a nervous impulse is transmitted allows us to appreciate the mode of action of some of the pharmacological agents used in practice that affect the nervous system. For example, neuromuscular blocking agents, used to provide muscle relaxation, act at the neuromuscular junction (where a neurone meets a muscle cell). They can act in one of two ways:

1. At the presynaptic neurone via inhibition of the synthesis of acetylcholine or by inhibiting its release
2. At the postsynaptic neurone via the blocking of the acetylcholine receptors (a non-depolarizing blockade), e.g. pancuronium (Pavulon®) or by persistent depolarization with an agonist that has a longer duration of action than acetylcholine, e.g. suxamethonium (Anectine®)

Muscle relaxant drugs are described as depolarizing or non-depolarizing depending on their actions. Depolarizing agents cause persistent depolarization of the muscle by inactivating the release of Na$^+$, thereby preventing the generation of an action potential. Paralysis is not reversed by giving an anticholinesterase agent. Non-depolarizing agents compete with acetylcholine for receptor sites and thereby inhibit the effects of the neurotransmitter. Their effects can be reversed by anticholinesterase agents such as neostigmine (Prostigmin®).

2.2 The nervous system

The central nervous system
The brain
The spinal cord
The peripheral nervous system
The autonomic nervous system

Introduction

As discussed in the introduction of this chapter, the nervous system is comprised of two parts, the central nervous system (CNS) and the peripheral nervous system (PNS). The CNS comprises the brain and spinal cord, and together, these control and co-ordinate the PNS. The PNS comprises all of the neural tissue that is outside the CNS. This includes the sensory nerves that send information from receptors (sensory structures) into the CNS (via **afferent neurones**) as well as the motor nerves that carry information from the CNS (via **efferent neurones**) to tissues and organs. Those connected to the brain are called cranial nerves whereas those that connect with the spinal cord are called spinal nerves. The efferent nerves can be divided into two classes; those that supply the skeletal muscles form the **somatic nervous system** (**SNS**) whereas those that supply smooth muscle, cardiac muscle, and glands, form the **autonomic nervous system** (**ANS**). The functioning of the ANS is completely involuntary whereas the SNS is usually under voluntary control. The only circumstances when the SNS is under some involuntary control are when the animal is unconscious (the muscles of respiration still function) or during a reflex response, such as standing on a sharp object. The limb is withdrawn as soon as the pain receptors are stimulated, without the need for conscious intervention. Throughout this chapter we will consider these basic concepts in more detail.

The central nervous system

Nervous tissue of the CNS can be classified as either grey or white matter, depending upon its appearance. Grey matter appears grey due to the presence of the cell bodies of the neurones in the tissue, while the white matter consists of the myelinated nerve cell processes (lipid within the myelin does not take up stains readily). In the following sections we will examine the structure and function of the CNS.

The brain

The brain is located in the cranial cavity. Its structure is such that it can be divided into three parts, the **forebrain**, **midbrain** and **hindbrain**. We will consider each of the areas in turn, referring to Figure 2.9.

The forebrain

The largest, rostral part of the forebrain is called the **cerebrum** and is thought to control learning, emotions, and behaviour in mammals. It is divided into the left and right **cerebral hemispheres** by a deep fissure or groove called the **longitudinal sulcus**. The hemispheres are connected by a thick band of neurones called the **corpus callosum**, which maintains a flow of information between the two halves of the cerebrum. Each cerebral hemisphere is divided into four topographical areas or lobes, the **frontal**, **parietal**, **occipital** and **temporal** lobes. The boundaries of these four lobes are not anatomically distinct. The outer layer of the cerebrum (the cerebral cortex) is comprised of numerous folds of tissue. The ridges of the folds are called **gyri** (sing = **gyrus**) and the indentations are called **sulci** (sing = **sulcus**). These act to increase the surface area and consequently the number of nerve cell bodies in this area of the brain. The cerebral cortex is composed of grey matter with underlying white matter beneath the cortex (this differs from the arrangement in the spinal cord where the grey matter is located on the inside, the white matter on the outside). Inside each

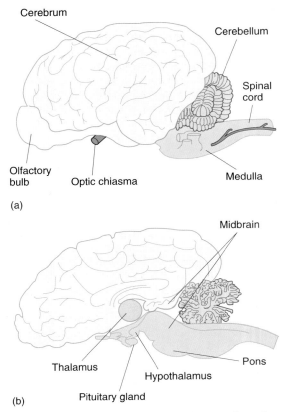

Figure 2.9 Lateral view and longitudinal section of the canine brain. (a) Lateral view; (b) longitudinal section.

hemisphere there is a cavity called the **lateral ventricle**. The brain has four ventricles in total, the remaining two being located in the middle of the forebrain (the third ventricle) and in the middle of the hindbrain (the fourth ventricle). The ventricles of the brain are connected with each other and also with the central canal of the spinal cord. They each contain a vascular projection of specialized secretory cells, collectively called the **choroid plexus**. This secretes **cerebrospinal fluid** (**CSF**) into the ventricles and central canal.

Cerebrospinal fluid

CSF is usually a clear, colourless, slightly alkaline fluid. It is similar in composition to plasma but only contains a small amount of protein. A few lymphocytes may be present but no red blood cells. Its function is to protect the brain and spinal cord by forming a fluid cushion between the delicate nerve tissues and the bones of the skull and vertebral column. It enables the pressure within the skull to remain constant and also carries waste and toxic substances away from the tissue to the interstitial fluid of the CNS. The CSF is capable of freely exchanging nutrients and waste products with the interstitial fluid of the CNS. Through the blood–brain barrier, it also has some protective function, although this is not yet fully understood.

The CSF circulates through the four ventricles of the brain. It also passes into the **subarachnoid space**, a space between the inner and middle of the three layers of connective tissue which surround the brain. There are three such layers and they are known as the **meninges**. The thin, inner layer that lies on the surface of the brain and spinal cord is known as the **pia mater**. Between this layer and the middle layer (the **arachnoid mater**) is the subarachnoid space containing the CSF. The outer layer (the **dura mater**) is a thick membrane and is composed of tough fibrous tissue. It lines the inside of the skull forming the **periosteum**. The epidural space lies between the dura mater and the spinal column, providing a suitable site for the administration of local anaesthetics. The structure of the meninges is illustrated in Figure 2.10.

Ventral to the cerebrum lies the thalamus, which acts as a relay station for information to and from

Samples of CSF may be collected for analysis from an enlargement of the subarachnoid space at the base of the skull called the **cisterna magna**. This site can also be used for injecting contrast agents for myelography in the dog, although the lumbar area between the 5th and 6th lumbar vertebrae is more commonly used in humans.

the cerebrum. Below the thalamus lie the hypothalamus and pituitary gland. These have a very close relationship that will be discussed further in the section on the Endocrine system below, although, broadly speaking, the hypothalamus is associated with the regulation of food and water intake and body temperature. It also controls the activity of the pituitary gland that in turn regulates the activity of many other endocrine glands.

The midbrain

Structures in the midbrain are associated with the transmission of impulses between the brain and spinal cord. They are also associated with the processing of impulses from the senses of sight and hearing.

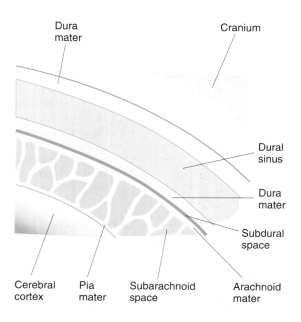

Figure 2.10 The meninges

The hindbrain

The hindbrain consists of three predominant areas. The most rostral area is the **pons** that lies between the midbrain and an area of the hindbrain known as the **medulla oblongata** (also referred to as the medulla). The pons and medulla lie at the level at which most cranial nerves enter the brain (see above). Both the pons and medulla are also responsible for the basic control of heart rate and respiration, known as the **brainstem reflexes**. The third area, the **cerebellum** controls the motor co-ordination of the body.

The limbic system

The limbic system is not an anatomically distinct area of the brain, unlike the other structures that have been discussed. It includes a large number of structures of the forebrain that are all inter-connected and associated with emotional response. The significance of this area is still under study, however it is likely to play an important role in the emotional aspects of behaviour.

The spinal cord

The spinal cord is continuous with the medulla of the brain. It runs within the protective vertebral column from the cisterna magna, terminating at the **cauda equina**, a group of nerves that run together in the region of the seventh lumbar vertebrae and the sacral region, resembling a mare's tail. The spinal cord is protected by the vertebrae, meninges and CSF against damage. A transverse section of the cord (see Figure 2.11) reveals that the grey matter is located centrally with the white matter forming the outer section. The central canal contains CSF.

Thirty-six pairs of spinal nerves leave the spinal cord, passing through the intervertebral foramina, each passing to a different part of the body (see section on Special senses). Each spinal nerve is surrounded by a layer of meningeal dura and has a dorsal and a ventral root. The dorsal root is comprised of sensory afferent fibres with their cell bodies located in a cluster or **ganglion** in the intervertebral foramen. The ventral root is com-prised of motor efferent fibres with the cell bodies located in the ventral horn of the grey matter. So sensory impulses enter the spinal cord via the dorsal root and motor impulses leave via the ventral root of the spinal nerve.

The peripheral nervous system

The PNS includes all other nervous tissue that is not within the brain or spinal cord. It includes all the nerves that pass out from the spinal cord to muscles and organs, as well as those that carry impulses back into the CNS for interpretation.

Efferent nerves can be divided into two broad categories, those which are part of the **somatic nervous system** (**SNS**), supplying skeletal muscle, and those supplying smooth muscle, cardiac

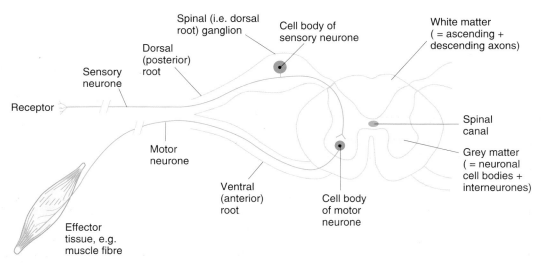

Figure 2.11 Transverse section of the spinal cord

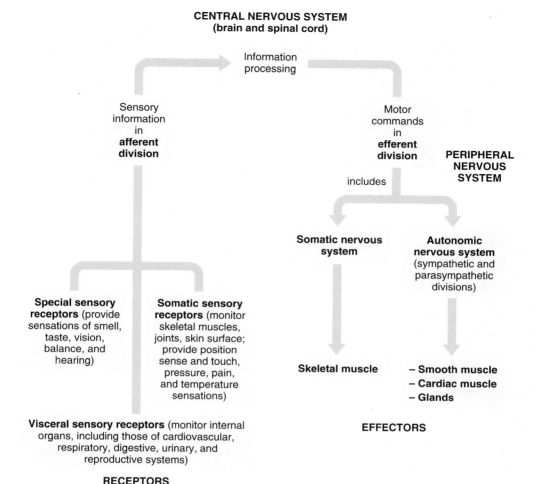

CENTRAL NERVOUS SYSTEM
(brain and spinal cord)

Information
processing

Sensory
information
in
**afferent
division**

Motor
commands
in
**efferent
division**

**PERIPHERAL
NERVOUS
SYSTEM**

includes

**Somatic nervous
system**

**Autonomic
nervous system**
(sympathetic and
parasympathetic
divisions)

**Special sensory
receptors** (provide
sensations of smell,
taste, vision,
balance, and
hearing)

**Somatic sensory
receptors** (monitor
skeletal muscles,
joints, skin surface;
provide position
sense and touch,
pressure, pain,
and temperature
sensations)

Skeletal muscle

– **Smooth muscle**
– **Cardiac muscle**
– **Glands**

Visceral sensory receptors (monitor internal
organs, including those of cardiovascular,
respiratory, digestive, urinary, and
reproductive systems)

EFFECTORS

RECEPTORS

Figure 2.12 Relationship between aspects of the nervous system

muscle and glands from the **autonomic nervous system (ANS)**. This is illustrated in Figure 2.12 and will be considered in the following sections.

The somatic nervous system

Efferent nerves of the SNS carry impulses from the CNS to skeletal muscle. Somatic sensory receptors are responsible for providing feedback to the brain from the skeletal muscle. The majority of the nerves of this system are under voluntary control, except in the cases of unconsciousness and reflexes when their action is involuntary. Nerves of the SNS can be further subdivided into cranial and spinal nerves, depending upon the part of the body that they innervate.

Cranial nerves

There are 12 cranial nerves in the dog (see Table 2.2), each originates or terminates within the brain, depending on whether it is a sensory or motor nerve. Some cranial nerves have both a motor and a sensory function and can be called 'mixed' nerves.

Spinal nerves

Spinal nerves supply the entire musculoskeletal system. We have examined the structure of the spinal cord earlier and have seen how the nerves on each side of the spinal cord divides into two roots, **dorsal** and **ventral**. The dorsal root carries sensory nerve fibres into the spinal cord whereas the

Table 2.2 Cranial nerves of the dog

Nerve	Type	Function
1 Olfactory	Sensory	Smell (impulses sent to the olfactory bulb in the brain)
2 Optic	Sensory	Sight
3 Oculomotor	Motor	Eye movements
4 Trochlear	Motor	Eye movements
5 Trigeminal	Mixed	Motor – movement of jaw muscles Sensory – from the skin of the facial region
6 Abducens	Motor	Eye movements
7 Facial	Mixed	Motor – muscles of facial expression Sensory – muscles of the tongue
8 Auditory (vestibulocochlear)	Sensory	Hearing and sense of balance
9 Glossopharyngeal	Mixed	Motor – to the pharynx Sensory – taste from the tongue
10 Vagus	Mixed	Supplies the larynx, thoracic and abdominal viscera including the digestive tract, controlling its movement and secretions
11 Accessory	Motor	Movements of the neck, pharynx and soft palate
12 Hypoglossal	Mixed	Movement of the tongue

ventral root carries motor fibres to the musculoskeletal system. In certain areas of the body the nerves interweave to produce a complex network of fibres known as a **plexus**. For example, in the dog, the **brachial plexus** is a network of nerve fibres that gives rise to the **radial**, **ulnar** and **medial** nerves supplying the forelimb. Figure 2.13 illustrates the brachial plexus in the forelimb of a dog. As can be seen from the figure, the detailed aspects of the nervous system are complex and not within the bounds of this text. Those wishing to study the nervous system in greater anatomical detail are referred to appropriate references at the end of this text.

It is worth noting that the nerves associated with the senses of sight/balance, taste, and smell are all dedicated nerves that supply special information about the surroundings of the animal, therefore they are entirely afferent in nature. Nerves that lead to skeletal muscle, e.g. cranial nerve VII, will also have some sensory fibres that transmit information back to the CNS from the muscle. However, despite this, they tend to be classified as motor nerves.

Reflexes

A reflex reaction is an inborn, involuntary response towards an external stimulus that is mediated by the nervous system. Let us consider a dog that is being fed. Such a dog will salivate when food is placed in the mouth – this is an inborn, involuntary action, known as a reflex response. A famous Russian scientist, Pavlov, trained dogs to anticipate food by ringing a bell prior to feeding. Over a period of time, the dogs would start to salivate as soon as the bell was rung, even if there was no other evidence of feeding. Every dog owner sees a similar response when they pick up the tin opener. Their dog starts to salivate in anticipation of being fed. Salivation in response to the bell (or the tin opener) is called a **conditioned reflex response**. It is a response that has been conditioned by training to be associated with a certain stimulus. This illustrates the difficulty faced when trying to ascertain whether or not a response is a true reflex action. In the example of the dog, salivation in response to food placed directly in the mouth is a true reflex action. Although salivation in response to bell ringing has the same end result or response, the triggering stimulus is different and has been learned as a predictor of an event.

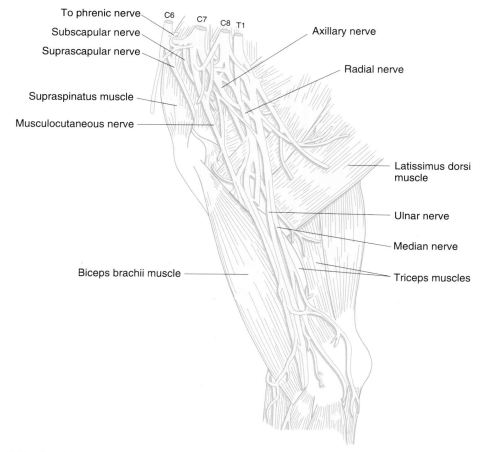

To phrenic nerve
C6
C7
C8 T1
Axillary nerve
Subscapular nerve
Suprascapular nerve
Radial nerve
Supraspinatus muscle
Musculocutaneous nerve
Latissimus dorsi muscle
Ulnar nerve
Median nerve
Biceps brachii muscle
Triceps muscles

Figure 2.13 The brachial plexus

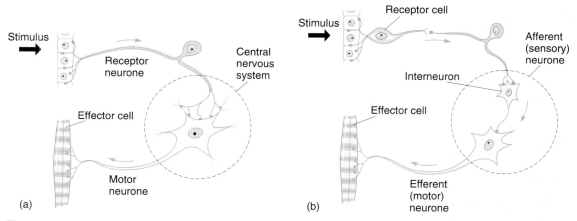

Stimulus
Receptor neurone
Central nervous system
Effector cell
Motor neurone
(a)

Stimulus
Receptor cell
Afferent (sensory) neurone
Interneuron
Effector cell
Efferent (motor) neurone
(b)

Figure 2.14 The simple reflex arc. (a) monosynaptic; (b) including several synaptic relays

Reflex responses can be from internal or external stimuli. Those arising from external stimuli are perhaps more easy to appreciate, for example, the reaction to standing on a sharp object. Those that arise internally include coughing, swallowing, vomiting, and, as discussed above, salivation. Whatever the stimulus, the reflex pathway is similar to that illustrated in Figure 2.14.

Let us consider the withdrawal reflex stimulated by standing on a sharp object. In addition to the reflex that occurs at spinal level, other nervous pathways are stimulated that help to maintain balance and perhaps to cause the animal to vocalize in response to the pain. These are not part of the reflex, however they are part of the overall behavioural response. Reflex reactions always involve the CNS. In simple responses this may only be at the level of the spinal cord, however more complex reflexes may also involve the brain. The receptor is stimulated by the stimulus and triggers an impulse to pass along the sensory afferent nerve fibre towards the CNS. On reaching the CNS the sensory neurone synapses with an interneurone that then transmits the impulse to the motor efferent nerve fibre. The stimulus is carried to the effector, in this case the muscle of the limb, to cause retraction of the limb away from the sharp object.

Sensory receptors

In order that information from both the internal and external environment can be translated into impulses that can be propagated to the brain and spinal cord for processing, specialized sensory neurones are required, distributed throughout the body. These form the afferent system of the PNS. **Somatic sensory neurones** provide information about the external environment of the animal whereas **visceral sensory neurones** monitor the internal environment and organs. Some sensory neurones have specialized terminals or cells known as receptors. Receptors can be classified in a number of ways, depending on their structure and function.

One method of classification is to consider from where they receive their stimulus, for example:

- **exteroceptors**, which are stimulated by information from the external environment such as touch, sight, smell, hearing, taste, pressure and temperature.
- **proprioceptors**, which monitor movements and position of the skeletal muscles and joints.
- **interoceptors**, which monitor the internal environment such as the respiratory, digestive, urinary, cardiovascular and reproductive systems. They are also stimulated by deep pressure and pain.

Others prefer to classify receptors by taking their structure into consideration, for example, those with:

- **unspecialized free nerve endings**, which are involved in detecting touch and painful stimuli and are located in the skin, muscles, and viscera. Nerve endings in the cornea are also stimulated by touch pressure and temperature.
- **specialized or encapsulated nerve endings**, which are located in the dermis of the skin and respond to touch and pressure.
- **specialized non-neuronal receptor cells**, which are located in the ear and eye, as well as the taste buds.

The method of classification that appears in most textbooks, however, is based on the type of stimulus to which the receptor responds. This is similar to the first example but a little more specific:

- **Chemoreceptors**, which detect chemical changes in the local area around the receptor. For example, in the brain there are chemoreceptors that detect the levels of oxygen and carbon dioxide in blood and osmoreceptors that detect changes in salt concentration. Receptors associated with taste and smell can also be considered chemoreceptors.
- **Mechanoreceptors**, which respond to touch and pressure and are predominantly located in the skin. There are also receptors that detect the degree of 'stretch' of muscles, for example, in the stomach, lungs and blood vessels.
- **Thermoreceptors**, which are stimulated by changes in temperature and are located in the skin.
- **Pain receptors or nociceptors**, which are usually triggered by any stimulus that may cause tissue damage or injury. Release of chemicals in an area of inflammation may also trigger these receptors.

- **Electromagnetic receptors**, which are stimulated by light and are found in the retina of the eye.
- **Proprioceptors**, which is a collective term used to group together all the receptors that relay information about the position of the body and its movements.

Whichever classification is chosen, the underlying function of the receptor is to detect a stimulus to allow information to be transmitted to the CNS for processing.

Adaptation

Some receptors show a reduced response in the presence of a constant stimulus, i.e. they become less sensitive. When the stimulus first occurs the receptor responds fully, however, if the situation persists the level of response declines until the receptor is no longer stimulated. This process is known as adaptation and helps to prevent the unnecessary waste of energy responding to stimuli that are insignificant to the individual. For example, thermoreceptors show adaptation. On entering a house, a dog may be aware that the temperature is warmer, however, the thermoreceptors adapt and are no longer stimulated.

Pain

Pain receptors (or nociceptors) show little adaptation. This helps the survival of the animal in that as long as pain persists, the animal will perform behaviours that minimize the pain. This will aid the healing process, the residual pain from an injured site will tend to prevent the animal from using the injured site and/or encourage the animal to protect the injured area.

The autonomic nervous system

We have examined that part of the nervous system over which an animal has some form of conscious control over the SNS. The autonomic nervous system (ANS) controls those parts of the body that are part of an animal's unconscious actions. These are usually the processes that are essential to life. For example, when an animal is anaesthetized its heart still beats and breathing still occurs, if a little more slowly than when conscious. This is possible because of the activity of the ANS, which co-ordinates the activities of the cardiovascular and respiratory systems, as well as the digestive, urinary and reproductive systems.

The structure of the ANS

The ANS can be divided into two parts, the **sympathetic nervous system** and the **parasympathetic nervous system**. Usually, the two parts have opposite effects, one is excitatory and the other inhibitory. However, this is not always true as sometimes they may work independently, some organs being innervated by one and not the other, and sometimes the two parts may work together. When comparing the somatic nervous system with the ANS it can be seen that whilst they both consist of neurones, neuroglia and connective tissue, the somatic nervous system has an upper motor neurone in the brain or spinal cord that controls the activity of a lower motor neurone. This lower motor neurone has direct contact with the skeletal muscle. When the lower motor neurone is stimulated it always has an excitatory effect on the muscle cells.

The ANS has a second visceral motor neurone between the brain and spinal cord, known as a **preganglionic neurone**. Fibres from the preganglionic neurone leave the CNS and form synapses with postganglionic neurones in the periphery, e.g. muscle of the heart, glands, and smooth muscle. Stimulating the postganglionic neurones may result in excitation or inhibition of the effector, in contrast to the lower motor neurones of the somatic nervous system.

The sympathetic nervous system

This part of the ANS prepares the body for activity. It is often referred to the system that prepares the body for a 'fight or flight' response. Consider a cat, sunning itself in the garden. It hears a dog approaching. It will immediately become more aware of its surroundings, i.e. there will be an increase in the level of alertness. Its metabolic rate will increase rapidly, it will start to breathe faster and more deeply, and its heart rate and blood pressure will increase. Blood flow to skeletal muscles will also increase whilst digestive and urinary functions will be temporarily put on hold. This ensures that the cat is prepared for the extra physical activity that may be required to either run away from the dog or stand its ground, as some cats do!

The sympathetic division has its preganglionic neurones in the thoracic and lumbar regions of the spinal cord. The postganglionic neurones with which they synapse are located in three different locations:

1. **Sympathetic chain ganglia or lateral ganglia** are located on either side of the vertebral column and their neurones affect the head, body wall, limbs, and inside the thorax.
   Stimulation of these ganglia causes:

   - constriction of the blood vessels in the skin
   - increased blood flow to the skeletal muscles and brain
   - release of lipid from fat store
   - dilation of the pupils
   - acceleration of heart rate and strength of cardiac contraction
   - bronchodilation

2. **Collateral ganglia** are located anterior to the bodies of the vertebrae and their neurones affect the tissue and organs of the abdomen and pelvis.
   Stimulation of these ganglia causes:

   - reduction of blood flow to visceral organs
   - decreased activity of digestive system
   - release of glucose from glycogen reserves in the liver
   - reduction in the rate of formation of urine
   - stimulation of release of lipids from fat stores

3. The **adrenal medulla**, found in the centre of each adrenal gland, is a modified ganglion of the sympathetic nervous system. It has postganglionic neurones with very short axons which, when stimulated, release their neurotransmitters into the blood stream. In this case the site of release of the neurotransmitter is not at a synapse but directly into the circulation. This mechanism allows the neurotransmitters, adrenaline (epinephrine) and noradrenaline (norepinephrine) to have an effect as hormones on many target cells throughout the body.

In general, the preganglionic neurones are relatively short as they are near to the spinal cord. The postganglionic fibres are longer as they innervate the effectors. The exception to this is the adrenal medullae, in which the postganglionic fibres are short as they release their neurotransmitters directly into the circulation.

Neurotransmitters of the sympathetic nervous system

On stimulation of the preganglionic neurones, acetylcholine is released at the synapse between the preganglionic and postganglionic neurones. These are called **cholinergic** synapses as they use acetylcholine as the neurotransmitter. The effect of the acetylcholine on the postganglionic neurones is always excitatory. The postganglionic neurones, once stimulated, carry the impulse to the effector, e.g. smooth muscle, and at the junction between the neurone and the effector (the neuro-effector junction), another neurotransmitter is released. This is usually noradrenaline, in which case we call the synaptic terminals **adrenergic**. A small number of neuro-effector junctions release acetylcholine (those of the body wall, skin and skeletal muscle); these are called **cholinergic**.

The effects of the noradrenaline are dependent upon the type of receptors within the effector. Alpha (α) receptors are stimulated more by noradrenaline than beta (β) receptors, whereas adrenaline stimulates both types of receptors equally, Alpha receptors can be classified as one of two types, alpha -1 (α_1) or alpha -2 (α_2); α_1 receptors are the more common and they generally have an excitatory effect. In contrast, α_2 receptors generally have an inhibitory effect. Beta (β) receptors can also be classified as one of two types, beta-1 (β_1) or beta-2 (β_2); β_1 receptors cause an increase in metabolism of cells, e.g. causing an increase in heart rate, while β_2 receptors tend to have inhibitory effects, e.g. causing relaxation of smooth muscle in the case of bronchodilation.

The parasympathetic nervous system

In contrast to sympathetic activity, the parasympathetic nervous system predominates when the animal is in a relaxed state, for example when

---

Some postganglionic fibres are cholinergic, releasing acetylcholine at the neuro-effector junction. These stimulate the production of sweat and dilate the blood vessels supplying skeletal muscle and the brain. Another neurotransmitter, **nitric oxide**, is released in some areas of the sympathetic nervous system; this acts on smooth muscle, primarily causing dilation of the blood vessels in skeletal muscle and the brain.

the cat was initially sunning itself in the garden before the dog arrived. Energy demands are minimal and the animal has a low respiratory and heart rate. Digestion is stimulated and smooth muscle contractions stimulate the production of faecal material and urine. It can be seen that in this way the effects of the parasympathetic are very different from those of the sympathetic nervous system.

The parasympathetic division has its preganglionic neurones located in the brain and spinal cord (sacral region). Postganglionic neurones are peripheral and are located either within or close to the relevant organs. The major nerve that carries information from most of the parasympathetic division is called the **vagus nerve** and supplies all the organs and structures within the thorax and abdomen.

Neurotransmitters of the parasympathetic nervous system

One neurotransmitter predominates within the parasympathetic nervous system, acetylcholine. However, there are two different types of receptor that are found on the postsynaptic membrane (both between neurones and at neuro-effector junctions).

Nicotinic receptors are found in both the sympathetic and parasympathetic nervous systems as well as at the junctions between nerves and muscles (neuromuscular junctions) in the somatic nervous system. Acetylcholine always causes excitation of the postsynaptic membrane or muscle.

Muscarinic receptors are found in the parasympathetic nervous system at neuro-effector junctions; a few are also located at the neuro-effector junctions of the sympathetic nervous system. Stimulation of these receptors may cause an excitatory or an inhibitory response.

Integration of the actions of the parasympathetic and sympathetic nervous systems

As mentioned briefly on page 53, in most cases the parasympathetic and sympathetic divisions have opposing but complementary actions as this permits a wide range of control. Most of the visceral organs are innervated from both divisions. When considering the heart, for example, nervous activity in the sympathetic division increases heart rate whereas activity in the parasympathetic division causes it to decrease. Similarly, the parasympa-

thetic system causes an increase in gastro-intestinal function whereas the sympathetic system causes its inhibition.

Not all organs have dual innervation, however. The spleen and adrenal medullae, for example, have only sympathetic innervation, while the ciliary muscles of the eye are only innervated by the parasympathetic division.

The ANS usually exists in a state of **tone** that can be described as a base level of activity that can increase or decrease, depending upon the situation. For example, the parasympathetic system exerts a basal tone on the activity of the heart via the vagus nerve. If this is severed, the heart rate increases as the inhibiting effects of the parasympathetic nervous system are no longer present. Levels of activity within the two divisions are controlled by areas within the brain and spinal cord. Similar to the somatic nervous system, visceral reflexes are processed within the spinal cord to provide a rapid feedback mechanism. More complex processes require the use of higher levels in the brain and are co-ordinated within the **medulla oblongata**. The medulla oblongata contains both the cardiac and respiratory centres, as well as those areas involved with salivation, digestive secretion, movement of the intestine, and urinary function. The medulla oblongata is regulated by the hypothalamus, which is discussed later in this chapter.

2.3 Special senses

Vision
Optic chambers
The lens
Rods and cones
Protection of the eye
Audition
Gustation
Olfaction

Introduction

Traditionally, there are five special senses, sight (vision), hearing (audition), touch, taste (gustation), and smell (olfaction). These are in contrast to the more general senses such as those that provide the animal with information regarding the position of its muscles and functioning of its visceral organs. In this chapter we shall consider the senses of vision, audition, gustation and olfaction. The senses of touch will be discussed with the skin (integumentary system) in Chapter 6.

Vision

As humans, our sense of vision is highly evolved and we probably rely on this sense far more than any other. This situation is different from that of other species, where senses such as olfaction and audition play a more important role. We need to bear this in mind when considering sight in the cat and dog; all we can do is examine the similarities and differences that exist in the visual structures and 'imagine' what it must be like to see the world through their eyes.

The eye

The organ of vision, the eye, is located in the orbital cavity and is surrounded by a protective padding of fat. It is interesting to note that the position of the eye in the head varies among different species of animal. Those that have evolved to be predators have their eyes situated at the front of their heads. This allows them to judge speed and distance effectively. Prey species, on the other hand, have their eyes situated more to the side. This allows them to be more vigilant in looking out for predators and allows a greater field of vision, i.e. they can see more detail to their sides without turning their heads. The anatomical structure of the mammalian eye is illustrated in Figure 2.15.

The gross structure of the eye of the cat or dog is very similar to that of our own. The eye is divided into three layers, each with anatomically distinct features and functions:

1. **The outer, fibrous layer (or fibrous tunic)**
   This can also be divided into two parts. The caudal part of the outer layer is white and opaque. It is referred to as the **sclera** or more commonly the 'white of the eye'. It is firm and fibrous, consisting of dense fibrous connective tissue and helps to maintain the shape of the eye. The rostral part of the outer layer is transparent, allowing light rays to enter the eye. It is called the **cornea** and it helps to bend the light rays to help focus them on the retina. The process by which the cornea bends the light is known as **refraction**. Refraction also occurs as light passes through the lens.

> Refraction is defined as the bending of light rays as they pass from one medium to another with a different density, for example, from air through the tissue of the cornea. It is the phenomenon responsible for the illusion that a stick, when placed in a glass of water, appears to bend where the air meets the water.

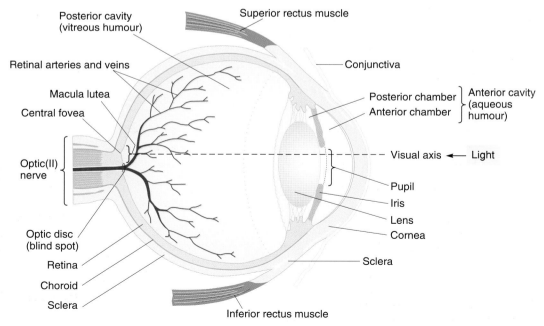

Figure 2.15 Structure of the mammalian eye

The junction between the sclera and the cornea is called the **limbus**.

2. **The middle, vascular layer (or vascular tunic)**

The middle vascular layer can also be called the **uvea** and is considered in three parts. The **choroid** lines all but the front of the eye. It is a vascular layer, supplying blood to other areas of the eye. The caudal inner surface of the choroid has a specialized area of light-reflecting cells called the **tapetum**. This area acts like a mirror and, in dim light, reflects light rays back into the eye to improve vision. This is why the eyes of some species, particularly cats, appear to shine at night (usually circular with a green or blue colour). The dog also has a tapetum although it is smaller and less reflective than in the cat. It is triangular and appears yellow, gold, or pink when reflecting light in the dark.

The **ciliary body** joins the choroid with the **iris** via the **suspensory ligaments**. It consists of both muscular and glandular tissue. The smooth muscle tissue controls the shape of the lens by pulling on the suspensory ligaments that attach it to the lens. This allows the eye to focus on close or distant objects, a process called **accommodation**. Glandular tissue of the ciliary body produces a thin watery fluid called the **aqueous humour**. This fills the rostral chamber of the eye and helps to maintain intra-ocular pressure.

The **iris** forms the most rostral part of the uvea and is the vascular, coloured, part of the eye. It divides the rostral chamber into two parts, the anterior and posterior chambers. The muscular tissue of the iris is arranged in circular and radial fibres that allow the opening and closure of the pupil (the opening in the centre) in response to light intensity. The size of the pupil controls the amount of light that enters the eye. When light intensity is high, the circular muscle fibres contract, causing the pupil to constrict, thereby protecting the inner layer of the eye from damaging light waves. If light intensity is low, the radial muscle fibres contract and the pupil dilates. This allows the maximum amount of light to enter the eye, improving vision in poor light conditions. Both types of muscle are under the control of the autonomic nervous system, parasympathetic activity causing constriction of the pupils and sympathetic activity causing dilation.

3. **The inner layer (or neural tunic)**

The inner layer contains the light-sensitive cells (photoreceptors) and is the layer adapted for the reception of light waves. A thin outer layer is pigmented and absorbs light that passes through the inner layer containing the photoreceptor cells. There are two types of photoreceptor cells, **rods** and **cones**. Rods are light sensitive and allow vision in poor light conditions (night vision). They are not able to distinguish between different colours of light. In contrast, cones allow detailed colour vision and are used predominantly in daylight. The area of the retina that has the highest concentration of cones is known as the **fovea** and is the area of greatest visual perception.

Rods and cones synapse with **bipolar cells** located in the centre of the retinal layer that in turn synapse with ganglion cells (see Figure

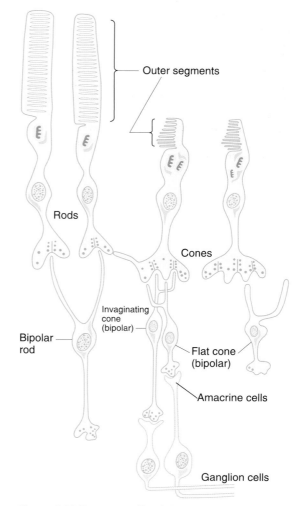

Figure 2.16 Receptor cells of the retina

The blind spot is also called the **optic disc**. This is an area on the retina where the optic nerve is formed from the axons of the ganglion cells, carrying nervous impulses to the brain. As there are no photoreceptor cells at this site, any light waves hitting this area are not 'seen', hence the name blind spot.

2.16). **Amacrine cells** are located where the bipolar cells synapse with the ganglion cells and help to change the sensitivity of the retina by facilitating or inhibiting impulses from the photoreceptor cells.

Note that the rods and cones are located at the furthest point from the incident light source.

Optic chambers

As illustrated in Figure 2.14 the eye is divided into a large posterior cavity containing a gel-like substance called **vitreous humour** and a smaller anterior cavity containing a more fluid-like substance, the **aqueous humour**. The anterior cavity is further subdivided by the iris into a posterior and anterior cavity and the aqueous humour circulates between the two smaller chambers.

As discussed previously, the aqueous humour is constantly secreted by the glandular tissue of the ciliary body. Its composition is similar to that of CSF and it provides a means of transporting nutrients and waste products. Fluid within the eye also allows the eye to retain its shape and helps in keeping the photoreceptors of the retina in contact with the pigmented layer (separation of the two layers is known as a detached retina and can lead to

a loss of vision). Aqueous humour is removed at approximately the same rate as it is manufactured by passing through the **canal of Schlemm** that passes completely around the eye at the site of the limbus. From the canal, the fluid passes in channels to veins in the sclera and so returns to the general circulation.

Vitreous humour is contained within the large posterior chamber of the eye. It is more gelatinous than the aqueous humour, containing fine fibres of collagen. Vitreous humour is not constantly manufactured and replaced, unlike aqueous humour, so consequently it cannot be replaced if lost due to injury.

The lens

The lens is supported by the suspensory ligaments and is located behind the iris, between the large posterior and anterior chambers. It is transparent, contraction of the muscles of the ciliary body changing its shape. Bi-convex in nature, the lens allows the light waves to be focused onto the area of the retina known as the fovea where visual acuity is at its greatest. The lens can change its shape via the action of the ciliary muscles upon the suspensory ligaments. In this way, the eye is able to focus on near and distant objects, a process known as **accommodation**. This is illustrated in Figure 2.17.

When the ciliary muscles contract they cause the suspensory ligaments to slacken which in turn allows the lens to become more spherical in shape. This allows the light to be focused from close objects onto the retina. Relaxation of the ciliary muscles cause tightening of the suspensory ligaments that pulls the lens into a more flattened shape. This allows the light from objects in the distance to be focused on the retina. Refraction of

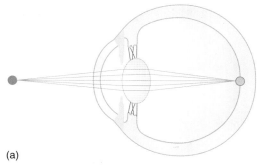
(a)

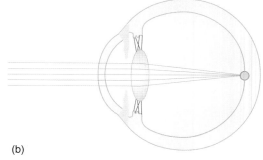
(b)

Figure 2.17 Illustration of the process of accommodation. (a) Contracted ciliary muscle, lens rounded for near vision; (b) relaxed ciliary muscle, lens flattened for distant vision

light as it passes through the lens also complements the focusing of light on the retina.

Formation of an image on the retina

We have seen how, when light from an external object enters the eye it is refracted at the cornea (and to some degree the aqueous humour) and focused by accommodation of the lens. Light rays are then refracted further by the vitreous humour before reaching the retina. On arrival at the retina,

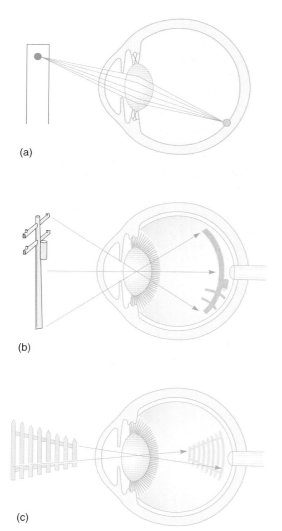

(a)

(b)

(c)

Figure 2.18 Inversion of the image on the retina. (a) and (b) shows that light from an object is focused on a different part of the retina with the resulting image (c) arriving inverted and backwards

the image is inverted and backwards. This is illustrated in Figure 2.18.

When an animal, ourselves included, sees an object, we are not aware of this phenomenon. The brain interprets the image as though it were in the correct orientation.

Rods and cones

Both rods and cones have many discs that contain substances known as **visual pigments**. These are derived from a compound called **rhodopsin**, sometimes known as **visual purple**. Rhodopsin is formed from a protein, **opsin**, bound to a pigment called **retinal**. Retinal is derived from vitamin A, so the myth that carrots (a good source of vitamin A) help you to see in the dark is not without foundation! Cones also contain retinal as a pigment, however in this case it is bound to other forms of opsin. Different types of opsin determine which colour of light is detected by the cones.

Impulses from the stimulated rods and cones are carried in the optic nerve to the brain. Each eye has its own optic nerve and they converge at the optic chiasma, where impulses cross over, resulting in stimuli from the right side of each retina travelling to the left side of the brain and **vice versa**. This is illustrated in Figure 2.19.

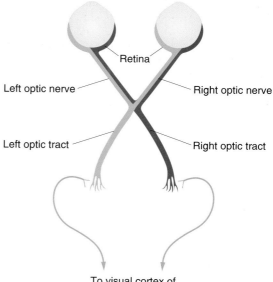

Retina

Left optic nerve

Right optic nerve

Left optic tract

Right optic tract

To visual cortex of cerebral hemispheres

Figure 2.19 The optic chiasma

Protection of the eye

The eye has several protective structures that help to protect it from damage from foreign bodies and physical trauma.

The eyelids or palpebrae

The eyelids protect the eye against intense light, physical damage, and the entry of small foreign bodies such as dust and grit. The blink reflex is initiated as soon as the eye is exposed to bright light or the threat of physical damage. The eyelids themselves are composed of a plate of fibrous tissue known as the tarsal plate that is covered with skin and lined with a mucous membrane. This membrane also covers the surface of the eyeball where it is known as the conjunctiva. The eyelids meet at the corners of the eye, known as the medial and lateral canthi (sing = canthus). The upper eyelid has a protective layer of hairs (cilia) or eyelashes. It is interesting that, in the dog and cat, there are no eyelashes on the lower lids as in humans. Modified sebaceous glands known as tarsal or meibomian glands secrete a fatty material that contributes to the tear film. Ducts to these glands open along the inner margins of the eyelids.

Both entropion and ectopion (turning in and out of the eyelids, respectively) are conditions commonly encountered in certain breeds of dog in veterinary practice. Surgical correction is possible. Distichiasis (additional cilia growing from the edge of the tarsal plate, pointing inwards and irritating the cornea) can also be encountered.

The third eyelid or nictitating membrane

The nictitating membrane consists of a plate of cartilage that projects from the medial canthus. Its main function is one of protection in the cat and dog, providing additional protection to the eye when the eyelid is closed. In the dog, the nictitating membrane is composed of hyaline cartilage, smooth muscle, and elastic cartilage, whereas in the cat there is no hyaline cartilage. The nictitans gland (or membrana nictitans) lies inside the third eyelid and contributes secretions to the tear film. Failure of the nictitating membrane to retract fully when the eye is open can often be a sign of illness in cats.

The lacrimal apparatus

This is the term given to the glands and associated structures that are associated with the production,

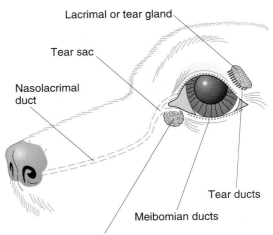

Figure 2.20 The lacrimal apparatus showing the eye and tear glands

dispersal and drainage of tears. Tear fluid is important in that it helps to maintain a healthy cornea. In addition to fats, proteins and an oily secretion, it contains a bactericidal enzyme called **lysozyme**. The structure of the lacrimal apparatus is illustrated in Figure 2.20.

The lacrimal gland produces tear fluid and is located on the dorsolateral surface of the eye. Other glands such as the tarsal (or meibomian) gland, the membrana nictitans gland of the nictitating membrane and goblet cells also contribute secretions to the tear film. Aided by blinking, the tear film is distributed over the surface of the eyeball and drains through the punctae, the openings to the lacrimal or tear sac located at the medial canthus. They drain through the lacrimal canaliculi to the lacrimal sac and from there into the nasolacrimal duct.

Audition

The sense of hearing is the primary sense in the cat and dog, dogs being able to distinguish sound at approximately four times the distance of humans. In addition to hearing, the ear has a second function, that of balance. These will both be discussed in the following section.

The structure of the canine ear is illustrated in Figure 2.21. Those structures associated with hearing include the pinna and external acoustic meatus (ear canal) of the outer ear, the ear ossicles of the middle ear and the cochlea of the inner ear. Those associated with balance include the

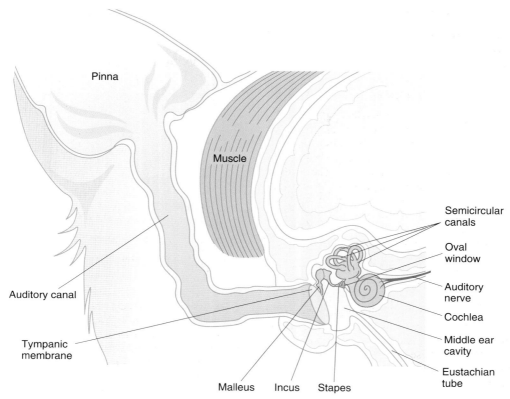

Figure 2.21 Structure of the canine ear

semicircular canals, utricle and saccule, all located within the inner ear.

Hearing

The sense of hearing or audition involves the structures of the outer, middle and inner ear. The function of each will be considered in the following section.

The external ear

The external ear has two parts, the **pinna** and the **external acoustic meatus**. The pinna consists of fibroelastic cartilage covered with skin. Its primary function is to assist the funnelling of sound waves into the ear. This is the case for species and breeds of animal with pricked ears, such as the cat and some breeds of dog, e.g. the German Shepherd. Other breeds of dog have been selected to have low-set, 'dropped' ears that lie close to the head, e.g. the Cocker Spaniel. These breeds primarily belong to the gundog group and it is thought that

the position of the ear may help to muffle the sound of the gun, making such breeds less reactive to gun shots. In addition to the funnelling of sound, the position of the ear in both the cat and the dog is used as a form of expression and communication. A dog with ears laid back close to the head and its body close to the ground is showing a submissive posture, although if accompanied by growling this posture may indicate that the dog is fearful.

The external acoustic meatus is the canal that runs from the base of the pinna to the **tympanic membrane**, or ear drum. It has a vertical and horizontal auditory canal, the walls of which are formed from cartilage covered with a type of modified skin that has very few hair follicles. Ceruminous glands secrete wax or cerumen that helps to prevent the access of foreign bodies and dust particles and slows bacterial growth. Individual animals may have large numbers of hair follicles within the auditory canals that may cause problems with the accumulation of excess wax and provide a suitable environment for ear mites

(**Otodectes cynotis**) or the development of ear infections.

The tympanic membrane is located at the end of the horizontal auditory canal. It is a semitransparent membrane that is composed of three layers, an outer layer of hairless skin, a middle layer of fibrous tissue, and an inner layer of mucous membrane. It is a drum-like structure that soundwaves cause to vibrate. These vibrations are transmitted to the middle ear.

The middle ear

The middle ear lies within the tympanic bulla (or cavity) of the temporal bone of the skull. It is an air-filled cavity lined with mucous membrane. Air enters via the auditory canal or Eustachian tube that opens into the nasopharynx. This allows the air pressure on either side of the tympanic membrane to be equalized, preventing rupture of the ear drum. Three small bones, or auditory **ossicles**, lie within the middle ear. These are illustrated in more detail in Figure 2.22.

The **malleus** (or hammer) articulates with the tympanic membrane and the second of the auditory ossicles, the **incus** (or anvil). This in turn articulates with the **stapes** (stirrup) that attaches to the oval window of the inner ear. Through these articulations the vibrations of the tympanic membrane are carried across the middle ear and are at the same time magnified in amplitude. Consequently a small vibration of the ear drum causes a significant vibration of the membrane of the oval window.

The inner ear

The inner ear lies within a cavity of the temporal bone that is called the **bony labyrinth**. This is lined with a membrane called the **periosteum**. Inside the bony labyrinth is the membranous labyrinth. The structure is similar to that of a tube within a tube. The space between the two labyrinths is filled with fluid called perilymph. The bony labyrinth contains the organs of both hearing and balance. Balance will be considered later in this chapter. The bony labyrinth can be divided into three parts, the **vestibule, semicircular canals** and **cochlea**.

The **vestibule** joins the middle ear at two windows, the upper **oval window** and lower **round window** (see Figure 2.22) and opens into the semicircular canals and cochlea. It contains the **utricle** and the **saccule** that are associated with the sense of balance.

There are three **semicircular canals** that are orientated perpendicular to each other in different planes. They are associated with the sensation of balance and will be discussed later in this chapter.

The **cochlea** is the organ of hearing. It contains the cochlear duct, an extension of the membranous

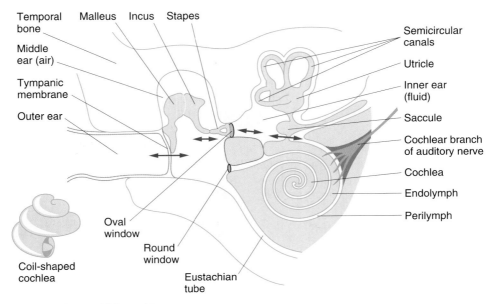

Figure 2.22 Detail of the middle and inner ear

labyrinth and is spiral in shape, filled with fluid called endolymph. The cochlear duct is enclosed by two surrounding chambers that are filled with fluid known as perilymph. Within the cochlear duct are the receptor cells for audition, contained within an area of the cochlea known as the organ of Corti. They contain hair cells and respond to changes in force applied to them, e.g. by movement of the fluid in the cochlear duct. Sound vibrations are transferred to the inner ear by the movement of the oval window (caused by the movement of the auditory ossicles of the inner ear). The vibration of the oval window causes movement of the fluid within the inner ear. The round window provides a mechanism whereby the fluid in the ear can move, as fluid is relatively incompressible. As the membrane of the oval window moves toward the fluid it pushes it around the inner ear to the round window that bulges outwards slightly and 'gives'. Movement of perilymph within the inner ear causes a distortion of the hair cells causing depolarization and stimulation of the sensory neurones of the auditory nerve. As the intensity of the sound increases so does the number of hair cells distorted and the degree of distortion. This provides information regarding the intensity of the sound.

Balance

The sensation of balance and position is achieved through a combination of feedback from receptors in the semicircular canals, utricle and saccule of the inner ear. The semicircular canals are responsible for detecting rotation of the head. They contain ducts filled with endolymph and a swollen base called the ampulla contains sensory hair cells. The hair cells are embedded in a gelatinous mass called the cupula that projects into the ampulla (see Figure 2.23).

Movement of the endolymph causes movement of the ampulla and distortion of the hair cells that stimulates depolarization and generates a nervous impulse. Movement of fluid in one direction only causes stimulation of the hair cells. Should fluid move in the opposite direction, the hair cells are inhibited. Via the presence of the semicircular canals in three planes, impulses are sent to the brain determining the movement of the head in every direction.

The utricle and the saccule contribute to the sensation of balance by sending impulses to the brain regarding the position of the head. They contain sensory hair cells that are grouped into maculae. These lie under a thin layer of calcium carbonate crystals called otoliths. When the head is upright, the otoliths push down on the maculae rather than to one side. If the head is tilted, gravity pulls the otoliths and the maculae are distorted triggering an impulse to the brain to indicate that the head is no longer level. This also helps to contribute to the sense of acceleration, as the otoliths lag behind again bending the maculae. When combined with visual information, the brain

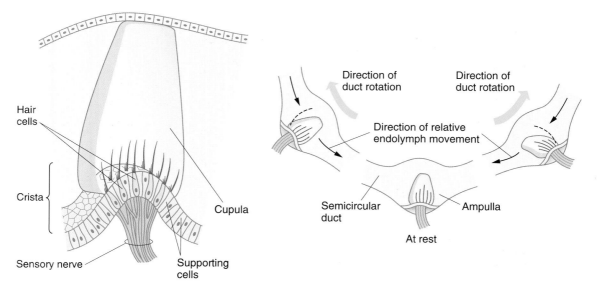

Figure 2.23 Ampulla of the semicircular canal

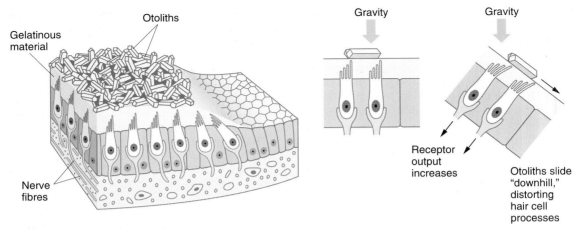

Figure 2.24 Structure of the maculae within the utricle and saccule

can distinguish between the two scenarios. The structure of the maculae is shown in Figure 2.24.

Gustation

Taste or gustation relies on sensory cells that are located in groups within the epithelium of the tongue, soft palate, pharynx and epiglottis, known as the taste buds. Stimulation of these receptor cells is carried to the brain via the glossopharyngeal, facial, vagus and cranial nerves, where it is interpreted by the temporal lobe along with the corresponding smell. There are traditionally thought to be four sensations of taste, sweet, bitter, salt and sour, although more recently other sensations are under investigation. Comparison of the sensory cells in the dog, cat and human reveals that it is likely that dogs are not as sensitive to taste as humans and that cats are unable to taste 'sweet' primarily due to their evolution as obligate carnivores; however, this is thought to be changing as there is recent evidence that a taste for sweetness is evolving in the domestic cat.

Olfaction

The sense of olfaction or smell is the most highly evolved sense in the dog and cat. Comparison of the number of receptor cells indicates that humans have approximately 5 million receptors whereas the cat has approximately 19 million and dogs 147 million receptors. Receptor cells lie within the mucous membranes of the nasal cavity and transmit impulses to the olfactory bulb that lies underneath the cerebrum of the brain and along the olfactory tract to the olfactory cortex of the temporal lobe.

Some animals, e.g. horses, may be seen to perform a Flehmen response to strong or sexual odours. Described as a 'strange, nose-wrinkling grimace' it serves to draw the odour over a specialized organ in the roof of the mouth known as the Jacobson's organ. This structure seems to be associated with both taste and smell and in animals such as the snake, is highly evolved to allow detection of the smell/taste of prey.

2.4 The endocrine system

Hormones
The hypothalamus
The pituitary gland
The pineal gland
The parathyroid glands
The thyroid gland
The thymus
The heart
The digestive tract
The kidneys
The adrenal glands
The pancreas
The gonads

Introduction

Every cell in the body must be able to communicate, not only with neighbouring cells but also with cells in other parts of the body, in order to function effectively and maintain homeostasis. There are several types of communication, some of which have already been discussed in this chapter.

Direct communication is the means whereby neighbouring cells in direct contact with each other, communicate by the exchange of ions and molecules through gap junctions in the cell membrane. This is a local type of communication acting over extremely small distances.

Paracrine communication also occurs over small distances, but uses chemical messengers that are used to carry information from cell to cell within the same tissue. The concentrations of the chemical messengers are so low that they do not affect neighbouring tissues.

Synaptic communication has already been examined in some detail within this chapter. A specialized cell, the neurone, releases a neurotransmitter very close to the target cell (the effector) at the synapse. The effects of synaptic communication are usually short-lived.

Endocrine communication involves the release of hormones, produced by specialized endocrine cells, into the circulatory system where they are carried to the target cells, tissues or organs. The target cells, tissues or organs have specialized receptor sites to which the hormone must bind before it exerts its effects. The target cells, tissues or organs can be located anywhere in the body and are usually some distance from the endocrine tissue that releases the hormone. A single hormone may have effects on multiple tissues or organs that may be long-acting, whereas the nervous system has a more rapid response that is shorter in duration.

In the following section we will consider the latter type of communication, the endocrine system and the effects that the various hormones have upon their target tissues within the body.

Hormones

A hormone is defined as a chemical messenger released by a tissue which is carried in the circulation to reach specific target cells in other tissues around the body. Hormones can be divided into three categories depending upon their structure:

1. **Those derived from amino acids**
   These hormones are very similar in structure to and are derived from amino acids. They include hormones such as adrenaline, noradrenaline, the thyroid hormones and melanin.
2. **Peptide hormones**
   Peptide hormones are formed from peptides, or longer chains of amino acids. Those formed from short chains include antidiuretic hormone (ADH) and oxytocin, while growth hormone and prolactin have longer chains and are classified as small proteins. Other hormones within the grouping include those formed from an amino acid chain with a carbohydrate molecule attached. They are known as glycoprotein-based hormones. This grouping includes follicle-stimulating hormone (FSH) and luteinizing hormone (LH), as well as several others.
3. **Those derived from lipids**
   Hormones derived from lipids belong to one of two groups, those similar in structure to cholesterol are known as **steroid hormones** whereas those derived from the essential fatty acid arachidonic acid are called **eicosanoids**. Steroid hormones include the reproductive hormones, e.g. oestrogens and testosterone, as well as corticosteroids released by the adrenal gland and calcitriol by the kidneys. They differ from other hormones in that they are transported in the blood bound to carrier proteins rather than as free molecules. Consequently they remain within the circulation longer than other hormones. Eicosanoids, mentioned above, act as important paracrine molecules, co-ordinating cellular activity and enzyme reactions in extracellular fluid, e.g. blood clotting.

Effects of hormones

Each hormone has a specialized effect upon the target cell, tissue, or organ and these will be discussed later in this section. First, however, we will consider hormonal effects in a more general way. A hormone alters the function of its target cells by changing the type, or quantity of certain enzymes or structural proteins within the cell. In this way, a hormone may activate genetic material to cause the production of an enzyme or structural protein that did not previously exist in the cell. It

---

Remember the difference between endocrine and exocrine glands. Endocrine glands release their secretions into extracellular fluid, e.g. the thyroid gland, whereas exocrine glands release their secretions into ducts that open onto epithelial surfaces, e.g. the salivary gland.

may activate or deactivate an existing enzyme within the cell, or it may affect the rate of synthesis of a structural protein or enzyme. It is possible that some hormones may use one or more of these methods to change the properties of the target cell. Hormones only have these effects when the target cell has specialized receptor sites for that particular hormone. These sites are usually located within the cell membrane or inside the cell. Any cell that does not have the specific receptors will not be affected by the hormone.

Hormone secretion

Hormones are usually released in areas that have a large capillary network in order that they can quickly enter the circulation, where they may circulate either freely or be bound to a carrier protein (as is the case with steroid and thyroid hormones). The stimulus that triggers the secretion of hormones is usually one of the following: a change in the composition of the extracellular fluid, the secretion or removal of another hormone, or the release of a neurotransmitter that affects the endocrine gland. The majority of the hormones within the body are controlled by a negative feedback mechanism. Let us take as an example the regulation of thyroid-stimulating hormone (TSH) which stimulates the production of the

thyroid hormones by the thyroid gland. When levels of TSH increase, so do the levels of circulating thyroid hormones within the circulation. The increased levels of thyroid hormones cause suppression of the production of TSH and of the hormone that stimulates its production (thyrotropin-releasing hormone (TRH), which is produced by the hypothalamus). This effect is illustrated in Figure 2.25.

Blood levels of most hormones operate through a negative feedback mechanism maintaining homeostasis.

> The secretion of most hormones is under a negative feedback method of control. Oxytocin secretion, however, is controlled by a positive feedback effect in which the contractions of the uterus during birth stimulate secretion of oxytocin which further increases the uterine contractions.

Other hormones are regulated by a more direct control mechanism, for example, the lowering of blood glucose levels by the pancreatic hormone insulin. As blood glucose levels rise following a meal, the production of insulin is stimulated and the blood glucose levels start to fall. The fall in blood glucose results in a fall in the secretion of insulin from the pancreas.

The more complex methods by which hormone secretion is controlled, such as those involving negative feedback mechanisms, involve the hypothalamus. This central area will be discussed, along with other important endocrine glands, in the following section.

The hypothalamus

The hypothalamus is located beneath the thalamus of the brain and has many important functions associated with control and integration. It plays a critical role in controlling the release of many of the hormones with the body. It secretes regulatory hormones that control the hormonal activity of the anterior pituitary, so affecting the activity of the thyroid gland, the cortex of the adrenal gland and the reproductive organs. It has autonomic nervous control over the hormones secreted by the medulla of the adrenal glands, in addition to acting as an endocrine organ itself, releasing hormones into the circulation via the posterior pituitary gland. These three functions are illustrated in Figure 2.26.

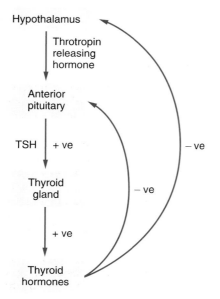

Figure 2.25 Negative feedback control of TSH secretion

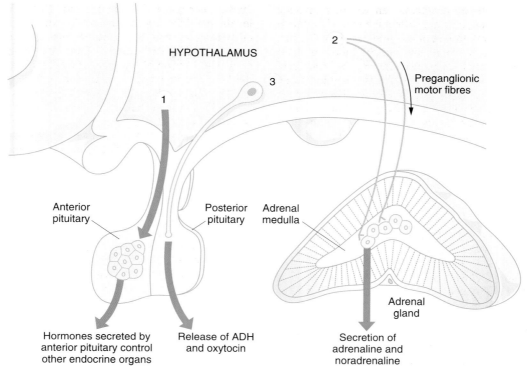

HYPOTHALAMUS

2

3

1

Preganglionic
motor fibres

Anterior
pituitary

Posterior
pituitary

Adrenal
medulla

Adrenal
gland

Hormones secreted by
anterior pituitary control
other endocrine organs

Release of ADH
and oxytocin

Secretion of
adrenaline and
noradrenaline

Figure 2.26 Endocrine role of the hypothalamus. 1, Secretion of regulatory hormones to control activity of anterior pituitary; 2, control of sympathetic output to adrenal medullae; 3, production of ADH and oxytocin

The pituitary gland

The pituitary gland or hypophysis can be considered in two parts, the posterior pituitary or **neurohypophysis** and the anterior pituitary or **adenohypophysis**.

The posterior pituitary gland (or neurohypophysis)

The posterior pituitary acts as a storage site for two hormones, **oxytocin** and **antidiuretic hormone** (ADH) or vasopressin. These are both synthesized in the hypothalamus by specialized secretory neurones and are stored in the posterior pituitary prior to release. ADH has effects on the kidneys, causing an increase in the absorption of water by the tubules (refer to Chapter 5). This reduces the volume of urine produced and increases water retention by the body. Oxytocin causes contraction of the smooth muscle of the uterus during labour and stimulates milk production or 'let down' during lactation. In the male animal it stimulates contraction of the smooth muscle of the ductus deferens and

prostate gland. These will be discussed in more detail in Chapter 6.

The anterior pituitary gland (or adenohypophysis)

The anterior pituitary secretes a total of seven different hormones, all of which are under the control of regulatory hormones secreted by the hypothalamus.

Thyroid-stimulating hormone (TSH or thyrotropin) exerts its effects upon the thyroid gland and stimulates the production of the thyroid hormones, thyroxine (T4), tri-iodothyronine (T3) and calcitonin (thyrocalcitonin). The role of each of these is discussed later in this section. The production of TSH is regulated by thyrotropin releasing hormone (TRH), which is produced by the hypothalamus.

Secretion of adrenocorticotropic hormone (ACTH or adrenocortin) is regulated by corticotropin releasing hormone (CRH) from the hypothalamus. ACTH regulates the production of glucocorticoids (cortisol and corticosterone) from the cortex of the adrenal gland. These are steroid-based hormones that affect cellular metabolism and will be discussed later in this section.

Follicle-stimulating hormone (FSH) is secreted in response to the production of gonadotropin releasing hormone (GnRH) from the hypothalamus. FSH acts on the ovarian follicles in the female animal to stimulate its development and maturation. In the male animal it promotes the maturation of sperm. Luteinizing hormone (LH) is another hormone regulated by GnRH. It stimulates ovulation and development of the corpus luteum in the female, while in the male it regulates production of the hormone testosterone by the interstitial cells of Leydig in the testes. In the male it may sometimes be referred to as interstitial cell stimulating hormone (ICSH).

The hormone prolactin (PRL) stimulates the development of the mammary glands of the pregnant female animal, as well as playing an active role in lactation following parturition. There are two hypothalamic hormones that control its secretion, prolactin releasing factor (PRF) and prolactin

> Growth hormone (GH, or somatotropin) plays a critical role in all cellular growth. It regulates the production of proteins by cells and controls the energy used within the body. During times of poor food supply it will stimulate the utilization of lipid as an energy source in order that essential glucose can be conserved for the nervous system. It is particularly important in young, growing animals. Its production is regulated by growth hormone releasing hormone (GH-RH) and growth hormone inhibiting hormone (GH-IH) produced by the hypothalamus.

inhibiting hormone (PIH). The role of prolactin in the male animal is not well understood.

The final hormone produced by the anterior pituitary is melanocyte-stimulating hormone (MSH). MSH is particularly important in the production of skin pigments in fish, amphibia, reptiles and many mammals, although not in

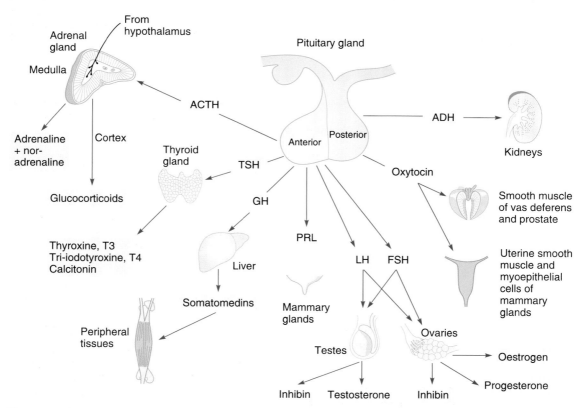

Figure 2.27 Schematic representation of the pituitary hormones

primates. Its target cells are the melanocytes within the epidermis of the skin and it stimulates these to produce a skin pigment known as melanin. The secretion of MSH is regulated by melanocyte-stimulating-hormone inhibiting hormone (MSH-IH), produced by the hypothalamus.

A summary of the pituitary gland hormones is illustrated in Figure 2.27.

The pineal gland

Sometimes called the 'third eye' for reasons that will become apparent, the pineal gland lies in the posterior part of the third ventricle of the brain. It contains neurones, neuroglia and specialized secretory cells called pinealocytes. The pinealocytes secrete a hormone called melatonin that forms the basis for a neurotransmitter molecule known as serotonin. Activity in the visual pathways from the brain has a direct effect on the production of melatonin. During periods of darkness, the production of melatonin is high while during daylight its production is low. It is thought that the levels of melatonin, and consequently serotonin, provide the animal with a means of determining the time of year. Consequently it is likely that melatonin is linked with the timing of sexual maturation, oestrus, and possibly with the maintenance of circadian rhythms.

The parathyroid glands

There are two parathyroid glands in the cat and dog that lie close to the thyroid gland. Endocrine cells called **chief cells** produce parathyroid hormone (PTH or parathormone) in response to falling levels of calcium ions in the blood. PTH secretion causes an increase in the circulating calcium ion concentration by the following mechanisms:

1. It stimulates the activity of osteoclasts within the bone that causes a breakdown of the bone matrix, releasing calcium ions into the circulation.
2. Osteoblast activity is inhibited, with the effect of reducing the rate of calcium ion deposition as bone. This prohibits the removal of any calcium ions from the circulation, thereby preventing the blood calcium levels deteriorating further.
3. Urinary secretion of calcium ions is greatly reduced.
4. It stimulates the secretion of calcitriol by the kidney; this increases the efficiency with which calcium is absorbed from the digestive tract.

Through these mechanisms, PTH acts as the major regulator of the concentration of calcium ions in the blood of healthy adult animals, working in conjunction with calcitonin (see later) to maintain homeostasis.

A condition known as hyperparathyroidism may occasionally be seen in practice. It can occur in one of three ways:

1. **Neoplasia of the gland** (abnormal growth) can cause over-production of PTH. This causes demineralization of bone and may cause the bones to weaken and fracture.
2. **Secondary indirect hyperparathyroidism** can be seen in cases of chronic renal failure. The kidneys are unable to regulate the loss of calcium ions in the urine; the body attempts to compensate for the loss by absorbing more from the bone into the circulation. The bones affected are usually the maxillae and mandibles, producing a condition known as 'rubber jaw'.
3. **Secondary nutritional hyperparathyroidism** is not seen as frequently now as it was formerly, due to the development of complete diets for dogs and cats. It occurs due to the feeding of butcher's meat to young animals. As the meat is very low in calcium the animal's daily requirements cannot be met and so growth and development of bone is affected.

The thyroid gland

The thyroid gland lies just below the larynx and secretes three thyroid hormones, thyroxine (T_4),

Hyperthyroidism is commonly seen in cats and is a consequence of over-production of T4 and T3, usually as a consequence of enlargement of the gland itself. Signs may include loss of weight and increased appetite due to an increase in the metabolic rate of cells within the body. Increased heart rate may also be evident, along with overactivity and increased irritability.

In contrast, hypothyroidism is more commonly seen in dogs. Underactivity of the thyroid gland results in the production of low levels of T4 and T3. In severe cases production can cease altogether. Signs of hypothyroidism may include sluggishness, with a tendency to put on weight due to the lowered metabolic rate. Skin and coat condition may also be poor.

tri-iodothyrodine (T_3) and calcitonin (or thyro-calcitonin). T_4 and T_3 have very similar effects, regulating cellular metabolism via the mitochondria and the production of ATP. Calcitonin assists with the regulation of calcium ion concentration in the blood and is secreted when there is an increase in the concentration of calcium ions above the threshold level. Opposite in its effect to PTH, it causes a fall in the calcium ion concentration by inhibiting osteoclast activity in bone (thereby increasing bone deposition) and by promoting the secretion of calcium ions by the kidney in urine. Calcitonin is also thought to be important in the regulation of bone growth in young animals and in maintaining the balance of calcium ions between mother and foetus during pregnancy.

The thymus

The thymus is located in the mediastinum of the thorax. In newborn animals it is quite large, although its size decreases with age. It produces a hormone called thymosin that promotes the development and maturation of lymphocytes. In this way it is thought to be a major contributing factor to the immune response in the young animal and its deterioration with age may account for the fact that animals become more prone to disease as they grow older.

The heart

Primarily associated with the circulatory system, the heart is often not considered to be an endocrine organ. However, the walls of the atria contain endocrine cells that secrete a hormone, atrial natriuretic peptide (ANP), when over-stretched. Over-stretching of the atrial walls occurs when the circulating blood volume is too high. ANP helps to reduce the circulating blood volume by the following mechanisms:

1. The secretion of sodium ions, and consequently water, is increased by the kidney.
2. The suppression of thirst.
3. The release of renin is suppressed, along with ADH and aldosterone. This further promotes the excretion of water.
4. Angiotensin II and noradrenaline cause vaso-constriction of the peripheral blood vessels. ANP prevents these effects and consequently promotes vasodilation, which helps to reduce blood pressure.

The digestive tract

There are several endocrine secretions associated with the digestive tract. These will be discussed along with the digestive system in Chapter 5.

The kidneys

The kidneys secrete two hormones, calcitriol and erythropoietin. The effects of calcitriol have already been discussed in relation to PTH. The secretion of PTH stimulates the production of calcitriol (from cholecalciferol or vitamin D_3), which increases the efficiency of absorption of calcium and phosphorus from the digestive tract. Calcitriol is also thought to have effects on muscle contraction, insulin release, and secretion of testosterone, although these are not yet fully understood. It is also thought to have other effects that have still to be determined.

Erythropoietin (EPO) is released by the kidney when circulating blood oxygen levels are low. It stimulates the bone marrow of long bones to increase the rate of production of red blood cells in an attempt to increase the oxygen-carrying capacity of the blood. It has recently become a substance that is used by some athletes to enhance their performance, although its use is banned. The function of EPO will be discussed further in Chapter 4.

The adrenal glands

Located on the dorsal aspect of each kidney, the triangular-shaped adrenal glands have an outer cortex and inner medulla that secrete different hormones.

The adrenal cortex

The outer cortex produces more than 24 different hormones which are all steroid-based (sometimes referred to as corticosteroids). They are all carried in the circulation bound to carrier proteins and consequently have a longer duration of action than other hormones. Steroid hormones affect the genes of cells that control the production of enzymes. Therefore their overall effects are upon cellular metabolism as a whole. They can be classified into one of three groups that are secreted by different regions of the adrenal cortex.

Mineralocorticoids such as **aldosterone** contribute to the regulation of electrolytes within the body, primarily sodium and potassium. The release of aldosterone is triggered by a number of different circumstances: a fall in the levels of sodium ions in the circulation below the threshold level, a fall in blood volume or blood pressure, or a rise in potassium ions in the extracellular fluid. Aldosterone is then secreted in order to conserve sodium ions within the body and excrete potassium ions. The action of aldosterone will be discussed further in Chapters 4 and 5, when we consider the circulatory and urinary systems.

> Hypoadrenocorticism is a condition known as Addison's disease that may be encountered in veterinary practice. It occurs when the adrenal cortices cannot produce adequate levels of aldosterone, resulting in an increase in the retention of potassium in the circulation (as it is not excreted by the kidneys). The animal may show vomiting, diarrhoea, lethargy and weight loss with general weakness, progressing to collapse, and, in severe cases, coma and death.

Glucocorticoids such as **cortisol** and **corticosterone** are secreted at times of stress. They help to spare glucose by mobilizing other sources of energy such as amino acids and lipids. This is particularly important during the resistance period of the stress response. Once the initial 'fight or flight' response has occurred (mediated primarily by adrenaline and noradrenaline), the stressor may still be present. This may include situations such as lack of food, chronic illness, or inappropriate living conditions, for example, if an animal is constantly under threat from a more dominant individual within the pack or is unaccustomed to being housed in a kennel environment. When the animal is unable to escape the stressor, a more long-term method of control is required. Mobilization of lipid and protein for metabolism as energy allows glucose to be spared for critical functions. For example, during prolonged starvation, blood glucose levels can remain within normal ranges for a considerable time due to the use of alternative energy sources. The resistance phase may be maintained for prolonged periods, providing that reserves of lipid and protein are adequate, however, as time passes, the animal will lose fat and also muscle mass. If the stressor continues, then the exhaustion phase of the stress response follows. Once the exhaustion phase is reached, it becomes likely

> Hyperadrenocorticism is a condition known as Cushing's disease. The adrenal cortices produce excessive amount of glucocorticoids, in particular cortisol, either due to the over-production of ACTH or due to the production of excess cortisol as a consequence of neoplasia of the gland. Symptoms may include polyphagia, polydypsia, polyurea, hair loss, pot belly and thinning of the skin.

that, if the stressor is not removed, death may occur.

Adrenal sex steroids (e.g. androgens such as testosterone) are also produced in small quantities by the adrenal cortex in both male and female animals. Some are converted into oestrogen, again in both the male and the female. Levels of these hormones are too low to have any effect upon the sexual characteristics of an animal and their exact purpose is not known. It is thought that they may have some effect in the neutered animal and might explain why some entire male dogs may try to mount castrated males. It is possible that they can detect low levels of oestrogens in the castrated male.

The adrenal medulla

The adrenal medulla is stimulated by neurones from the sympathetic nervous system to produce adrenaline and noradrenaline (sometimes referred to as epinephrine and norepinephrine, respectively). These are traditionally thought of as the 'fight or flight' hormones, preparing the animal to meet emergencies. They cause an increase in heart rate, blood pressure, and rate and depth of respiration. Blood glucose levels increase due to the increased breakdown of glycogen and blood vessels supplying skeletal muscle are dilated. All these mechanisms ensure that the animal can react to any emergency if required.

The pancreas

The pancreas can be considered a mixed gland, having both exocrine and endocrine functions. The endocrine function is through the secretion of hormones, and an exocrine function via the secretion of an enzyme-rich fluid into the digestive tract. The exocrine function of the pancreas will be considered in Chapter 5 and the endocrine function will be discussed in the following section.

Only 1% of pancreatic cells are endocrine in function and these are called the **Islets of Langerhans**. The Islets contain four different types of cells that secrete different hormones.

Alpha cells secrete a hormone called **glucagon**. This causes an increase in the blood glucose levels by stimulating the breakdown of glycogen in muscle and the liver. It is secreted in response to a fall in blood glucose which is detected by the alpha cells themselves.

Beta cells secrete **insulin** in response to a rise in blood glucose, for example, following a meal. Insulin promotes the uptake of glucose by cells and the conversion of glucose into glycogen by the liver and muscle tissue. Whilst the beta cells of the pancreas can detect a rise in blood glucose, insulin production is also affected by the autonomic nervous system, activity in the parasympathetic nervous system stimulating its release and the sympathetic nervous system inhibiting its production.

Delta cells produce a hormone called **somatostatin**, which is secreted in response to peaks of insulin or glucagon production suppressing their release, thereby avoiding dramatic 'swings' in the levels of blood glucose. Somatostatin also acts to slow the digestive process by reducing the speed with which food moves along the digestive tract and decreasing the rate of enzyme secretion.

F cells of the islets produce a hormone called **pancreatic peptide**. It is thought to affect the production of some of the pancreatic digestive enzymes and inhibit the contraction of the gall bladder, although this is an area that requires much more research before its precise functions can be determined.

Diabetes

There are two forms of diabetes that are seen in veterinary practice, **diabetes mellitus** ('sugar diabetes') and **diabetes insipidus**.

Diabetes insipidus is associated with the inability of an animal to produce adequate amounts of ADH, the hormone that causes retention of water within the body. Consequently, animals with diabetes insipidus cannot control the amount of water secreted in the urine, and produce copious quantities of dilute urine. Diabetes insipidus can be controlled by the administration of exogenous ADH, usually via nasal drops that are readily absorbed by the highly vascular nasal epithelium.

Diabetes mellitus is caused by the inability of an animal to produce insulin or to a decreased sensitivity of the insulin receptors in the pancreas. As a consequence, the animal cannot regulate its blood glucose levels, which rise beyond the renal threshold resulting in glucose appearing in the urine. This type of diabetes can be treated by the injection of exogenous insulin at regular intervals to help to reduce glucose levels to within normal ranges.

The gonads

The male and female gonads are the testes and ovaries, respectively. Their endocrine function is discussed in detail in Chapter 6 in relation to reproduction. However, a brief summary is included here.

In the male animal, following puberty, the testes produce two hormones, **testosterone** and **oestrogen**. **Testosterone** is the predominant hormone and is secreted by cells of the testis called the interstitial cells of Leydig. The function of the testosterone is to develop and maintain the production of viable spermatozoa, to maintain the secretory cells of the reproductive tract, and to determine male secondary sexual characteristics such as increased musculature, and male behaviours such as territorial scent marking. **Oestrogens** are produced in much smaller quantities by the Sertoli cells of the testis and contribute towards the maturation of the spermatozoa. Occasionally, tumours of the Sertoli cells may develop, causing 'feminization' of the male dog. This may cause an increase in nipple size, a soft pendulous prepuce and a soft 'puppy-type' coat. The secretion of testosterone in the male is controlled by LH or ICSH from the anterior pituitary gland while that of oestrogen is controlled by FSH, again from the anterior pituitary gland. The hormone **inhibin**, produced by the testis and ovary, has a negative feedback upon the production of FSH from the anterior pituitary in both the male and the female animal.

The ovaries of the female animal produce two hormones in different amounts, depending upon the stage of ovulation. **Oestrogens** are produced by the developing cells of the follicle, prior to ovulation. This is under the direct control of the anterior pituitary hormone FSH. Oestrogens act to support the maturation of the oocyte and help to prepare the reproductive tract for mating and conception. Following ovulation (which is triggered by a surge in the production of LH from the anterior pituitary), **progesterone** is produced by the corpus luteum of the ovary. This helps to sustain pregnancy (pro = for, gesterone = gestation) by ensuring that the uterus is maintained in a suitable condition to support a developing embryo.

A third hormone is produced by the female during pregnancy in the corpus luteum, placenta and uterus. This hormone is called **relaxin** and its function is to help to prepare the body of the female for the birth process. It causes relaxation of the joints between the bones of the pubic symphysis, thereby allowing a degree of laxity. It also contributes towards the development of mammary tissue. During the early stages of pregnancy its production is stimulated by LH from the anterior pituitary gland. However, as the pregnancy progresses, additional stimulation is received from chorionic gonadotropin, which is produced by the placenta.

Review questions

1. The efferent part of the parasympathetic nervous system
   (a) brings sensory information to the CNS
   (b) carries motor commands to smooth and cardiac muscle and glands
   (c) processes and integrates sensory data
   (d) controls the higher functions of the body
2. Voluntary control of skeletal muscle is provided by the:
   (a) somatic nervous system
   (b) autonomic nervous system
   (c) visceral motor system
   (d) parasympathetic nervous system
3. Smooth and cardiac muscle are both under control of the
   (a) somatic nervous system
   (b) autonomic nervous system
   (c) voluntary nervous system
   (d) sensory neurones
4. What increases the speed of transmission of nervous impulses by the neurone?
   (a) increase in length of the neurone
   (b) myelination
   (c) increase in diameter of the neurone
   (d) absence of Schwann cells
5. Myelin is produced by:
   (a) Myelinocytes
   (b) Ranvier cells
   (c) Schwann cells
   (d) The nerve axon
6. Which cells are thought to be responsible for maintenance of the blood–brain barrier?
   (a) oligodendrocytes
   (b) microglia
   (c) neurones
   (d) astrocytes
7. The sodium/potassium pump uses what transport mechanism in the transport of ions across cell membranes?
   (a) passive transport
   (b) active transport
   (c) diffusion
   (d) osmosis
8. Which one of the following neurone types is predominantly found on the CNS?
   (a) anaxonic neurones
   (b) bipolar neurones
   (c) unipolar neurones
   (d) multipolar neurones
9. Which type of neurone would relay impulses from within the animal to the CNS?
   (a) somatic motor
   (b) somatic sensory
   (c) visceral motor
   (d) visceral sensory
10. Which are the two ions that play a major role in the generation of an action potential?
    (a) K^+ and Cl^-
    (b) K^+ and Na^+
    (c) Na^+ and Cl^-
    (d) Cl^- and PO_4^{2-}
11. When classifying neurones according to structure what four classifications can be made?
12. List the four different types of glial cell within the CNS.
13. State the two types of glial cell in the PNS.
14. Describe what is meant by the transmembrane, or resting, potential of a nerve.
15. Describe what an electrochemical gradient is.
16. Give details of what causes the generation of an action potential.
17. Describe the term saltatory conduction.
18. What is the region called where a nervous impulse transfers from one neurone to the next?
19. Describe the all-or-none principle regarding the generation of action potentials.
20. Describe how the action potential is transmitted from one neurone to the next across the synapse.
21. Which one of the following is not one of the meninges?
    (a) pia mater
    (b) arachnoid mater

    (c) sub mater
    (d) dura mater

22. CSF can be sampled from the:
    (a) pia mater
    (b) subarachnoid space
    (c) dura mater
    (d) arachnoid mater

23. Which one of the following is not a part of the hindbrain?
    (a) cerebrum
    (b) pons
    (c) cerebellum
    (d) medulla oblongata

24. The spinal cord terminates at the:
    (a) obturator foramen
    (b) cauda equina
    (c) cisterna chyli
    (d) cisterna magna

25. Which cranial nerve carries the impulses associated with sight?
    (a) I
    (b) II
    (c) V
    (d) VI

26. Stimulation of the parasympathetic portion of the nervous system causes:
    (a) dilation of the airways in the lung
    (b) dilation of the pupil in the eye
    (c) increased gastrointestinal function
    (d) increased heart rate

27. Stimulation of the sympathetic portion of the nervous system causes all of the following except:
    (a) dilation of the blood vessels in skeletal muscle
    (b) dilation of the pupil in the eye
    (c) increased salivary secretion
    (d) piloerection

28. The autonomic nervous system is composed of:
    (a) somatic motor fibres
    (b) somatic sensory fibres
    (c) visceral motor fibres
    (d) visceral sensory fibres

29. Which type of receptor is responsible for the sensation of pain?
    (a) mechanoreceptor
    (b) chemoreceptor
    (c) proprioreceptor
    (d) nociceptor

30. Which nerve carries the majority of the impulses of the parasympathetic nervous system?

    (a) vagus
    (b) hypoglossal
    (c) trigeminal
    (d) abducens

31. Outline the function of the limbic system.

32. Name the two divisions of the somatic nervous system called.

33. Briefly describe the function of a plexus.

34. Describe what happens when a dog stands on a piece of glass.

35. Explain the term adaptation.

36. Explain/describe is the role of the sympathetic portion of the autonomic nervous system.

37. Describe the term neurotransmitter.

38. Describe how an impulse is transmitted across a synapse.

39. Describe how a neuromuscular blocking agent might exert its effects.

40. Describe the conditioned reflex.

41. Which one of the following represents the pathway of light through the eye?
    (a) cornea, aqueous humour, lens, vitreous humour, retina
    (b) cornea, vitreous humour, aqueous humour, lens, retina
    (c) cornea, vitreous humour, lens, aqueous humour, retina
    (d) lens, aqueous humour, cornea, vitreous humour, retina

42. What is the name given to the reflective area on the inner surface of the choroid?
    (a) sclera
    (b) retina
    (c) cones
    (d) tapetum

43. Refraction is associated with which ocular structure?
    (a) retina
    (b) ciliary body
    (c) conjunctiva
    (d) cornea

44. Where can the third eyelid of the dog be seen?
    (a) at the lateral canthus of the eye
    (b) under the upper eyelid
    (c) at the medial canthus of the eye
    (d) dogs do not have a third eyelid, only cats

45. What is the function of the iris?
    (a) to refract the light entering the eye
    (b) to focus the light entering the eye
    (c) to reflect the light entering the eye
    (d) to control the amount of light entering the eye

46. What is the name given to the white of the eye?
    (a) sclera
    (b) retina
    (c) conjunctiva
    (d) cornea
47. Which layer of the eye contains rods and cones?
    (a) choroid
    (b) cornea
    (c) sclera
    (d) retina
48. Rotary motion of the head is detected by which sensory structure?
    (a) the cochlea
    (b) the semicircular canals
    (c) the stapes
    (d) all of the above
49. The eustacian tube connects the pharynx to the:
    (a) nasal cavity
    (b) inner ear
    (c) outer ear
    (d) middle ear
50. The malleus is attached to:
    (a) the round window
    (b) the oval window
    (c) the stapes
    (d) the tympanic membrane
51. Describe the passage of light through the eye.
52. Describe the process of accommodation.
53. Name the component parts of the lacrimal apparatus.
54. Outline the function of the tapetum.
55. Describe/state the function of the nictitating membrane.
56. Describe the passage of sound through the ear during audition.
57. Outline the function of the eustachian tube.
58. Describe the processes involved in the sensation of balance.
59. Explain the function of the semicircular canals.
60. Outline the function of the Jacobson's Organ.
61. ADH (anti-diuretic hormone) is released by the:
    (a) adrenal glands
    (b) anterior pituitary gland
    (c) kidney
    (d) posterior pituitary gland
62. Regarding calcium balance, which one of the following statements is most accurate?

    (a) parathyroid hormone increases calcium deposition in bone
    (b) parathyroid hormone increases the calcium concentration in extracellular fluid
    (c) calcitonin increases the intestinal absorption of calcium
    (d) calcitonin increases the calcium concentration in extracellular fluid
63. Glucagon is secreted by which type of pancreatic islet cell?
    (a) alpha cells
    (b) beta cells
    (c) gamma cells
    (d) delta cells
64. Insulin is secreted by which type of pancreatic islet cell?
    (a) alpha cells
    (b) beta cells
    (c) gamma cells
    (d) delta cells
65. The adrenal medulla secretes:
    (a) adrenaline
    (b) epinephrine
    (c) norepinephrine
    (d) all of the above
66. Which one of the following hormones is produced by the anterior pituitary gland?
    (a) anti-diuretic hormone
    (b) calcitonin
    (c) luteinizing hormone
    (d) oxytocin
67. Which two hormones are produced by the anterior pituitary gland and have a direct effect on the ovary?
    (a) follicle-stimulating hormone and luteinizing hormone
    (b) follicle-stimulating hormone and progesterone
    (c) luteinizing hormone and progesterone
    (d) progesterone and oestrogen
68. Oxytocin and vasopressin are released from the:
    (a) adrenal glands
    (b) anterior pituitary
    (c) hypothalamus
    (d) posterior pituitary
69. Growth hormone is produced by the:
    (a) adrenal glands
    (b) anterior pituitary
    (c) hypothalamus
    (d) posterior pituitary
70. Calcitriol is secreted by the:
    (a) kidneys
    (b) parathyroid glands

(c) thyroid gland
(d) pituitary gland
71. List the hormones produced by the anterior pituitary gland.
72. Describe the function of parathyroid hormone.
73. Outline the effects of hyperparathyroidism.
74. Describe the function of calcitonin.
75. Name the three types of steroid hormones produced by the adrenal cortex.
76. Name the hormones secreted by the adrenal medulla.
77. Describe the functions of the three hormones secreted by the pancreatic islets.
78. Explain the difference between the causes of diabetes mellitus and diabetes insipidus.
79. Outline the role of inhibin.
80. List the hormones produced by the ovary.

3

Support and movement

3.1 The skeletal system

> The skeleton
> The formation and structure of bone
> Classification of bones
> Features of the surfaces of bones

Introduction

The skeletal system includes all the structures that give a rigid framework to the body, supporting and protecting the softer tissues within. It includes bones and cartilage as well as the tissues that form joints. In this chapter we will examine these aspects in detail, starting with a basic overview of the skeletal system and progressing to the muscular system and joints.

The skeleton

The skeleton has many functions within the body of an animal, some of which are more evident than others. These functions are listed below:

1. It provides a framework and support for the soft tissues of the body.
2. Articulations between the bones at the joints permit movement via the muscles that are attached at critical sites.
3. It protects delicate organs such as the brain, heart, and lungs.
4. The formation of blood cells occurs in the bone marrow of long bones such as the femur and humerus of the hindlimb and forelimb, respectively.

> The skeleton can be divided into three areas: the **axial** skeleton, the **appendicular** skeleton, and the **splanchnic** skeleton. The **axial** skeleton comprises the skull, vertebral column, ribs and sternum. The forelimbs and hindlimbs are part of the **appendicular** skeleton, which also includes the scapula and pelvis. The **splanchnic** skeleton includes those bones that develop in tissue and that are unattached to the rest of the skeleton. In the cat and the dog the only bone in the splanchnic skeleton is the os penis of the male animal. These areas of the skeleton are illustrated in Figure 3.1.

5. It acts as a storage site for minerals such as calcium and phosphorus. In times of need, these can be mobilized from the bone and released into the blood supply.

The formation and structure of bone

Bone is classified as a type of connective tissue consisting of a matrix of a substance that is secreted by specialized cells called **osteoblasts**. The matrix gives bone some degree of flexibility and the strength to support the body, due to deposition of mineral salts such as calcium and phosphorus within the matrix. Flexibility, as well as strength, is required in order to allow the bone to give when pressures are applied. If the bone were completely rigid it would be more inclined to fracture.

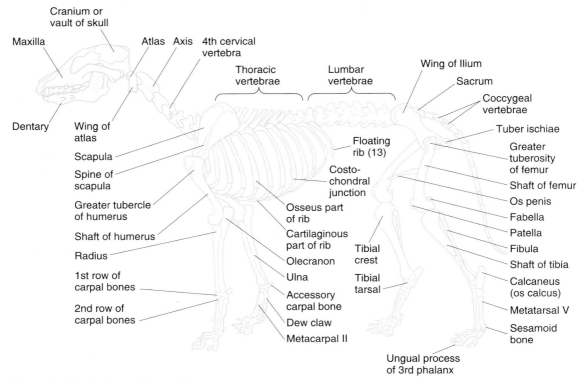

Figure 3.1 The skeleton of the male dog

Bone cells

In addition to their strength and flexibility, bones are also comparably light for their size. This is due to the presence of cavities within the bone that are filled with air, adipose tissue, or bone marrow, as well as 'spongy' bone located internally. These cavities allow the animal to move the skeleton via the muscles. If the bones were dense structures they would be too heavy to move!

Bone cells

There are several different types of cell present within bone. Those already discussed, osteoblasts, produce new bone matrix (often remembered by students as bone-building cells). These cells are particularly important in the initial development of bone in the growing animal and in the repair of fractured bone tissue. Once surrounded by bone matrix, the cell is referred to as an **osteocyte**.

Osteocytes are the main cells found within mature bone. They are unable to divide and help to recycle calcium salts in the surrounding bone matrix, as well as assisting in the repair of

damaged bone by converting themselves into osteoblasts when necessary. Osteocytes are located within the osteons in layers around the Haversian canal (see Figure 3.2).

Osteoprogenitor cells can also be found, although their numbers are usually small. They are mitotic cells that divide to produce daughter cells that will eventually differentiate into osteoblasts. Osteoprogenitor cells are responsible for the maintenance of the population of osteoblasts within bone, and are therefore critical to the repair of bone when fractured.

The final type of cell that can be found within the bone structure is the **osteoclast**. These cells have the opposite effects to osteoblasts and are responsible for the breakdown of bone matrix. By doing this they liberate calcium and phosphorus ions, helping to maintain levels of circulating calcium and phosphorus ions within acceptable limits. If the activity of osteoclasts is greater than that of osteoblasts, then bone demineralization will occur. This is seen in cases of hyperparathyroidism (see Chapter 2).

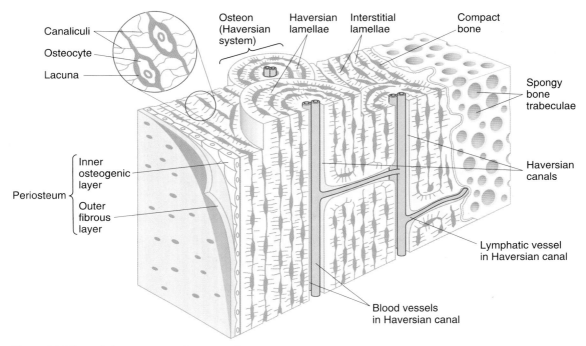

Figure 3.2 The cellular structure of compact bone

Compact bone

Compact bone is located on the outer surface of bones where the mechanical stresses on the bone are at their greatest. The overall strength of bone is due to the outer layers of compact bone, which is hard and dense. It is composed of units called **osteons** or **Haversian systems** that all lie in the same direction (hence the strength of compact bone), the structure of which is illustrated in Figure 3.2.

The **Haversian canal** that runs along the centre of the osteon contains the blood supply that is carried into the tissue of the bone. This blood supply passes from the outer surrounding membrane of the bone, the periosteum, through perforating canals (also called canals of Volkmann) to the osteons deep in the bone.

Spongy or cancellous bone

In contrast, spongy or cancellous bone does not contain a rigid structure of osteons. Instead it is comprised of trabeculae, thin spines of bone that branch out to form a loose network. Spaces in the network may be filled with red bone marrow. Spongy bone is not particularly strong, as is to be expected when considering its structure. It is much lighter than compact bone and is found where

mechanical stresses on the bone are low or where they are applied in many directions. It can be found in the vertebrae, flat bones, and at the end of long bones of the skeleton.

Development of bone

In the previous sections we have considered the different types of bone in the skeleton as well as the different kinds of cells that form the structure of bone. In this section we will examine the anatomical structure of bone in further detail and consider the development and growth of bone within the animal.

> Bone develops in one of two ways. The first route is through the ossification of hyaline cartilage that is deposited during development of the embryo. This is known as endochondral or interchondral ossification. The second route is through the replacement of fibrous connective tissue by bone and is known as intramembranous ossification. A long bone develops by the former method, endochondral ossification, and this is illustrated in Figure 3.4.

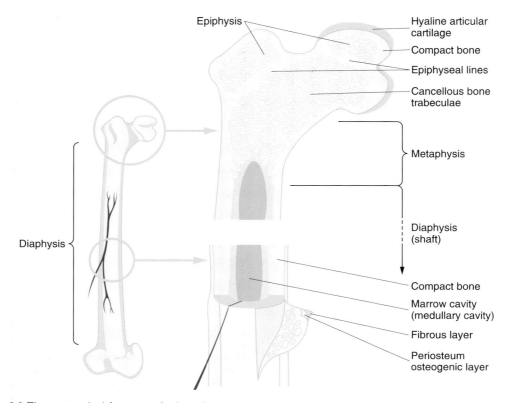

Figure 3.3 The anatomical features of a long bone

Figure 3.3 illustrates the typical anatomical features of a long bone such as the femur of the hindlimb.

The end of the bone is called the **epiphysis** (plural = **epiphyses**), while the shaft of the bone is known as the **diaphysis**. The end of the diaphysis, where bone growth takes place, is termed the **metaphysis**, growth plate, or epiphyseal plate. This becomes calcified once bone growth is complete and is visible on radiographs as the epiphyseal line. The outer surface of the bone is covered by a layer of fibrous connective tissue called the **periosteum** that provides a vascular and nervous supply to the bone.

Bones that develop by intramembranous ossification include the bones of the cranium, mandible and clavicle.

Innervation and blood supply

Bone can be described as a vascular connective tissue (compare this to cartilage in Chapter 1). It has an extensive blood supply, as illustrated in Figure 3.5. The nutrient artery and vein supply the diaphysis. The majority of bones have one nutrient artery and a vein, although some may have more. The vessels pass into the bones through small holes called foramina and carry the blood supply to the osteons. The metaphyseal blood vessels carry blood to the epiphyseal plates where bone growth occurs. The third type of blood vessels, the periosteal vessels, supply the surface of the bone and the secondary centres of ossification during bone formation. When the bone has finished growing the three types of vessels interconnect with each other.

Bones have a rich nerve supply, hence the pain felt when an injury occurs. The nervous supply is primarily located in the periosteum and branches travel with the artery into the cortex, providing innervation to the epiphyses, marrow cavity and endosteum (a layer of cells lining the marrow cavity).

Repair of fractures

Bone is a dynamic structure. The activity of osteocytes, osteoblasts and osteoclasts results in

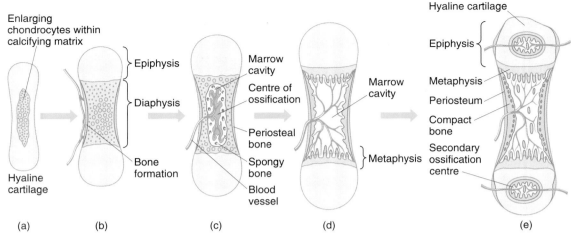

Figure 3.4 Endochondral ossification of a long bone. (a) Ossification of the hyaline cartilage that is deposited during development of the embryo; (b) blood vessels grow; (c) blood vessels penetrate the cartilage; (d) as growth continues, remodelling occurs, creating a marrow cavity; (e) capillaries and osteoblasts migrate, creating secondary ossification centres

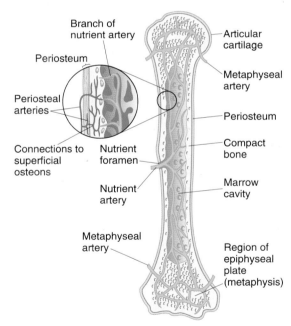

Figure 3.5 Blood supply of a developing and mature long bone

the constant formation and breakdown of the matrix, and recycling of the mineral salts. When a fracture occurs it is usually associated with bleeding, as the blood vessels within the bone are damaged. Due to a failure of circulation within the bone, osteocytes die around the injured area,

resulting an a significant area of dead bone around the injured site. In the adult animal, the endosteum and periosteum produce cells that move into the damaged area and form an area of cartilage and bone at the fractured site. Osteoblast activity replaces the cartilage with spongy bone as the fracture starts to heal. At this point a **callus** will be palpable at the site of the injury. Over time, the activity of osteoblasts and osteoclasts remodel the fractured site and, once complete, the spongy bone will have been replaced by compact bone. In many cases, the site of the original fracture may be indistinguishable from the rest of the bone.

Classification of bones

Bones of the skeleton are classified into one of five groups depending upon their shape:

1. **Short bones** are strong, compact, 'box-like' bones with limited motion. They have a thin layer of compact bone on the surface but are otherwise composed of cancellous bone with no medulla (or marrow cavity). Examples include the carpal bones of the forelimb and tarsal bones of the hindlimb.
2. **Long bones** form the system of levers in the skeleton that allow locomotion. They have a diaphysis and two epiphyses that are usually enlarged for muscle attachment and articulation

(see Figure 3.3). The outer layer of the bone is formed from compact bone and the inner medulla contains bone marrow. The epiphyses are formed from cancellous bone that gives some degree of strength in many directions without being too heavy. Long bones are usually curved to help them to withstand greater forces.

3. **Flat bones** are usually quite thin. They provide extensive protection in the areas where they are located and provide a broad surface for muscle attachment. They are composed of two outer layers of compact bone with an inner layer of cancellous tissue. They include the bones of the cranium, sternum, scapula, ribs, and pelvis.

4. **Irregular bones** are unusual in shape and have an outer layer of compact bone with cancellous bone within. Examples include the vertebrae, and the maxima, temporal and sphenoid bones of the skull.

5. **Sesamoid bones** are located near freely moving joints, e.g. of the stifle. They are small, flat bones that form in the tissue of tendons or ligaments. They alter the direction of tendons over bony prominences to prevent excessive wear and tear. Examples of sesamoid bones include the patella and fabellae of the stifle joint.

Features of the surfaces of bone

All bones have surface features – they are not smooth, even structures. Bones have many raised areas (eminences) and sunken areas (depressions). They also have articular surfaces, i.e. parts of the joints, and areas of tendon or muscle attachment. In this section we will consider some of the terminology that may be encountered when describing the external features of bones.

Terminology

A description of anatomical features, along with others that may be commonly encountered, can be found in Table 3.1. Figure 3.6 shows the femur of the hindlimb with several anatomical features of the bone labelled. For a more detailed overview of the anatomy of individual bones within the skeleton, the reader is referred to a specialized anatomical textbook.

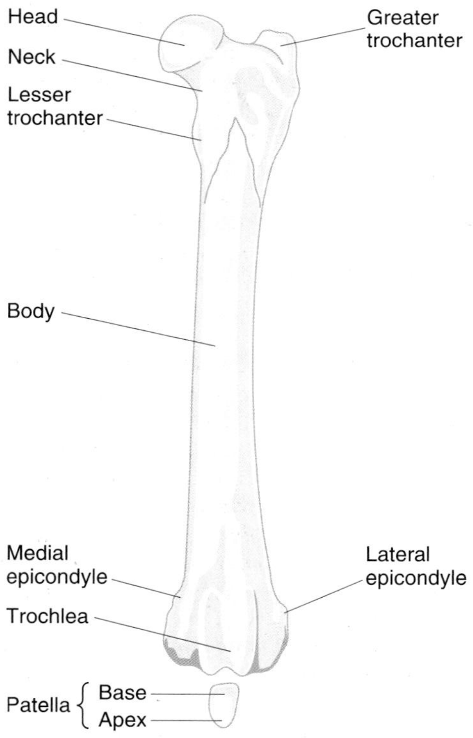

Figure 3.6 Anatomical features of a canine femur

Table 3.1 General anatomical features of bones

Condyle	A rounded enlargement at the end of a bone, usually covered with cartilage
Crest	A ridge or line running along the surface of the bone
Foramen	A small passage for blood vessels or nerves
Fossa	A small depression or pit in a bone
Groove	A long narrow depression
Process	A rough projection for muscle attachment
Sinus	A chamber within a bone
Spine	A sharp, slender pointed eminence
Trochanter	A large rough projection for muscle attachment
Tubercle	A small rounded projection for muscle attachment
Tuberosity	A smaller projection for muscle attachment

3.2 The muscular system

Muscle tissue
Striated (voluntary) muscle
Muscle contraction
Aerobic and anaerobic respiration
Smooth (involuntary) muscle
Cardiac muscle
Skeletal muscles

Introduction

The muscular system allows the skeleton to move. It also has functions that are less obvious, such as causing the heart to beat, allowing the lungs to expand and relax, and moving food through the digestive system. It is a critical component of every living animal in all aspects of daily existence, and although we will initially consider muscle as part of the skeletal system, controlling movement, we will also examine its other functions later in this chapter.

Muscle tissue

Muscle tissue constitutes between one third and one half of the total body weight of an animal. It is an extremely specialized tissue containing cells that are capable of contraction. It is classified into three different types: **striated** or **voluntary muscle, smooth** or **involuntary muscle**, and **cardiac muscle**. Each of these will be discussed in detail in the following sections.

Striated (voluntary) muscle

Striated muscle fibres are cylindrical in shape. The cells that make up the fibres are multi-nuclear and have a striped or striated appearance due to the presence of light and dark bands. Each muscle is surrounded by three layers of connective tissue. The outer layer or **epimysium** is composed of

Striated or voluntary muscle is often referred to as skeletal muscle, as it the muscle that determines and controls the movement of the animal, attaching to the bones of the skeleton, either directly or via tendons. It also acts to maintain posture, support and protects soft muscle tissue, and contributes to the maintenance of body temperature.

collagen fibres and protects the muscle. The middle layer or **perimysium** divides the muscle into sections of muscle fibres and contains the blood vessels and nerves that supply the muscle. The inner layer or **endomysium** surrounds the individual muscle fibres (the cells of the muscle). A diagram of the structure of skeletal muscle is shown in Figure 3.7.

The three layers of connective tissue join together at the end of the muscle forming a **tendon,** or in the cases of some muscles, a sheet of tendon called an **apneurosis**. The tendons attach the muscle firmly to bones of the skeleton.

Muscle contraction

Each muscle fibre or cell has a cell membrane called the **sarcolemma**. The characteristics of the sarcolemma are similar to that of the cell membrane of a neurone, i.e. it is an excitable membrane which is activated by a change in the transmembrane potential of the cell. Due to its relatively large size, the muscle fibre has an interconnecting series of tubes that run throughout the cell. This allows a stimulus to be rapidly transported throughout the cell and cause the fibre to contract. Also located within the muscle fibre are structures known as **myofibrils**. These contain bundles of **myofilaments** that are composed of two proteins, **actin** and **myosin**. The myofibrils within the cell shorten, causing the muscle to contract.

Myofilaments are organized within the muscle in repeated sections called **sarcomeres**, a myofibril containing approximately 10 000 sarcomeres. It is the relationship between the thick filaments (myosin) and the thin filaments (actin) that cause muscle contraction. The structure of a sarcomere is illustrated in Figure 3.8.

As can be seen, the sarcomere has different colour bands or zones due to the distribution of the actin and myosin. Dark bands are known as A bands while the lighter bands are known as I bands. Within the A band, the M line represents the site at which each thick filament (myosin) joins with adjacent filaments via proteins. The H band represents the area containing only thick filaments (myosin). The zone of overlap represents the area where thick filaments (myosin) overlap with thin filaments (actin).

The I bands contain only thin filaments (actin). The end of one sarcomere and the start of the next is termed the Z line.

Muscle contraction occurs as the thin filaments slide inwards toward the M line. This is known as

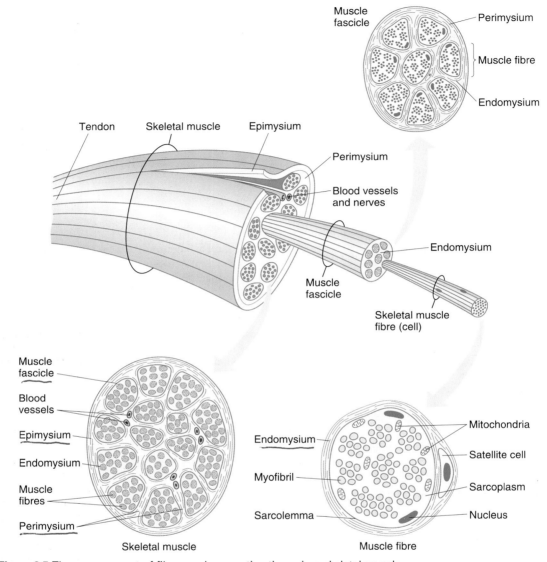

Figure 3.7 The arrangement of fibres and connective tissue in a skeletal muscle

the sliding filament theory of muscle contraction and is illustrated in Figure 3.9.

Release of the neurotransmitter acetylcholine at the neuromuscular junction causes the depolarization of the sarcolemma and the generation of an action potential. This stimulates the activation of the actin and myosin molecules within the sarcomeres. The thick fibres pull the thin fibres in towards the M line and the muscle contracts. Once the acetylcholine has been bro-

ken down at the neuromuscular junction, the stimulus to sustain the contraction of the sarcomeres stops. However, the sarcomeres are unable to return to their normal length passively and require an active external force to stretch them back to their original length. These external forces include the elastic forces stored through stretching the muscle, contraction of opposing groups of muscles (see later), and the effects of gravity.

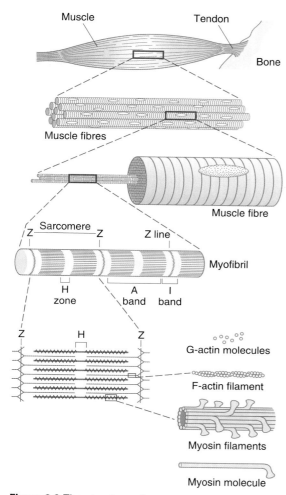

Figure 3.8 The structure of a sarcomere

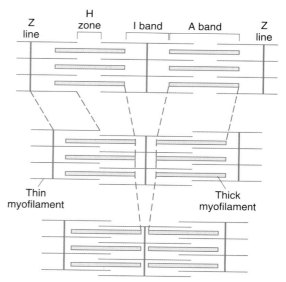

Figure 3.9 The sliding filament theory of muscle contraction

Isitonic and isometric muscle contraction

Muscle contraction can be described as either isotonic or isometric. Isotonic contractions cause the shortening of muscle, whereas isometric contractions do not involve a change in length of the muscle. Instead, the tension of the muscle increases but never enough to overcome the resistance. Consider two dogs playing tug of war with a rubber ring. If the two dogs are unequally matched, the stronger of the two will pull with sufficient strength to overcome the weaker dog and will pull the weaker along the floor. This is similar to isotonic muscle contraction, where the muscle contracts first to resist the force but then to overcome it and produce movement. However, if the two dogs are evenly matched, each will pull to resist the other but neither will overcome the initial force. This is similar to isometric muscle contraction, where the tension of the muscle builds to resist the force but never actually overcomes it.

Aerobic and anaerobic respiration

A muscle at rest can gain what little energy it requires from the aerobic metabolism of fatty acids by the mitochondria, producing adenosine triphosphate (ATP). On the other hand, the contraction of a muscle requires more energy, which is obtained by the metabolism of glucose (from glycogen reserves in the muscle). Active muscle breaks down glucose (a process known as glycolysis) into pyruvic acid from which the mitochondria can generate ATP, which is then available as an energy source for the contracting muscle fibre. Moderate activity causes an increased requirement for ATP by the muscle and this is synthesized by the aerobic respiration of the mitochondria (aerobic = using oxygen). If activity levels increase to the point that it is no longer possible to supply the tissue with the amount of oxygen required from the quantity of ATP available, a supplementary route for the production of ATP is necessary. This is produced through the glycolytic pathway and is known as anaerobic respiration. In situations of very high muscle activity the glycolytic pathway produces more pyruvic acid than can be used by the mitochondria to generate ATP. The excess pyruvic acid is converted into lactic acid that builds up within the tissues. Excess lactic acid is toxic and can cause the sensation of muscle cramps as the muscle becomes unable to contract in the increasingly acidic environment. Once the period of muscular contraction has come to an end, the excess lactic acid that has built up is converted into ATP and glucose, using the oxygen that is inhaled as the result of the intense period of heavy breathing following strenuous exercise. The amount of oxygen that is required to convert the excess lactic acid and restore the pre-exercise condition of the muscle is known as the oxygen debt.

Muscle hypertrophy and atrophy

Repeated exercise stimulates the development of the muscle fibres to adapt to increasing demands. They develop more mitochondria and are able to store greater levels of glycogen as an energy reserve. The muscle filaments also enlarge, causing an increase in size, or hypertrophy, of the muscle. The number of muscle fibres remains constant, although each fibre increases in diameter. The development of muscle fibres is also stimulated by the male hormone testosterone. Consequently, entire male animals are usually more muscular then females. Muscular atrophy occurs in a muscle that is not exercised. Muscle fibres become small and weak and the muscle itself becomes flaccid. Animals that are prevented from using a limb for a period of time, for example, due to a fracture or pain from arthritis, will show muscle atrophy in the affected limb. Physiotherapy is critical in maintaining the muscle mass of an animal that may be unable to walk for a period of time due to injury or illness.

> Smooth muscle tissue is located within many of the different systems of the body. It forms a lining around the blood vessels, thereby controlling the amount of blood that is supplied to different areas by contraction and relaxation. It lines the respiratory tract and can dilate or constrict the airways. It controls the movement of food through the digestive system, as well as moving gametes along the reproductive tracts. It also facilitates the movement of urine along the ureters and surrounds the bladder.

Smooth (involuntary) muscle

In the previous sections we have examined the structure and function of skeletal muscle. The second type of muscle found in the body is smooth or involuntary muscle. As the name suggests, the contraction of this type of muscle is not under the voluntary control of the animal. It is innervated by the autonomic nervous system and may also be influenced by the secretion of hormones in some parts of the body. In contrast to the cylindrical, striped, appearance of the striated muscle fibre, smooth muscle cells are spindle-shaped with one nucleus.

Although actin and myosin are still the proteins that cause smooth muscle to contract, they are not arranged in blocks or sarcomeres and are more loosely distributed throughout the sarcoplasm of the cell. Consequently, smooth muscle is also referred to as non-striated muscle.

Cardiac muscle

Intercalated discs lie between each muscle cell. They provide stability of structure within the tissue and allow the rapid transmission of the nerve impulse from one cell to another throughout the tissue. **Purkinje fibres** further facilitate this speed of transmission. They are specialized nerve fibres that spread out within the cardiac muscle of the heart and help to co-ordinate muscle contraction. The myofibrils themselves are also interconnected, again facilitating the co-ordinated contraction of the muscle. The mechanism of heart muscle contraction is discussed in further detail in Chapter 4.

Skeletal muscles

In this section we shall consider the skeletal muscles of the body. Detailed anatomy will not be

> Cardiac muscle, as the name suggests, is found exclusively in the walls of the heart. Similar to the smooth muscle cells, those of the cardiac muscle are also under the control of the autonomic nervous system. Cardiac muscle is similar in some ways to striated muscle as it does contain sarcomeres, which are aligned to give a striped appearance. However, there are some structural differences that are unique to cardiac muscle.

discussed, as this text is primarily concerned with physiology of animals. However, there are some basic terms and principles that we need to consider.

Most muscles of the skeletal system are attached to bone or cartilage by **tendons**, which are formed from specialized connective tissue. In some cases, the connective tissue may be in the form of a flat, sheet-like structure. This is called an **apneurosis**. Some muscles may also attach directly to the bone itself.

All muscles have a point of origin and a point of insertion. The origin is the end of the muscle that remains more fixed during a muscular contraction while the insertion is the area that is more moveable.

Muscles are classified depending upon the type of movement that they cause. These are summarized in Table 3.2.

Opposing muscle groups

Muscles of the body usually exist in opposing groups that together produce a range of movement around a joint. These two groups are usually termed **agonistic** and **antagonistic** (as described in Table 3.2) and together, usually act to flex and extend a joint. For example, in bending the elbow, the biceps brachii acts as the agonist whilst the triceps brachii opposes its action and is therefore the antagonist.

There are also some structures that are commonly associated with muscles, known as accessory structures. These include **sesamoid bones**, **synovial tendon sheaths**, **bursae** and **fascias**.

Sesamoid bones

Sesamoid bones were discussed in the previous section. They usually develop in tendons or ligaments. They protect tendons in vulnerable areas, increase the surface area for the attachment of tendons, and re-direct the direction of pull of the tendon in order that it can function more efficiently.

Synovial tendon sheaths

Synovial tendon sheaths are sac-like structures containing synovial fluid. They pass around tendons, protecting them and reducing the effects of friction.

Bursae

A bursa is a sac of fluid that is located between a tendon, ligament, or muscle and a projection of bone. It acts to reduce friction at the point of contact with the bone

Fascias

Fascias are formed from connective tissue and may separate, surround, or connect muscles, blood vessels, and nerves. They may also act as a site for fat storage.

Table 3.2 Classification of muscles according to their action

Classification	Action	Example
Extensor	Increases the angle between two bones	*Triceps brachii* of the forelimb
Flexor	Decreases the angle between two bones	*Biceps brachii* of the forelimb
Adductor	Moves a limb towards the body	*Pectineus* of the hindlimb/pelvis
Abductor	Moves a limb away from the body	*Pectoralis* of the forelimb/chest
Circumduction	Movement of the limb in a plane representing the surface of a cone	Groups of muscles work together to achieve this movement
Rotation	Movement of a limb around the long axis	*Infraspinatus* of the shoulder
Agonist	The muscle(s) that causes the prime movement of the joint	In the forelimb, the *Biceps brachii* and *Triceps brachi* act
Antagonist	The muscle(s) responsible for the opposite action	as agonist and antagonist, respectively

3.3 Joints

Joint classification
Movement of a synovial joint
Ligaments
Tendons

Introduction

In addition to the bones and muscles of the skeleton, there is one other important area that we need to examine in order to have a full understanding of support and movement of the body. Joints, or articulations as they are sometimes called, are crucial to the movement of the skeleton, giving the flexibility to permit movement. In the next section we shall consider the types of joints that are present and determine their structure and function within the skeletal system as a whole.

Joint classification

Fibrous joints

Fibrous joints or synarthroses (sing = synarthrosis) are immovable and are located where the surfaces of the bones are in almost direct contact, separated only by dense connective tissue. In some cases the surfaces may interlock. They form stable joints and are usually found where the movement of the bones is undesirable. They can be one of four types:

1. **Syndesmoses** (sing = syndesmosis)
   This type of joint occurs where bones are united by fibrous tissue forming an interosseus membrane or ligament that allows a small degree of movement, e.g. the attachment of the **hyoid apparatus** to the temporal bone of the skull.
2. **Sutures**
   Sutures are the joints between the different bones of the skull. The edges of the bones are

A joint or articulation is defined as the region where two or more bones are united by fibrous, elastic, or cartilaginous tissue (or a combination of any of the three). They are classified into three main groups: **fibrous joints (synarthroses)**, **cartilaginous joints (amphi-arthroses)**, and **synovial joints (diarthroses)**. These three types of joint are discussed in this section.

interlocked and held together by a layer of dense connective tissue.
3. **Gomphoses** (sing = gomphosis)
   A gomphosis is the joint between the teeth and the alveolar sockets of the mandible and maxilla. The fibrous periodontal ligament connects the tooth to the bone of the socket.
4. **Synostoses** (sing = synostosis)
   This is sometimes referred to as an additional classification of fibrous joint and is a term used to describe any normal or abnormal union of two bones by osseus material.

Cartilaginous joints

Cartilaginous joints or amphi-arthroses (sing = amphi-arthrosis) are those that permit only a limited movement such as compression or stretching. They can be formed by hyaline cartilage, fibrocartilage, or a combination of the two.

1. **Hyaline cartilage joints**
   These are usually temporary joints that disappear with age. They are present in the fetus and within growing bone, and occur where the epiphysis unites with the diaphysis at the cartilaginous epiphyseal plate. In adulthood, the region becomes ossified, although a faint line may be seen on radiographs. This ossification would be an example of a synostosis, discussed previously. One hyaline joint that remains throughout the adult life of the animal is at the costochondral junction of the osseus and cartilaginous rib.
2. **Fibrocartilage joints**
   Examples of these can be found in the joints of the mandibular symphysis, the pelvic symphysis, the **sternebrae** and the bodies of the vertebrae. In some cases the joints may have an intervening plate of hyaline cartilage at each end and some may ossify with age.

Synovial joints

Synovial joints or diarthroses (sing = diarthrosis) facilitate a wide range of movement and are usually located at the ends of long bones, particularly the forelimb and hindlimb. Their basic structure is illustrated in Figure 3.10.

The joint is contained within the joint capsule, composed of an outer fibrous membrane and an inner synovial membrane. In the stifle it is strengthened by collateral ligaments. The joint cavity is lined with a synovial membrane that

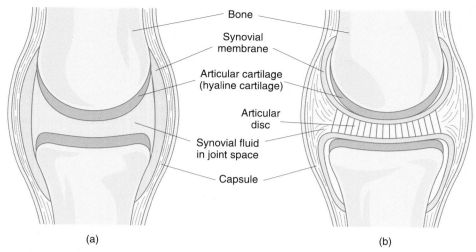

Figure 3.10 The structure of (a) a typical synovial joint, (b) a synovial joint containing articular cartilage

secretes synovial fluid into the cavity to act as a lubricant, reducing friction within the joint. It also carries nutrients and waste products to the hyaline cartilage within the joint. The hyaline cartilage reduces the effects of stress on the joint, acting like a shock absorber.

Some synovial joints have additional structures that facilitate their function. These may **include intra-articular ligaments, menisci,** and **fat pads.** **Intra-articular ligaments** act to stabilise the joint, preventing excessive movements that may cause damage. **Menisci** (sing = meniscus) are pads of

fibrocartilage that lie between the articular surfaces. Their function is to protect areas that are subject to a great deal of physical stress. Fat pads are masses of adipose tissue that protect the articular cartilage and act as a packing substance within the joint. They are found in similar areas to menisci.

Movement of a synovial joint

Synovial joints can exhibit several different types of movement. These are outlined, with some examples, in Table 3.3.

Table 3.3 Movement of synovial joints

Movement	Description	Example
Flexion	The angle of the joint between the two bones is decreased to less than 180°	Bending the stifle of the hindlimb
Extension	The angle of the joint between the two bones is increased towards 180°	Extending the stifle of the hindlimb
Gliding	The surface of one bone slides over the surface of another	Movement of the bones in the carpus and tarsus
Abduction	Movement of the limb away from the body	A dog cocks its leg to urinate
Adduction	Movement of the limb towards the body	As the dog returns to standing from the previous example
Circumduction	Movement of the limb following the surface of the cone	This movement does not occur naturally, although the joint can be manipulated in this way
Rotation	Movement of the limb around its long axis	As above

We can classify synovial joints according to their structure and range of movement into the following five groups:

1. **Hinge joints**
   Hinge joints allow flexion and extension. They have limited rotational movement. An example of a hinge joint is the elbow.
2. **Ball and socket joints**
   Ball and socket joints are the most freely moving type of synovial joint. The rounded head of a bone fits into the cavity (or fossa) of another. Examples of this type of joint include the hip and shoulder, although in the dog and cat the movement of the shoulder is more similar to that of a hinge joint due to the presence of two capsular muscles that stabilize the joint.
3. **Pivot joints**
   Movement of pivot joints is described as a movement along the longitudinal axis of the joint, an example being the atlanto-axial joint of the atlas and axis (vertebrae C1 and C2). The joint between the radius and ulna at the proximal end of the lower forelimb is also a pivot joint.
4. **Plane (or gliding) joints**
   A plane or gliding joint is found where the articular surfaces of the bones are flattened and the bones glide over each other as the joint is mobilized. Examples of plane joints include those between the bones of the carpus and tarsus (i.e. the intercarpal and intertarsal joints).

> Ligaments are bands of fibrous connective tissue that connect bones or cartilage within joints. They act to stabilize the joint, giving it support and strength. The illustration in Figure 3.11 shows clearly that there are collateral ligaments that help to stabilize the stifle joint. These are described as extracapsular ligaments as they join with the articulating bones and pass outside the joint capsule.

5. **Condylar joints**
   A condylar joint has a movement resembling that of a hinge joint, however the articular surfaces are condylar (see Table 3.1). Examples of condylar joints include the stifle and temporomandibular joints.

This is a greatly simplified classification system; it should be remembered that each joint may differ slightly in its structure and range of movement from those listed above.

Ligaments

There are other ligaments within the joint itself that further assist stabilization and prevent extreme movement of the joint. These are known as the cruciate ligaments and can be ruptured or damaged during exercise (see Figure 3.11). This type of

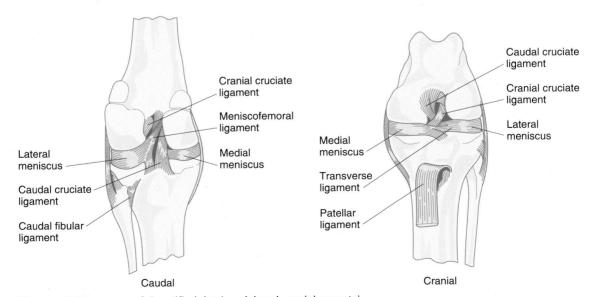

Lateral meniscus

Cranial cruciate ligament

Meniscofemoral ligament

Medial meniscus

Caudal cruciate ligament

Caudal fibular ligament

Caudal

Caudal cruciate ligament

Cranial cruciate ligament

Lateral meniscus

Medial meniscus

Transverse ligament

Patellar ligament

Cranial

Figure 3.11 Ligaments of the stifle joint (caudal and cranial aspects)

ligament is also known as an intracapsular ligament, as the ligaments are located within the joint capsule.

Tendons

The terms ligament and tendon are often confused. A tendon is described as a sheet or band of white fibrous connective tissue that connects muscle to bone or other structure. Note that a ligament connects bones to each other, rather than to muscle. Whilst tendons are not directly involved in the joint structure they can have stabilizing effects if they pass around or close to joints.

Review questions

1. Intramembranous ossification occurs when:
   (a) the femur develops from a hyaline cartilage model
   (b) the femur develops from primitive connective tissue
   (c) the frontal bone develops from primitive connective tissue
   (d) the parietal bone develops from transitional epithelial tissue
2. In young animals, growth in length of a long bone occurs at the:
   (a) epithelium
   (b) periosteum
   (c) diaphysis
   (d) epiphyseal plate
3. The calcaneus is found:
   (a) in the hock
   (b) in the stifle
   (c) in the elbow
   (d) in the carpus
4. The femur is an example of a:
   (a) long bone
   (b) short bone
   (c) irregular bone
   (d) flat bone
5. The scapula is an example of a:
   (a) long bone
   (b) short bone
   (c) irregular bone
   (d) flat bone
6. During endochondral ossification, the primary centre of ossification develops:
   (a) in the epiphysis
   (b) in the diaphysis
   (c) at the epiphyseal plate
   (d) in the growth cartilage
7. Secondary centres of ossification then develop:
   (a) in the epiphysis
   (b) in the diaphysis
   (c) at the epiphyseal plate
   (d) in the growth cartilage
8. Within bone, blood vessels are situated:
   (a) within the lacunae
   (b) in the Haversian canals
   (c) only within the marrow cavity
   (d) nowhere, bone is avascular
9. Which bone articulates with the proximal end of the humerus?
   (a) radius
   (b) ulna
   (c) scapula
   (d) tibia
10. What is the name given to the articular depression of the scapula?
    (a) acetabulum
    (b) obturator foramen
    (c) glenoid fossa
    (d) spine
11. List the five functions of the skeleton.
12. Name the three parts of the skeleton.
13. Identify the two types of bone.
14. Describe the role of osteoblasts and osteoclasts in the modelling of bone.
15. How are bones classified? Give an example for each classification.
16. Define the term 'foramen'.
17. Define the term 'condyle'.
18. Draw a diagram to illustrate the anatomical features of a long bone.
19. Outline how hyperparathyroidism affects the structure of bone.
20. Describe the processes involved in the healing of a fracture.
21. Without available oxygen, working muscles continue to contract through a biochemical pathway known as:
    (a) aerobic respiration
    (b) anaerobic respiration
    (c) muscle tone
    (d) photosynthesis
22. What is the name of the outer layer of connective tissue that surrounds skeletal muscles?
    (a) epimysium
    (b) endomysium
    (c) perimysium
    (d) sarcolemma
23. Which of the following is not formed from striated muscle?

(a) the biceps femoris
(b) the gastrocnemius
(c) the muscles of the rib cage
(d) the muscle of the intestine

24. Which muscle type is found in the walls of blood vessels?
    (a) cardiac
    (b) striated
    (c) skeletal
    (d) smooth

25. What is the name of the carbohydrate that acts as a storage product found in skeletal muscle?
    (a) triglyceride
    (b) glycogen
    (c) glucose
    (d) lipid

26. What is the term given to the enlargement of muscle due to repeated exercise?
    (a) atrophy
    (b) hypotrophy
    (c) hypertrophy
    (d) hyperenlargement

27. During anaerobic respiration there is a build-up of a substance that can be toxic at high levels. This is known as:
    (a) pyruvic acid
    (b) sulphuric acid
    (c) acetic acid
    (d) lactic acid

28. A joint known as a gomphosis can be classified as a:
    (a) fibrous joint
    (b) cartilaginous joint
    (c) synovial joint
    (d) fixed joint

29. Cartilaginous joints are located:
    (a) at the joint of the tooth with the periodontal ligament
    (b) between the vertebral bodies
    (c) between the flat bones of the skull
    (d) in the stifle

30. The movement of one articular surface over another, as in the case of movement of the carpus, is known as:
    (a) flexion
    (b) rotation
    (c) gliding
    (d) circumduction

31. Describe the three types of muscle.

32. Name the two proteins involved with muscle contraction.

33. State which neurotransmitter is released at the neuromuscular junction, stimulating muscle contraction.

34. Explain the difference between isometric and isotonic muscle contraction.

35. Give an example of a muscle that acts as an extensor.

36. Outline the difference between an abductor and adductor muscle.

37. State the purpose of sesamoid bones.

38. Name the two types of cartilaginous joint.

39. Draw a diagram to illustrate the structure of a synovial joint.

40. Describe the difference between a tendon and a ligament.

Transport

4.1 Blood

```
Blood
Plasma
Blood corpuscles (cells)
Haemopoiesis
Haemostasis
Fibrinolysis
```

Introduction

As multicellular organisms, all mammals require a transport mechanism that allows substances to be transported to tissues and cells in every area of the body. In Chapter 1 we discussed the need for systems whose functions are adapted to ensure that homeostasis is maintained. The transport system that has evolved in mammals is a highly specialized body system that carries vital components to all cells in the body, e.g. glucose, oxygen, and hormones. It also transports waste products, e.g. urea and carbon dioxide, away from the cells to the organs responsible for their elimination and excretion.

We shall consider the transport system in two sections, although one would not exist without the other. In the first section of this chapter we shall discuss the important features and functions of the transport medium, the blood, and in the second section we shall examine the importance of the transport system, consisting of the heart and blood vessels, commonly known as the cardiovascular system.

Blood is the major transport medium of the body and in the dog and cat accounts for 9% of body weight or 90 mls/kg. It carries nutrients, oxygen and water to the tissues whilst removing waste products to the organs responsible for their elimination and excretion. The blood is also responsible for the circulation of hormones and enzymes, as well as distributing body heat from the core to the extremities, thus helping to maintain body temperature. As well as its transport function, blood also has a role to play in the protection of the body. White blood cells and antibodies help in the fight against infection and invasion, while the clotting mechanism helps to protect against severe haemorrhage, thereby maintaining homeostasis. The blood also helps to protect the body tissues against changes in pH by the buffering action of some proteins and mineral salts.

Blood

Blood consists of two components, **plasma** and **corpuscles** (or cells). These will be considered in the following sections.

Plasma

Plasma is a clear, straw-coloured fluid that forms approximately half the volume of whole blood,

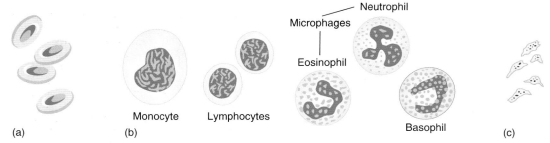

Figure 4.1 The different types of blood cells. (a) Erythrocytes (red blood cells); (b) leucocytes (white blood cells); (c) thrombocytes (platelets)

accounting for approximately 7% of the total body weight of an animal. It is slightly alkaline with a pH of approximately 7.4 and consists of about 90% water. It is very similar in composition to that of interstitial fluid except that it contains a larger quantity of proteins. Constituents include mineral salts (e.g. sodium chloride, calcium carbonate and potassium phosphate), plasma proteins (e.g. albumin, globulin and fibrinogen), dissolved gases (e.g. oxygen, carbon dioxide and nitrogen), waste products (e.g. urea and creatinine), and nutrients (e.g. glucose and amino acids). It also contains varying levels of antibodies, hormones, and enzymes, depending upon the physiological status of the animal.

Blood corpuscles (cells)

There are a total of seven different types of cells that are found in the blood of all mammals. These are all derived from one single bone marrow cell that divides and differentiates into the different forms.

As can be seen in Figure 4.1, the seven different types of cells can be considered in three groups: **erythrocytes** (red blood cells), **thrombocytes** (platelets), and **leucocytes** (white blood cells). The latter group, leucocytes, can be further subdivided into **polymorphonuclear leucocytes, lymphocytes**, and **monocytes.** Lymphocytes and monocytes are also classified as **agranulocytes,** while the polymorphonuclear leucocytes, of which there are three different types, are classified as **granulocytes**, on the basis of the appearance of their cytoplasm following staining. We shall consider each type of cell in turn.

Erythrocytes

Erythrocytes (red blood cells) have no nucleus as they have become so specialized for their function

that they have lost the ability to directly reproduce themselves. Consequently, their shape is often described as that of a biconcave disc (see Figure 4.2).

They are the most numerous blood cells in a healthy animal and are relatively small compared to the leucocytes. Their function is to transport oxygen from the lungs to the tissues of the body and to carry carbon dioxide back to the lungs. They achieve this by means of a protein called haemoglobin, which has a high affinity for oxygen. In the lungs, the oxygen in the inspired air combines with the haemoglobin in the erythrocyte to form a compound called oxyhaemoglobin. This is bright

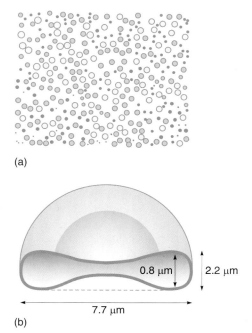

(a)

(b)

Figure 4.2 The structure of an erythrocyte (red blood cell)

red in colour and it is this compound that gives the characteristic bright red colour to arterial (oxygenated) blood. As the blood passes through the capillaries within tissues, the oxygen dissociates from the haemoglobin molecule and diffuses from a high concentration (in the blood cells) to a low concentration (in the tissues). In a similar way, carbon dioxide diffuses from the tissues (high concentration) to the blood (low concentration) and is returned to the lungs where it is exhaled. Deoxygenated blood appears a dull red colour when compared to the bright red colour of the oxygenated form. The efficiency of oxygen transport is directly dependent upon the number of circulating erythrocytes in the circulation and the amount of haemoglobin that each cell contains.

Erythrocytes made in the bone marrow (see the section on haemopoiesis below) and are active in the circulation for approximately 120 days, following which they are broken down, primarily by the spleen. Other sites are also involved in the breakdown of erythrocytes, e.g. the liver and bone marrow, so an animal can still function adequately without its spleen. Iron from the breakdown process is stored in the liver for re-use and the remaining components are converted into bile pigments and excreted in the faeces.

Thrombocytes

Thrombocytes, or platelets as they are more commonly called, are the smallest of the blood cells. They appear as non-nucleated fragments of variable shape on a blood film. Their primary function is to assist with haemostasis (blood clotting). This will be discussed later in this chapter.

Leucocytes

This group of cells, more commonly called white blood cells, are the largest cells found in the blood, although they are less numerous than either thrombocytes or erythrocytes. They can be subdivided into two types: (a) **granulocytes** (or **polymorphonuclear leucocytes**); and (b) **agranulocytes**. Agranulocytes can be further subdivided into lymphocytes and monocytes and are classified as such due to the absence of granules in the cytoplasm.

Polymorphonuclear leucocytes (or granulocytes)

Polymorphonuclear leucocytes are classified as granulocytes due to the appearance of small granules within their cytoplasm on staining. The

All leucocytes can be rapidly transported in the circulatory system to areas of tissue damage and can move out of the blood stream through the capillary walls into the surrounding tissues. Both polymorphonuclear leucocytes and monocytes are associated with the non-specific defences of the body, i.e. they can respond to a variety of invasive stimuli. In contrast, lymphocytes are involved primarily with specific immunity, responding to an attack from a particular pathogen. This concept will be expanded further in Chapter 6.

term polymorphonuclear reflects the shape of the nucleus, which has several lobes (poly = many, morph = shaped). This group of cells is the most numerous among the leucocytes, forming approximately 70% of the total white cell count. The group can be further subdivided into three kinds of cell (see Figure 4.3) on the basis of their staining properties.

Neutrophils are the most numerous of the granulocytes and are difficult to stain by either acidic or alkaline dyes (hence the name neutrophil, 'neutro' meaning neutral). The nucleus and granules within the cytoplasm appear purple. The nucleus is dense and segmented into up to five lobes that resemble beads on a string. The granular appearance of the cytoplasm is due to the presence of small lysosomes containing lysosomal enzymes. These cells ingest particles such as bacteria and cell debris by the process known as phagocytosis. They are capable of squeezing out through capillary walls and accumulate rapidly where there is a

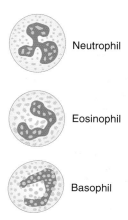

Figure 4.3 Polymorphonuclear leucocytes (granulocytes)

source of infection. Most neutrophils only last in the circulation for approximately 10 hours. This time may be reduced if the cell is active at an infected site.

Eosinophils are only stained by acid-based dyes, the granules within the cytoplasm appear red and the nucleus purple. They are similar in size to neutrophils, but fewer in number (approximately 2–4% of the total white blood cell population). They have a bi-lobed nucleus and strongly staining granules in the cytoplasm. These cells increase in number during allergic reactions and also in response to a nematode infection. They are also active at injury sites when they attack antibody marked bacteria either by engulfing them or by releasing toxic substances that destroy them. They may also release enzymes that help to prevent the spread of inflammation.

Basophils are the least common of the granulocytes and are stained by alkaline dyes. The nucleus stains purple whereas the cytoplasmic granules stain blue. They are smaller than either neutrophils or eosinophils and are relatively rare, representing only approximately 1% of the total white blood cell count. Basophils manufacture histamine and heparin which they release at the site of injury to promote inflammation. Inflammation causes an increase in the supply of blood to the tissue, which results in an improved supply of oxygen, nutrients and neutrophils, and also facilitates the removal of toxins and waste products, and promotes tissue regeneration at the injured site (see Chapter 6 for further details).

Lymphocytes

As discussed previously, lymphocytes are agranular (i.e. they do not possess cytoplasmic granules). They have a large nucleus with a small surrounding region of cytoplasm (see Figure 4.4).

They are produced in the lymph nodes and lymphatic tissue of the spleen, liver and other organs and constitute approximately 20–30% of the total white blood cell count. They are classified primarily into one of two types, although these two types cannot be distinguished using a light microscope:

B-Lymphocytes (or B-cells) are associated with the production of antibodies that attack specific **antigens** (foreign bodies that illicit an immune response) that may enter the body. When activated, they produce and secrete the specific antibody for the invading antigen. The antibodies produced can attack the antigen in any region of the body. An immune response based on the production of

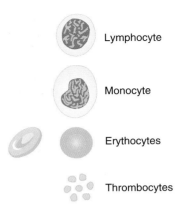

Figure 4.4 Agranulocytes

antibodies is also known as humoral immunity (see Chapter 6).

T-Lymphocytes (or T cells) are associated with the defence response to invading cells and tissues, e.g. bacteria, viruses and protozoa. This is known as cellular immunity. T-Lymphocytes attack and destroy the invading cells directly.

Monocytes

Monocytes are the largest of the leucocytes, representing approximately 5% of the total white blood cell population. They have a large nucleus that can vary in shape, sometimes resembling that of a kidney bean (see Figure 4.4). They are phagocytic and enter the tissue at the site of injury to engulf foreign objects. Whilst doing this they release chemicals that attract neutrophils and monocytes to the site.

Haemopoiesis

Haemopoiesis (sometimes referred to as haematopoiesis) is the term given to the production of blood cells. As we discussed previously, all the blood cells originate from one cell in the bone marrow. In this section we shall consider the development of each type of cell and the factors that may affect their development.

Erythropoiesis

Erythropoiesis (or the production of erythrocytes) occurs in the red bone marrow of cancellous (or spongy) bone. As discussed in Chapter 3, this is located in flat bones such as the ribs and bones of the cranium, irregular bones such as the vertebrae, and the epiphyses of long bones such as the femur

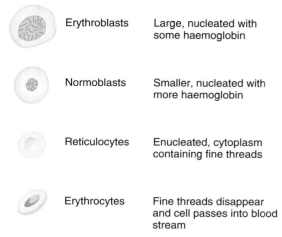

Erythroblasts	Large, nucleated with some haemoglobin
Normoblasts	Smaller, nucleated with more haemoglobin
Reticulocytes	Enucleated, cytoplasm containing fine threads
Erythrocytes	Fine threads disappear and cell passes into blood stream

Figure 4.5 Development of an erythrocyte

Occasionally, immature erythrocytes (reticulocytes and normoblasts) may enter the circulation. This can occur in cases of regenerative anaemia following acute haemorrhage.

and humerus. The blood cell develops along the pathway illustrated in Figure 4.5.

The developmental process requires amino acids, and vitamins C, B_6, and B_{12}, as well as iron and folic acid. If any of these are deficient in the diet of the animal, symptoms of anaemia may develop. The process of erythropoiesis is affected by several hormones (e.g. thyroxine, testosterone, and growth hormone), although the major hormone having direct effects is **erythropoietin**. Erythropoietin is produced by the kidneys in response to a fall in the circulating levels of oxygen in the blood (hypoxia). It stimulates the rate of cell division within the erythroblast and in the stem cells that produce the erythroblasts, as well as speeding up the rate of red blood cell maturation by increasing the rate of synthesis of haemoglobin.

Thrombopoiesis

Thrombopoiesis (or thrombocytopoiesis) is the term given to the formation of thrombocytes (platelets). It occurs in the bone marrow from large cells called **megakaryocytes**. The megakaryocytes shed small portions of cytoplasm enclosed in cell membrane. These are the platelets that enter the circulation. The rate of thrombopoiesis is controlled by a peptide hormone called thrombopoietin, which is secreted by the kidneys and stimulates the production of megakaryocytes. The controlling mechanisms for this hormone are still unknown.

Leucopoiesis

Leucopoiesis, or the production of leucocytes, also occurs within the bone marrow. Progenitor cells (or myeloid stem cells as they are sometimes called) differentiate to produce all the different types of leucocytes except lymphocytes. All of those that develop from the progenitor cells complete their development within the bone marrow, with the exception of monocytes. Monocytes enter the circulation and complete their development once they enter the body tissues. In some cases, the **band cell** stage of the other leucocytes may enter the circulation. Lymphopoiesis (the formation of lymphocytes) occurs primarily within the lymphoid tissue of the spleen, thymus and lymph nodes, although it may also occur within the lymphoid tissue of the bone marrow.

Our understanding of the factors controlling the formation of leucocytes is still incomplete. In the immature animal, the thymus produces hormones known as **thymosins** that assist in maintaining the required number of T-lymphocytes. In the adult animal it would appear that their production is related to the animal's exposure to antigens. This is discussed in more detail in Chapter 6.

Haemostasis

The initial phase is triggered when a blood vessel is damaged. Initial responses are for localized constriction of the smooth muscle surrounding the vessel that slows, or may even stop, blood flow at the damaged site. The endothelial cells lining the

Haemostasis, or blood clotting as it is more commonly called, is a complex process that involves many factors. Haemostasis is vital to the maintenance of homeostasis within the animal, and when blood loss is severe the animal may enter into a state of shock and ultimately die. The process of homeostasis can be considered as a series of steps, although it is likely to be a more complex chain reaction within the living tissue.

vessels become 'sticky' and platelets adhere to their surface (platelet adhesion) and to each other, eventually forming a 'platelet plug' at the damaged site which may cover the site completely if the damage is minor. This usually occurs within 15 seconds of the injury occurring. As the platelets adhere and aggregate, they start to change shape and release various substances, including calcium ions, that promote the aggregation of further platelets. In addition to the substances released by the platelets, the damaged tissues releases a tissue factor. This combines with the calcium ions and a clotting factor present in the blood to produce tissue thromboplastin. A second route for the production of thromboplastin is from the activation of some of the substances released by the platelets. When thromboplastin from either route enters the plasma, an enzyme called prothrombinase (or thrombokinase) is formed, which converts pro-thrombin into thrombin. Thrombin then converts

the plasma protein fibrinogen into insoluble strands of fibrin and it is this that forms a mesh-like structure across the wound. Blood cells become trapped in the mesh of fibres and a blood clot is formed. This cascade of reactions is illustrated in Figure 4.6.

Both calcium ions and vitamin K are necessary for the above cascade reaction. Calcium ions are required for the formation of thromboplastin and vitamin K is required for four clotting factors, including prothrombin. A deficiency in either of these two components will impair the clotting sequence.

Once the clot has been formed it starts to shrink slightly, due to the contraction of the platelets. This pulls the edges of the wound closer together to stabilize the injured site and promote healing. At this stage a clear, colourless fluid may be seen. This is known as serum and is formed from plasma but does not contain clotting factors.

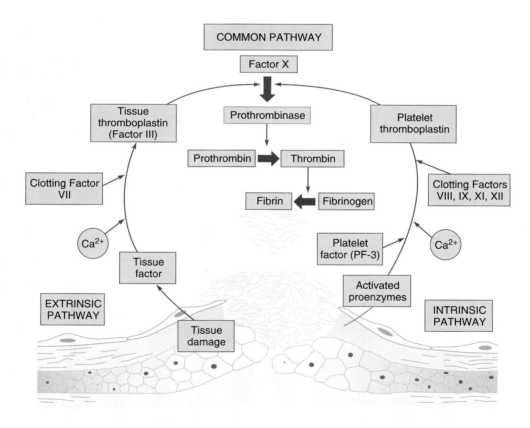

THE COAGULATION PHASE

Figure 4.6 Cascade of reactions involved in coagulation

Fibrinolysis

Fibrinolysis is the process whereby the clot gradually dissolves as the wound heals. The fibrin that formed the clot is broken down by an enzyme called plasmin or fibrinase. This is produced from plasminogen, the inactive form that circulates within the plasma and body fluids. Plasminogen activators are produced by red and white blood cells locally and also by the body tissues.

4.2 The cardiovascular system

Anatomy of the heart
Cardiac muscle
Heart valves
Heartbeat and conduction
The vascular system
Heart rate and cardiac output
Blood pressure
Shock

Introduction

We have examined the transport medium of the body, blood, but we now need to consider how it is carried around the body in order to reach tissues and cells. The structure of the cardiovascular system can be considered to be similar to that of the central heating system of a house. Both have a pump (in the case of the cardiovascular system, the heart) that pumps water (or blood) through a system of pipes (or blood vessels) to the radiators (or organs), where the exchange of heat occurs (similar to the capillary beds within the tissues where the exchange of nutrients, oxygen and carbon dioxide occurs). The water is then re-heated by the boiler (and the blood is oxygenated in the lungs) before being pumped back around the body. Whilst this is something of a simplification, it does allow us to appreciate the function of the cardiovascular system at a basic level before progressing to the finer detail.

Anatomy of the heart

The heart is situated within the **pericardial cavity** located in the **mediastinum** of the thorax. The cavity is enclosed by a membranous sac, the pericardium, which is composed of two layers of tissue. The outer layer, or **parietal pericardium**, is comprised of tough, dense, connective tissue that serves to protect the heart and attach it within the thoracic cavity. The inner membrane, or **serous pericardium**, forms a double layer and secretes a lubricating pericardial fluid into the space between the membrane and the heart (the pericardial cavity). This fluid helps to reduce the friction of the beating heart against the walls of the pericardium.

The heart itself is composed of three layers of tissue. The outer layer, or **epicardium**, is really the inner layer of the serous membrane discussed in the previous paragraph. The middle layer, or **myocardium**, consists of the cardiac muscle of the heart. This will be discussed in more detail later in the chapter. Finally, the inner layer, or **endocardium**, is a delicate membrane formed from endothelial cells that are continuous with those of the blood vessels entering and leaving the heart.

As discussed in the introduction, the heart can be considered as a pump. It is divided into four chambers with the right side being separated from the left side by a wall of cardiac muscle known as the **septum**. The basic anatomy of the heart is illustrated in Figure 4.7.

The upper chambers are the right and left **atria** (sing = atrium). These pump blood into the right and left **ventricles**, respectively, through the **tricuspid** and **bicuspid** (or mitral) valves. The tricuspid and bicuspid valves are also known as the right and left atrioventricular valves. The ventricles then pump blood to one of two destinations. The left ventricle, with its thickened muscular wall, contracts and propels blood into the aorta, the major artery that supplies the body with blood. The thinner-walled right ventricle pumps blood to the lungs. The wall of the right ventricle is thinner than that of the left ventricle, as the force of contraction required to pump the blood the relatively shorter distance to the lungs, is less than that needed to get all round the body. In the lungs, the exchange of oxygen and carbon dioxide occurs (see Chapter 5) and oxygenated blood returns to the left atrium of the heart, before being pumped around the body.

Consequently, it can be seen that the circulation of blood in mammals can be described as a double circulation, i.e. blood passes twice through the heart in one circuit around the body. Any expert in plumbing will realize that the circulatory system differs from the central heating systems in this way, as a central heating system is a single circulation system, water passing through the pump only once in its full circuit. We can describe the two parts in the circulation of blood within a

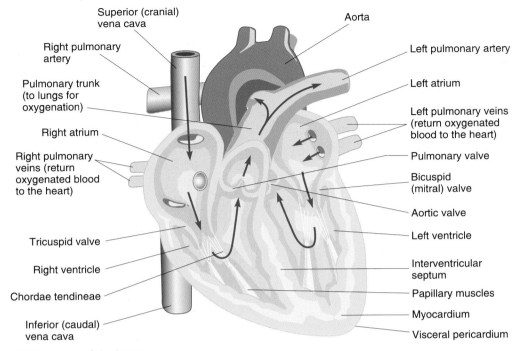

Figure 4.7 Anatomy of the heart

mammal as the **pulmonary circulation** (that to the lungs) and the **systemic circulation** (to the body). The circulation of blood around the body is illustrated in Figure 4.8.

In the pulmonary circulation, deoxygenated blood is pumped from the right side of the heart to the lungs in the pulmonary arteries. It is oxygenated at the lungs before being returned to the heart in the pulmonary veins. As a rule, blood vessels known as arteries carry blood away from the heart, whereas blood vessels known as veins carry blood towards the heart. Many use another rule that veins always carry deoxygenated blood whereas arteries carry oxygenated blood. Whilst this is usually the case, there are exceptions. The example illustrated above is one such exception, where the pulmonary arteries carry deoxygenated blood and the pulmonary veins, oxygenated blood. Another exception occurs in the blood supply to the foetus. The umbilical artery carries deoxygenated blood away from the foetus whereas the umbilical vein carries oxygenated blood to the foetus.

The systemic circulation is responsible for the passage of blood from the left side of the heart to the body tissues, via arteries and capillaries, where it becomes deoxygenated before returning to the right side of the heart in veins. In this way we can see that the circulation of blood around the mammalian body occurs in a figure-of-eight pattern, passing twice through the heart on each circuit round the body.

Cardiac muscle

The contact between the cells via the intercalated discs allows the cells to contract simultaneously, and the heart appears to act like one large muscle cell.

Cardiac muscle is unique in that it is the only muscle that does not fatigue following repeated contractions (unlike skeletal muscle that tires relatively quickly). It is also capable of rhythmic contraction without any nerve supply, a property known as **automaticity**. The intercalated discs that lie between the branching muscle cells (see Chapter 3) allow the contraction of one cell to stimulate the contraction of adjacent cells by facilitating the transfer of action potentials between cells. The structure is illustrated in Figure 4.9.

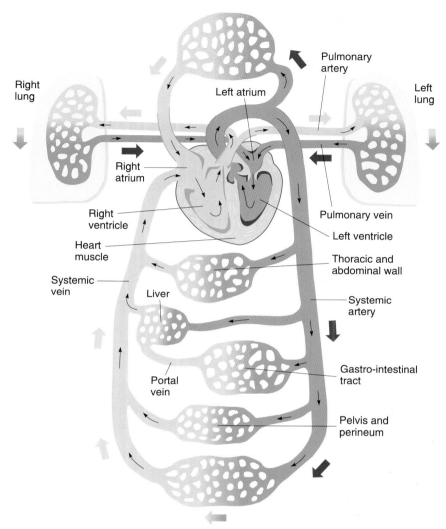

Figure 4.8 Schematic representation of the systemic and pulmonary circulation around the body of a mammal. A, Deoxygenated blood; B, capillary blood; C, oxygenated blood

Heart valves

Figure 4.7 shows that there are four valves in the heart. Their function is to facilitate the flow of blood through the heart by preventing the blood flowing in the wrong direction as the heart chambers contract. The **mitral** valve (sometimes referred to as the **bicuspid** valve) is located between the left atrium and ventricle, and the **tricuspid** valve is located between the right chambers. These can also be called the atrioventricular valves. Their function is to prevent blood flowing back into the atria as the ventricles

contract. During ventricular diastole or relaxation, the valves are open and the ventricles fill with blood. However, as the ventricles enter systole contraction, the blood forces the valves to close. The papillary muscles, which attach to the chordae tendinae, contract and prevent the cusps of the valves being pushed back into the atria.

Other valves are located at the junctions of the pulmonary artery and aorta with the right and left ventricles. These are known as the pulmonary and aortic **semi-lunar valves**, respectively, and prevent the flow of blood into the ventricles following systole.

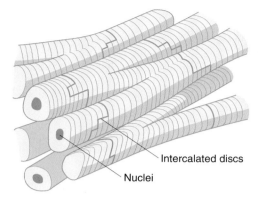

Figure 4.9 The structure of cardiac muscle

There are many problems that can develop with the valves of the heart that may be seen in practice. Congenital defects, i.e. those that are present at birth, include pulmonic stenosis and aortic stenosis. Both of these conditions are due to a deformity of either the pulmonary or aortic semi-lunar valve of the heart, leading to a narrowing in the valvular region. In the case of pulmonic stenosis, the narrowing obstructs the flow of blood from the right ventricle to the lungs. If the condition is severe, the animal may be incapable of sustaining exercise and becomes breathless (dyspnoea). In the case of aortic stenosis, the narrowing causes an obstruction of the blood flowing from the left ventricle to the systemic circulation. The animal may appear normal at rest but may not be tolerant of exercise. Some individuals may collapse and even die if over-exerted or over-excited.

Acquired heart disease develops with age, in adult animals. Acquired valvular diseases arise when the cusps of the valves thicken and lose their elasticity. This causes the valve to leak, a term often called valve incompetence. The most common valve disease, mitral valve disease, is usually first evident as a general slowing down of the animal during exercise that may be accompanied by breathlessness. The animal may start to cough and, if left untreated, the animal will progress into heart failure, as the heart is unable to pump sufficient blood around the body. Blood accumulates in the left atrium and may flow back into the lungs in severe cases, causing pulmonary congestion. This may lead to pulmonary oedema and dyspnoea, even in an animal at rest.

In a minority of cases the tricuspid valve may be affected by incompetence and/or stenosis. The animal may show accumulation of fluid in the body tissues (particularly the abdomen) as the pressure of the blood in the systemic circulation increases. Weight loss may also occur.

Heartbeat and conduction

The heartbeat cardiac cycle is described in two phases, a contraction phase known as **systole** and a relaxation phase known as **diastole**. When listening to the heart through a stethoscope, a practice known as auscultation, the untrained ear hears two sounds in each heartbeat. These are the first and second heart sounds and are sometimes referred to as 'lub' and 'dup'. They are the sound of the heart valves closing, the 'lub' being produced as the atrioventricular valves close (as the ventricles contract) and the 'dup' occurring as the semi-lunar valves close (as the ventricles start to fill following contraction). In some circumstances, a third and fourth heart sound may be audible, although they are usually very faint. The third sound is associated with blood flowing into the ventricles and the fourth with atrial contraction.

The initial stimulus for the heartbeat arises spontaneously by depolarization of specialized muscle cells in the area of the heart known as the sino-atrial node (often referred to as the pacemaker of the heart). This is located in the wall of the right atrium (see Figure 4.10). The wave of depolarization then spreads across the left and right atria as they contract, emptying their contents into the lower ventricles. On reaching the atrioventricular node, located in the septum (see Figure 4.10), the wave of depolarization then travels along the bundle of His within the septum, spreading out along the Purkinje fibres that radiate upwards from the bottom of both ventricles. The ventricles then contract, pumping blood into the pulmonary artery and aorta to circulate to the pulmonary and systemic circuits, respectively.

Whilst the initial stimulus arises spontaneously at the sino-atrial node, the sympathetic and parasympathetic regions of the autonomic nervous system can modify the nature of the heartbeat, in terms of its frequency and force of contraction. The central area of control, the cardiac centre, lies in the area of the brain known as the medulla oblongata (see Chapter 2). This area receives and processes information from other areas of the brain, in particular the parasympathetic and sympathetic areas of the hypothalamus. It also receives feedback from baroreceptors that detect levels of blood pressure and chemo-

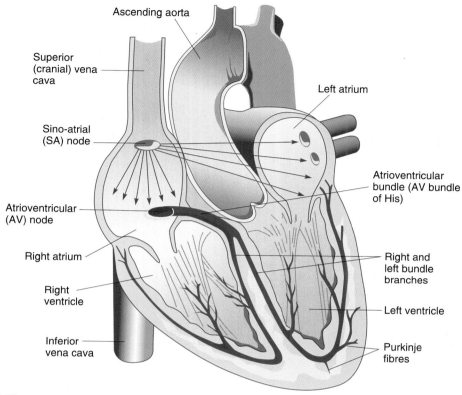

Figure 4.10 The cardiac conduction system

receptors that detect the chemical composition of the blood. Consequently, should there be a fall in blood pressure or in circulating levels of oxygen, or an increase in the circulating levels of carbon dioxide, the cardiac centre stimulates the heart to increase its output. This increases the supply of blood to the tissues at the periphery and will lead to an increase in blood pressure and in the oxygen content of the blood, with a corresponding decrease in the circulating levels of carbon dioxide. The theories underlying control of the cardiovascular system are discussed in detail later in this chapter.

An electrocardiogram (ECG) measures the electrical activity of the heart associated with activity of the cardiac conduction system and can be taken by placing electrodes at specific points on the body of an animal. A typical ECG taken from a healthy dog is illustrated in Figure 4.11.

Different areas of the tracing represent the electrical activities that are occurring in each region of the heart. The P-wave represents the depolarization and subsequent contraction of the atria. This is followed by the QRS complex, as the action potential is propagated down the bundle of His to the Purkinje fibres and the ventricles depolarize and contract. The T-wave represents the period of the recovery of the ventricles prior to the commencement of another heartbeat. It is not uncommon for an irregularity in the trace to be detected (as indicated at point A in the tracing in Figure 4.11). This is related to inspiration and known as sinus arrhythmia. It occurs regularly in healthy dogs, and is no cause for concern.

The ECG can also be used to detect cardiac dysrhythmias (disturbances in the heart rate). As these can only be intermittent, however, it may be necessary to monitor the heart for 24 hours, or even longer in some cases. The ECG can also be used to detect enlargement of a heart chamber in conjunction with radiographic techniques.

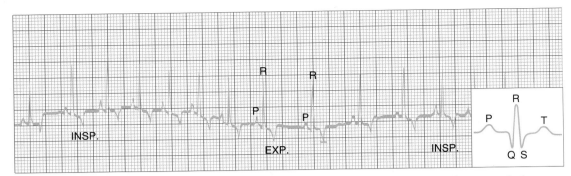

Figure 4.11 The ECG of a healthy dog. The rate increases during inspiration (INSP) and decreases during expiration (EXP)

The vascular system

As well as the pump itself, the cardiovascular system requires a network of vessels to deliver the blood to the tissues. Blood vessels that leave the heart are called arteries. These are relatively large in diameter and branch into smaller vessels known as **arterioles**. The arterioles branch further, leading to a network of very fine vessels known as **capillaries**.

The capillaries are contained within the tissues and are the site of all chemical and gaseous exchange between interstitial fluid and blood. Eventually the capillaries join larger vessels known as **venules**. These form the part of the vascular system that returns blood to the heart. The venules link and become larger, forming **veins**, as they get closer to the heart. Figure 4.13 illustrates the relationship between the blood vessels of the body.

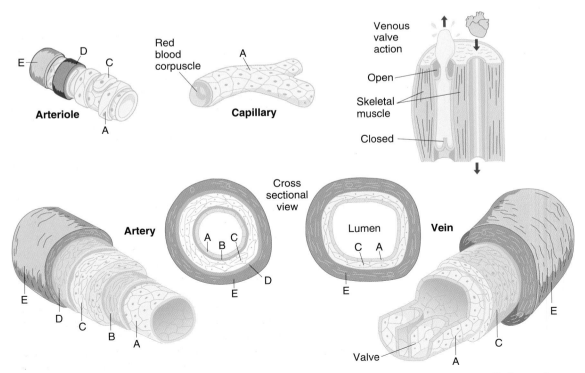

Figure 4.12 Structure of a typical artery, vein and capillary. Key: **tunica intima**: A, endothelium; B, internal elastic lamina; **tunica media**: C, smooth muscle; D, external elastic lamina; **tunica adventitia**: E, fibrous tissue

Arteries and veins are composed of three layers of tissue in differing proportions. The outer coat or **tunica adventitia** is formed from collagen and elastic fibres. It serves to protect the vessel. The middle layer or **tunica media** contains smooth muscle and elastic fibres. The smooth muscle is innervated by the sympathetic nervous system and can contract or relax to determine the amount of blood that flows through the vessel. The inner layer or **tunica intima** consists of a single layer of elastic fibres and flattened endothelial cells. These provide a smooth surface to facilitate the circulation of blood. The relative proportions of the differing layers of tissue described varies, depending upon the type of blood vessel concerned.

Arteries

The walls of arteries are thicker than those of veins or capillaries. They have a thick **tunica media** containing muscle and elastic fibres. This allows the vessel to resist the pressure of the blood as it is pumped around the body. Due to their elastic nature, arteries usually retaining their tube-like structure are far more resilient to physical damage than capillaries or veins, as they stretch and recoil when the heart ejects blood. The smooth muscle

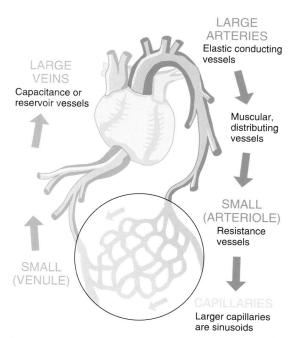

Figure 4.13 The different types of blood vessels in the body

within the arterial wall is innervated by the sympathetic nervous system and, when stimulated, contraction of the muscle causes vasoconstriction. Conversely, when the smooth muscle relaxes, vasodilation occurs. This provides an essential mechanism for the control of blood pressure in the body and will be discussed later in this chapter. The structure of an artery is illustrated in Figure 4.12.

The major artery of the body is the aorta. This travels from the left ventricle of the heart and branches into the brachiocephalic trunk and left subclavian artery. It then descends into the thoracic and abdominal regions. The brachiocephalic trunk branches into the left and right common carotid arteries (supplying the face and neck) and the right subclavian artery supplying the right fore limb. The left subclavian artery supplies the left fore limb. The thoracic aorta passes through the mediastinum in the thorax and supplies blood to the pericardium, oesophagus, bronchi of the lungs, and the intercostal muscles. It then passes through the diaphragm and supplies blood to the abdominal tissues and organs. Figure 4.14 illustrates the major branches of the aorta in the dog and cat.

Veins

Veins are usually more flaccid than arteries as their **tunica media** is thinner. They have less elastic fibres and consequently have less 'stretchability' than arteries. Most veins contain valves (see Figure 4.12). The valves facilitate the circulation of the blood by preventing it from flowing backwards into the capillaries, particularly in regions such as the limbs where the effects of gravity are predominant.

Blood samples may be taken from different veins, depending upon the size of the animal, the species, and reason for sampling (see Figure 4.15). Veins are safer sites than arteries as they are more accessible (arteries tend to run deeper than veins as this gives them more protection) and have thinner walls. Also, should the vessel be damaged during the procedure, the consequences are less severe if a vein rather than an artery is being used. Damage to an artery may compromise the blood supply to several tissues and organs. As the blood is under greater pressure there is also an increased risk of development of a haematoma in the area.

The major veins that return blood to the heart are the cranial (superior) and caudal (inferior) vena cavae. Blood returns from the head and neck in the left and right jugular veins that join the left and

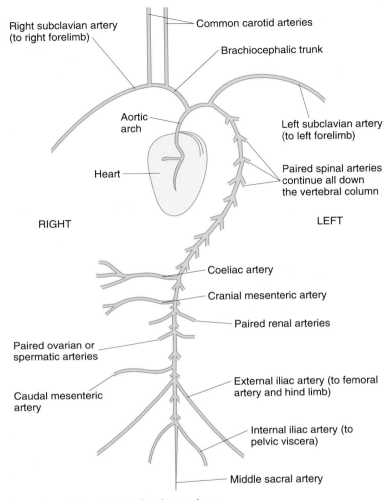

Figure 4.14 Major branches of the aorta in the dog and cat

right subclavian veins from the fore limbs to form the left and right brachiocephalic veins. These drain into the cranial vena cava. The caudal vena cava returns blood from the thorax, abdomen and hind limbs. It is usual for each artery supplying a tissue or organ to have a corresponding vein that returns blood back to the heart, e.g. the renal artery supplies blood to the kidney and the renal vein returns it from the kidney to the heart.

The azygos vein, that drains blood from the intercostal spaces of the thorax and the thoracic wall, is unusual in that it has no corresponding artery. Similarly, the hepatic portal vein carries the absorbed products of digestion from the intestine (as well as from the stomach, spleen, pancreas and gall bladder) to the liver for assimilation. There is no hepatic portal artery, the liver receiving its circulatory blood supply via the hepatic artery and vein. This will be discussed further in Chapter 5.

Capillaries

Capillaries are the smallest of the blood vessels and form a network between the arterial and venous systems. It is here that the exchange of interstitial fluid between the tissues and the blood occurs. This is because a capillary wall is formed from a single layer of flattened epithelial cells (note that capillaries do not have a **tunica media** or **tunica externa**). Capillaries divide and link within a tissue, to form a capillary network or bed (see Figure 4.16).

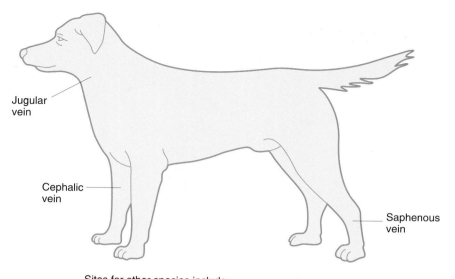

Sites for other species include:
    Brachial vein – wing of bird
    Ventral coccygeal vein – tail vein for lizards and snakes
    Dorsal coccygeal vein – tail vein for chelonians

Figure 4.15 Sites for taking a venous blood sample

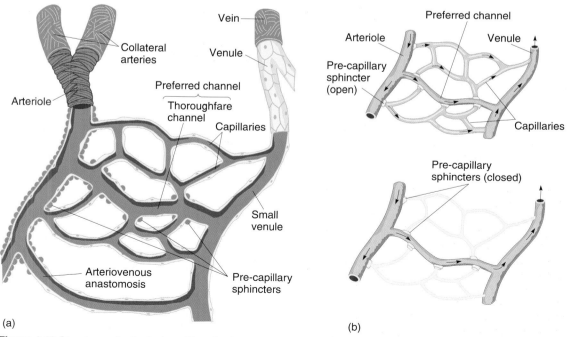

(a)

(b)

Figure 4.16 Structure of a typical capillary bed

Pre-capillary sphincters of smooth muscle surround the beginning of each capillary. These can contract or relax to decrease or increase the flow of blood through the capillary bed as required. For example, if an animal has lost a significant amount of blood, pre-capillary sphincters will contract, thereby reducing the flow of blood to the peripheral tissues and increasing the amount of blood available to supply the vital organs. An animal in this condition is said to be in 'shock'. Its mucous membranes will be pale and its extremities cold, due to the reduction in the flow of blood to the periphery.

Heart rate and cardiac output

Earlier in this chapter we discussed the properties of cardiac muscle and the generation and propagation of contraction resulting in the heartbeat. In this section we shall consider the modification of the heartbeat and control of cardiac output. The heart is innervated by the autonomic nervous system. Activity in the parasympathetic division, primarily the vagus nerve (cranial nerve X), causes the heart rate to slow, in addition to decreasing the force of contraction. This combined effect reduces cardiac output. The sympathetic division has the opposite effect and causes increased heart rate accompanied by an increased force of contraction. This increases cardiac output.

Heart rate can be measured either by listening directly to the heart or more routinely by taking the pulse. The pulse is taken where an artery passes over a bony prominence. This makes it easy to feel the pulsating blood through the vessel and this corresponds directly to the beating of the heart. Note that a pulse is not detectable in veins as the blood in these vessels is no longer under sig-

---

Normal values of heart rate in the cat and dog are:

Cat   110–180 beats/min
Dog   60–180 beats/min, depending upon size

(as a rule of thumb, the larger the animal, the lower its heart rate).

Cardiac output can be defined as the volume of blood pumped by the heart in a given time. Consequently:

Cardiac output = Stroke volume × Heart rate

If the heart pumps 10 ml of blood into the aorta at every beat and it beats at 180 beats per minute then:

Cardiac output = 10 × 180 = 1800 ml/min

---

nificant pressure, having passed through the capillary beds.

Some of the factors that may affect cardiac output include exercise, excitement, fear/stress, anaesthesia/sedation and heart disease.

Blood pressure

Blood pressure is defined as the force that the blood exerts upon the blood vessels in the body. It is at its greatest in the aorta where the blood leaves the heart and decreases as the blood vessels branch to different organs and tissues, becoming low in the capillary beds and very low in the veins returning to the heart. When monitoring blood pressure in the major arteries it fluctuates as the heart beats. We can therefore measure systolic pressure, coinciding with ventricular contraction and diastolic pressure, coinciding with ventricular relaxation.

The maintenance of blood pressure is critical to the circulatory competence of the animal. Should blood pressure fluctuate above or below the ideal range then circulation will be compromised, affecting the health of the animal. Arterial blood pressure can be maintained by the combination of a variety of mechanisms. We have already shown that cardiac output = stroke volume × heart rate. By increasing or decreasing cardiac output, blood pressure can rise or fall. This can be achieved by altering the stroke volume, the heart rate, or both.

Common sites for taking the pulse in the dog and cat are as follows:

Artery	Location
Femoral	Medial aspect of femur
Cranial tibial or pedal	Cranio-medial tarsus
Brachial	Medial aspect of humerus
Ulnar	Palmar aspect of carpus
Coccygeal	Ventral aspect of tail
Carotid	Neck
Sub-lingual*	Ventral aspect of tongue

*Note that this site is only suitable in an anaesthetized animal.

Changing the peripheral resistance of the blood vessels (i.e. resistance to the flow of blood in vessels at the periphery) also alters blood pressure. When the peripheral arterioles and capillaries are dilated, blood will flow freely through them. However, if the arterioles are constricted and the pre-capillary sphincters contract, blood will not be able to flow freely through the peripheral tissues as the resistance is increased. This will cause the blood pressure to increase. The activity of the sympathetic nervous system and/or certain vaso-constrictor hormones affects blood vessel dilation and therefore peripheral resistance and blood pressure.

Severe loss of blood causes a reduction in the circulating blood volume, which in turn causes a reduction in blood pressure. Medical conditions that result in a retention of body fluid may increase blood volume and also cause blood pressure to rise. Blood viscosity can also affect blood pressure. If viscosity increases, for example, due to an increased level of plasma proteins or erythrocytes, then blood pressure increases.

Neural control of blood pressure and blood volume

Changes in cardiac output and peripheral resistance are under the constant influence of the nervous system. Within the medulla oblongata of the brain lie two vital centres, the cardiac centre and the vasomotor centre, that are sometimes considered together as the cardiovascular centres. The cardiac centre has two regions, one that causes the acceleration of heart rate via the sympathetic nervous system and another that causes deceleration via the parasympathetic nervous system. The vasomotor centre also has two regions, one that causes vasoconstriction and the other vasodilation.

The cardiovascular centres of the brain monitor the chemical content and the pressure of the arterial blood. Specialized baroreceptors located in the carotid and aortic sinuses detect the degree of stretch of the vessel walls. This gives feedback about the level of blood pressure, allowing cardiac output and peripheral resistance to be adjusted accordingly. If blood pressure increases, this is detected by the baroreceptors. The cardiovascular systems respond by causing a decrease in cardiac output and vasodilation. The opposite effects occur if blood pressure falls.

The chemical content of the blood is monitored by specialized chemoreceptors located in the carotid and aortic bodies (located around and within the aortic arch). They detect changes in the levels of dissolved oxygen, carbon dioxide, and pH. There are also chemoreceptors located in the medulla oblongata of the brain that monitor the chemical composition of cerebrospinal fluid. If there is an increase in the carbon dioxide levels of the blood or a fall in pH, the cardiovascular centres are stimulated, increasing the cardiac output coupled with vasoconstriction. This facilitates the uptake of oxygen and removal of carbon dioxide from the blood. The respiratory rate is also stimulated to increase by the medullary chemoreceptors. A fall in the levels of circulating oxygen has the same effects.

The cardiovascular centres of the brain are also stimulated by other areas of the brain. When there is general stimulation of the sympathetic part of the autonomic nervous system, the cardiovascular centres increase the cardiac output and cause vasoconstriction. This prepares the animal to meet any emergencies that might occur, e.g. the need to run away from a dangerous situation – the 'fight or flight' response. In contrast, activity in the parasympathetic nervous system causes a reduction in cardiac output.

Hormonal control of blood pressure and blood volume

The effects on blood pressure discussed above are primarily under the control of the hormones of the sympathetic nervous system, adrenaline and noradrenaline. These regulate cardiovascular function in the shorter term. More long-term effects on blood pressure (and resultant effects on blood volume) are associated with other hormones.

Angiotensinogen is an inactive plasma protein produced by the liver. It is converted into **angiotensin I** by the renal hormone renin and is then converted into angiotensin II by angiotensin converting enzymes (ACE) which is secreted by the lungs.

The kidney is one of the major organs associated with longer-term control of blood pressure and blood volume. If blood pressure falls, the enzyme renin is produced by the juxtaglomerular apparatus (see Chapter 5). This initiates the cascade reaction illustrated in Figure 4.17, which results in the production of **angiotensin II**.

Renin   **ACE**

ANGIOTENSINOGEN → **ANGIOTENSIN I** → **ANGIOTENSIN II**

Figure 4.17 Cascade chain reaction following the production of renin by the kidneys

Angiotensin II is an active hormone with four major effects:

1. It causes the secretion of the hormone, aldosterone, by the adrenal cortex. This increases the retention of sodium ions in exchange for potassium ions which are excreted into the urine.
2. It stimulates the secretion of antidiuretic hormone (ADH). The effects of this hormone are discussed in detail in Chapter 5; briefly, it acts to increase water retention by the kidneys, by reducing the volume of urine produced.
3. It stimulates thirst, causing the animal to seek and drink water. This leads to an increase in blood volume.
4. It acts as a vasoconstrictor, reducing the blood flow to the periphery to ensure that blood flow to vital organs is maintained.

As a consequence of these four actions, the blood pressure increases; a longer-term effect is an increase in the circulating blood volume.

Erythropoietin is the major hormone controlling erythropoiesis, as discussed earlier in this chapter. It stimulates the production of more erythrocytes which causes an increase in the circulating blood volume and results in an increase in blood pressure.

Atrial natriuretic peptide also has effects on blood pressure (discussed in Chapter 2). Secreted by the heart in response to excessive atrial stretching, its long-term effects lead to a decrease in circulating blood volume and in blood pressure.

Shock

Now that we have examined the structure and function of the different components of the cardiovascular system, we can apply our knowledge to one of the more common emergencies seen in veterinary practice, circulatory shock.

Depending upon the degree of blood loss, the animal may show a number of clinical signs. Due

> Circulatory shock usually occurs in response to severe haemorrhage, such as that caused by injury during a road traffic accident, a ruptured splenic tumour, other internal bleeding, or severe burns. An animal that has lost less than 10% of the circulating blood volume will show few, if any signs. At a 25% loss, symptoms will include tachycardia (accelerated heart rate) and mild to moderate hypotension (low blood pressure) although few practices can measure the latter directly. Losses of 40% or greater of the circulating blood volume will result in severe hypotension and the animal may not recover if treatment is not carried out within two hours.

to severe blood loss its mucous membranes will be pale with a slower than normal capillary refill time. Its extremities may feel cold to the touch. Blood pressure will be low and the heart rate will be increased with a rapid weak pulse. The animal may appear depressed.

A priority should be to identify the cause of the blood loss and stop any further bleeding as soon as possible. The use of vasodilator drugs such as acepromazine or direct heat should be avoided, as both will cause dilation of the peripheral blood vessels. This is undesirable in this situation as a priority of treatment of the shocked patient is to ensure that blood is available for the vital organs, e.g. brain, heart and lungs. Further heat loss should be prevented by wrapping in blankets and laying the patient on an insulated surface, e.g. a vetbed. In severe cases, warmed crystalloid fluids, e.g. Hartmann's solution, should be administered to restore the circulating blood volume. It may be beneficial to administer a colloidal solution initially to reduce the amount of crystalloids required. Colloidal solutions remain in the circulatory system longer than crystalloids due to the larger molecules they contain, being less able to move between fluid compartments until the molecules are broken down over time. A blood transfusion may also be considered.

In milder cases of haemorrhage, fluid replacement by the intravenous route may not be necessary. Oral fluids containing electrolytes may be all that is required. However, in all cases, vital signs (temperature, pulse and respiration) should be monitored regularly to ensue that there is no further blood loss and deterioration.

Review questions

1. Which type of blood cell would you expect to see an increase in with a nematode infection?
   (a) lymphocytes
   (b) eosinophils
   (c) basophils
   (d) neutrophils
2. Name the term given to an increase in the production of white blood cells.
   (a) leucocytosis
   (b) leucopaenia
   (c) leukocytosis
   (d) leukopaenia
3. Identify which is the most numerous white blood cell in the healthy animal.
   (a) lymphocytes
   (b) eosinophils
   (c) basophils
   (d) neutrophils
4. State which of the following is not required for the formation of a blood clot.
   (a) fibrinogen
   (b) calcium ions
   (c) sodium ions
   (d) prothrombin
5. Name the blood cells that are involved in haemostasis.
   (a) eosinophils
   (b) monocytes
   (c) lymphocytes
   (d) platelets
6. State which hormone hypoxia triggers production by the kidneys.
   (a) erythropoetin
   (b) renin
   (c) aldosterone
   (d) thrombopoetin
7. Which of the following is not an agranulocyte?

(a) monocyte
(b) B-lymphoctye
(c) T-lymphocyte
(d) eosinophil
8. The most numerous blood cell is the
   (a) erythrocyte
   (b) neutrophil
   (c) monocyte
   (d) eosinophil
9. The formation of red blood cells occurs:
   (a) in the spleen
   (b) in the liver
   (c) in lymphatic tissue
   (d) in cancellous bone
10. Identify the following cells is not phagocytic.
    (a) lymphocyte
    (b) monocyte
    (c) neutrophil
    (d) erythrocyte
11. Describe the process of haemostasis.
12. Outline how an erythrocyte differs from other blood cells.
13. State where lymphocytes are produced.
14. Define the average lifespan of a red blood cell in the circulation.
15. Name the blood cells that are involved with the specific immune response.
16. Describe the composition of plasma.
17. Describe the difference between plasma and serum.
18. Name the tissue that is responsible for the manufacture of red blood cells.
19. Identify the three protective functions of blood.
20. Define the term eythropoeisis.
21. The blood vessels that communicate with the left atrium of the heart are called
    (a) the pulmonary arteries
    (b) the coronary arteries
    (c) the vena cavae
    (d) the pulmonary veins
22. The sino-atrial node (pacemaker of the heart) is located in the
    (a) wall of the right atrium
    (b) atrioventricular bundle (bundle of His)
    (c) septum
    (d) wall of the right ventricle
23. The name of the valve separating the left atrium and ventricle of the heart is the
    (a) tricuspid valve
    (b) mitral valve
    (c) pulmonary valve
    (d) semi-lunar valve

24. The junctions between adjacent cardiac muscle fibres are called
    (a) terminal bars
    (b) intercalated discs
    (c) motor end plates
    (d) synapses
25. Which one of the following statements is incorrect?
    (a) blood leaving the left ventricle is oxygenated
    (b) blood leaving the pulmonary vein is deoxygenated
    (c) blood leaving the liver is deoxygenated
    (d) blood entering the right atrium is deoxygenated
26. The first heart sound is produced by closure of which heart valves?
    (a) aortic and mitral
    (b) mitral and pulmonary
    (c) mitral and tricuspid
    (d) pulmonary and aortic
27. Which part of the myocardium is the thickest?
    (a) left ventricle
    (b) right ventricle
    (c) left atrium
    (d) right atrium
28. The serous membrane covering the outer surface of the heart is called the:
    (a) parietal pericardium
    (b) myocardium
    (c) endocardium
    (d) visceral pericardium
29. Heart muscle contraction is known as
    (a) systole
    (b) diastole
    (c) emptying
    (d) filling
30. The QRS complex of an ECG appears as the
    (a) atria depolarize
    (b) ventricles repolarize
    (c) ventricles depolarize
    (d) atria repolarize
31. Name the valves in the heart and describe their function.
32. Describe the pattern of electrical impulse through the heart.
33. Describe the four chambers of the heart in terms of their relation with the pulmonary and systemic circuits.
34. Compare and contrast the three types of blood vessels in terms of their structure and function.
35. State the average heart rate of the dog.
36. List five sites that can be used to monitor pulse in the conscious animal.
37. Describe the role of baroreceptors in the maintenance of blood pressure.
38. Describe the reaction that occurs when renin is produced by the kidney in response to a fall in blood pressure.
39. State where is ACE produced.
40. List the signs of circulatory shock.

5 Acquisition of nutrients and disposal of waste

5.1 The digestive system

The digestive process
The digestive or alimentary tract
Digestive secretions
The exocrine function of the pancreas
Bile
Absorption of the products of digestion
Defecation
Vomiting or emesis

Introduction

The digestive process allows complex foodstuffs such as fats, proteins and carbohydrates to be broken down, by catabolic processes, into simple compounds that can be absorbed by the digestive tract and utilized by the animal's body. Consider a piece of fillet steak. In its normal form, as bought from the butchers, it is of no immediate use to any animal. The cells within the intestine simply cannot absorb a huge chunk of fillet steak. When the animal eats the steak, however, the digestive processes break it down into small molecules. Proteins are digested into amino acids, fats are digested into fatty acids and glycerol, and carbohydrates are digested into simple sugars known as monosaccharides, e.g. glucose. These small molecules can be absorbed by the intestine and pass into the circulation, where they are available to the animal for energy, growth, and repair.

This describes the process of digestion in very simple terms. Now that we have an appreciation of the basic principles, we can consider the details of the digestive process.

The digestive process

The process of digestion can be considered in two distinct stages:

1. The mechanical stage.
   This involves the physical breaking down of the food into a form that can be swallowed. Essentially, this consists of chewing or mastication. The churning action of the stomach also contributes towards the mechanical process.
2. The chemical stage.
   This involves chemicals and enzymes within the digestive tract that break the food down further into its component parts, also known as nutrients, which can then be absorbed through the wall of the digestive tract into the circulation.

By far the majority of the digestive process is chemical in nature and occurs within the digestive tract, primarily in the stomach and small intestine for **monogastric** species such as the cat and the dog. Herbivorous animals have a large population of **symbiotic** organisms, such as protozoa and bacteria, within the digestive tract. These are usually found in an additional stomach (e.g. in ruminants such as the cow) or within a well-developed caecum, part of the large intestine (e.g. in the rabbit). They assist in the breakdown of plant cell walls, which are composed of a relatively indigestible carbohydrate, cellulose. In the case of the rabbit, in addition to a well-developed caecum, the end-products of the first passage through the digestive tract are eaten again and pass through the animal twice. The eating of the soft, caecal pellets, caecotrophs (or 'night faeces' as they are sometimes called), is termed coprophagia. This behaviour is normal in herbivorous species such as the rabbit and guinea pig.

The digestive or alimentary tract

In this section we will examine the basic anatomy of the digestive system before considering the chemical process of digestion. An appreciation of basic anatomy will help in understanding the digestive process. A simplified diagram of the monogastric digestive tract, similar to that of the dog and cat, is illustrated in Figure 5.1.

The oral cavity

The mouth or oral cavity contains the tongue and teeth (dentition). Its purpose is to take hold of and manipulate the food, chewing it to break it down. Both dog and the cat have teeth that have been developed in order to help them adapt to the diet and lifestyle of their wild ancestors.

The tongue

The tongue is muscular and is attached to the floor of the mouth. It manipulates food during mastication and swallowing (or deglutition as it is sometimes called). The process of mastication is thought to be less important in the cat and dog, however, as they tend to swallow large pieces of food whole rather than chewing them.

The tongue has several functions in addition to those associated with digestion. It is important in the sense of taste, as well as assisting with thermoregulation (via panting) and grooming. Cats in particular have tongues that are well adapted for grooming, having large papillae on the surface of the tongue which point backwards. These 'comb' the hair as the cat licks itself.

Dentition

The cat and dog, being predators, have evolved teeth that are specialized for capturing prey, and shearing meat from bones. The incisors and canine teeth all play a part in the initial capture phase, whereas the pre-molars and molars are adapted for shearing and cutting meat (rather than for grinding, as in herbivores). The last pre-molar in the upper jaw and the lower first molar are particularly well developed for this function and are known as the carnassial teeth. The dentition of the dog and cat is illustrated in Figure 5.2.

It can be seen from Figure 5.2 that the dog has four pre-molars on each side of the upper and lower jaws as well as two molars on each side of the upper jaw and three on the lower jaw. This is in contrast to the cat, which has fewer pre-molars and molars (three pre-molars and one molar on each side of the upper jaw and two pre-molars and a molar on each side of the lower jaw). If we were to consider representing dentition in terms of a formula, we could represent it as follows:

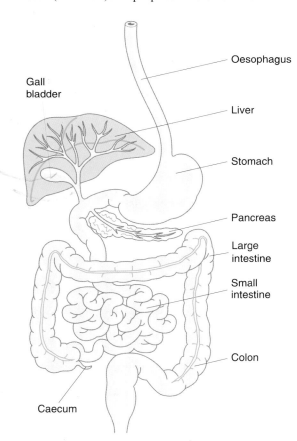

Adult dog $\dfrac{\text{I3, C1, P4, M2}}{\text{I3, C1, P4, M3}}$

or   I3/3, C1/1, P4/4, M2/3

Adult cat $\dfrac{\text{I3, C1, P3, M1}}{\text{I3, C1, P2, M1}}$

or   I3/3, C1/1, P3/2, M1/1

Oesophagus

Gall bladder

Liver

Stomach

Pancreas

Large intestine

Small intestine

Colon

Caecum

Figure 5.1 Diagram to illustrate the principal features of the monogastric digestive tract

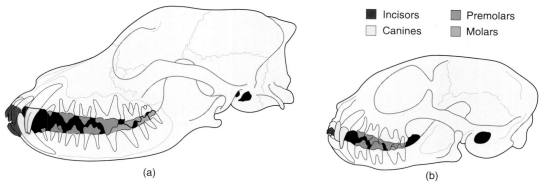

| ■ Incisors | ▨ Premolars |
| □ Canines | ▨ Molars |

Figure 5.2 Dentition of the (a) dog and (b) cat

where I stands for incisor, C for canine, P for pre-molar, and M for molar.

It is probable that the dog has more pre-molars and molars than the cat due to its omnivorous diet in the wild. Cats are obligate carnivores, i.e. they are unable to survive on a diet that is not based upon meat whereas dogs have evolved so that they can exist upon a more omnivorous diet and are therefore more likely to eat plant materials for which molars and pre-molars are better developed.

The structure of a tooth is illustrated in Figure 5.3. The majority of the tooth is composed of dentine, the structure of which resembles that of bone. Dentine is formed by cells known as odontoblasts and the structure is hardened by deposits of calcium phosphate. Both a blood supply and a nerve supply are contained within the pulp cavity of the tooth. The outer surface or the crown of the tooth is covered by enamel, a hard avascular deposit, harder even than bone. Cement lines the root of the tooth and helps to secure the tooth within its socket or alveolus, with the assistance of the periodontal ligament.

The palate and pharynx

The palate can be considered in two parts. The hard palate forms the roof of the mouth, separating it from the nasal cavity. The more caudal soft palate is involved with the mechanism of swallowing,

---

During early life, puppies and kittens have a deciduous set of teeth (also known as milk teeth) that fall out in preparation for the permanent adult teeth as they age. Milk teeth usually erupt at about 3–4 weeks of age, around the time of weaning, and are replaced at about 5–6 months old. The dental formulae for the deciduous teeth of the puppy and kitten can be represented as follows:

Puppy $\dfrac{\text{I3, C1, P3, M0}}{\text{I3, C1, P4, M0}}$

Kitten $\dfrac{\text{I3, C1, P3, M0}}{\text{I3, C1, P2, M0}}$

Note that molars are not present as deciduous teeth in either species.

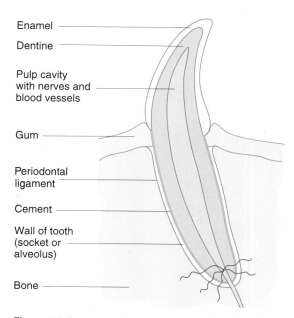

Enamel
Dentine
Pulp cavity with nerves and blood vessels
Gum
Periodontal ligament
Cement
Wall of tooth (socket or alveolus)
Bone

Figure 5.3 Structure of a tooth

during which it is raised to prevent food entering the nasopharynx (the rostral region of the pharynx, which as a whole joins the oral cavity with the oesophagus). A small piece of cartilagenous tissue called the epiglottis moves backwards to cover the larynx, preventing entry of food into the larynx and trachea. The pharynx is opened and food is propelled down and into the oesophagus. Following this, the soft palate is lowered and the epiglottis falls forwards, opening the larynx.

The salivary glands

We have concentrated primarily upon the function of the oral cavity with respect to the mechanical process of digestion. However, there is also a chemical process at work in the oral cavity; it is also the first site at which the breakdown of complex substances into simpler products occurs. There are four pairs of salivary glands, illustrated in Figure 5.4, that secrete continuously an alkaline secretion known as saliva. Secretion of saliva (salivation) increases in response to the sight, taste, smell, and anticipation of food. Its functions are to moisten, lubricate and soften food, as well as to moisten the oral cavity. In addition to these functions, saliva also contains the enzyme ptyalin (or salivary amylase) which is secreted by the parotid salivary gland. Salivary amylase starts to breakdown carbohydrates into smaller chains of saccharides.

The oesophagus

The oesophagus is the connecting tube between the pharynx and stomach. It carries the bolus of swallowed food rapidly to the stomach by waves of smooth muscle contraction known as **peristalsis**.

The stomach

The stomach acts as a storage organ for the ingested food. The mechanical process of digestion is continued in the stomach, through its churning movements, and it is also a site of chemical digestion via the production of acids and enzymes. Finally, a glycoprotein known as **intrinsic factor**, which is necessary for the animal to absorb the essential vitamin, B_{12}, is also produced by the stomach.

Often described as J-shaped, the stomach can be divided into four regions, the **cardia**, **fundus**, **body** and **pylorus**, as illustrated in Figure 5.5, although some texts simplify these to three, excluding the body.

The **cardia** is the smallest part of the stomach, located near the oesophagus. The **fundus** lies to the left of and dorsal to the cardia, whilst the **body** is the largest, middle portion located at the curve of the J. Gastric glands located in the body and the fundus produce most of the digestive secretions, such as enzymes and acid. The **pylorus** forms the upward curve of the J, being the distal third of the stomach. It narrows to form the **pyloric canal** before terminating at the pyloric sphincter.

The stomach wall is lined with a layer of secretory epithelial cells that secrete a protective layer of mucus which covers the lining of the stomach. This protects the stomach wall, preventing damage by the acidic secretions and auto-digestion by its own digestive enzymes. The stomach wall also contains three layers of smooth

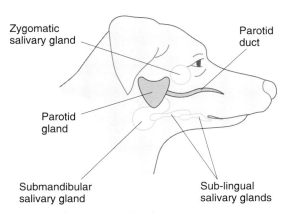

Figure 5.4 Salivary glands of the dog

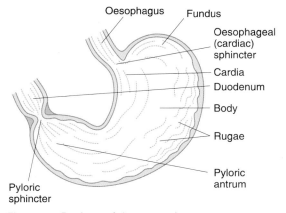

Figure 5.5 Regions of the stomach

muscle which are innervated by branches of the autonomic nervous system. These layers help to strengthen the wall of the stomach and help in the churning and mixing of stomach contents during the process of digestion. When the stomach is empty the inner mucosa lies in folds or **rugae**. These permit expansion of the stomach as it fills following a meal. The stomach capacity of individual animals varies, depending upon species and breed. In the dog it may range from 0.5 to 6.0 litres.

The small intestine

The small intestine can be considered in three regions from the proximal to the distal end: the **duodenum**, **jejunum**, and **ileum**.

The **duodenum** is relatively short and immobile compared to the other two regions. It is joined by the pancreatic and bile ducts and secretions from both the pancreas and gall bladder enter the small intestine at these junctions. The function of these secretions will be discussed later in this chapter. The prime function of the duodenal part of the small intestine is continuation of the digestive process. The **jejunum** is relatively mobile and lies in many coils, supported and held in place by mesentery (connective tissue joining the intestine to the body wall). The proximal region of the jejunum is associated with the continuation of digestive processes, while the absorption of electrolytes and some of the products of digestion occurs in the distal end. The **ileum** is located at the distal end of the small intestine where absorption of electrolytes and nutrients, the products of digestion, continues. When the food leaves the small intestine, the digestive process should be complete.

The wall of the small intestine consists of three layers of tissue. The inner tunica mucosa of the intestinal wall is folded into finger-like projections called **villi**. These are themselves lined with simple columnar epithelial cells that possess **microvilli**. Both the villi and microvilli act to facilitate the efficiency of digestion and absorption by increasing the overall surface area of the small intestine. The middle layer, the tunica muscularis is composed of smooth muscle that contracts in a 'wave-like' manner to move the contents of the intestine along the digestive tract. This type of contraction is called **peristalsis** and is under the control of the autonomic nervous system. The outer layer, known as the outer tunica serosa is concerned primarily with protection of the middle and inner layers.

The structure of a villus is illustrated in Figure 5.6.

Each villus contains an extensive capillary network, nerve endings and a lymphatic capillary

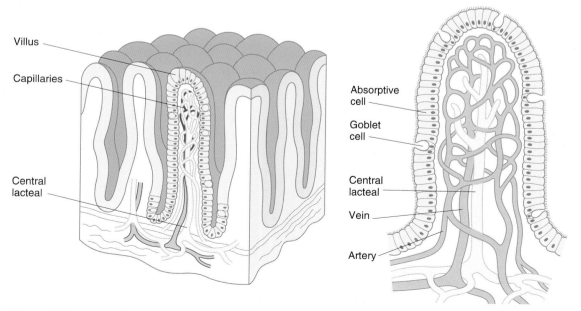

Figure 5.6 Structure of an intestinal villus

known as a **lacteal**. The lacteals are responsible for the absorption and transport of fatty acids that are too large to be transported in the circulation. They are converted into chylomicrons by incorporation with proteins that enter the lymphatic system (see Chapter 6) before passing into the bloodstream.

The large intestine

Although the name of the terminal part of the digestive tract may lead one to believe that it is bigger than the small intestine, this is not the case. The small intestine is approximately seven times longer than the large intestine in the cat and dog. The term 'large' does not refer to its length but to the diameter of its lumen, which is greater in the large intestine than in the small intestine.

The large intestine has three regions from the proximal to the distal end: the **caecum**, **colon**, and **rectum**. The caecum forms the proximal region of the large intestine and is linked to the ileum by the ileo-caecal valve. As discussed previously, the caecum of the dog and cat is relatively insignificant compared to that of herbivorous species such as the rabbit. Nevertheless, it is here that the process of digestion and absorption of nutrients is completed and compac-

tion of the remaining contents of the digestive tract commences. On leaving the caecum, the contents pass into the colon. This region of the large intestine is puckered and possesses pouches (or **haustra**) within its wall that allow the colon to expand considerably if required. Three anatomical regions of the colon can be identified: the ascending, transverse and descending colon. These are illustrated in Figure 5.7.

In the colon, the process of compaction through the absorption of water is continued. Certain vitamins (in particular, vitamin K and biotin) are produced by the action of bacteria within the large intestine and are also absorbed in the colon. The rectum forms the terminal part of the large intestine and acts as an expandable, temporary store for faecal material prior to defecation.

Digestive secretions

Now that we have an understanding of the anatomical structure of the digestive tract, we can examine the chemical processes of digestion that occur in each region.

The parotid salivary glands produce the first digestive enzyme, salivary amylase (or ptyalin) (note that the ending -ase usually indicates that the

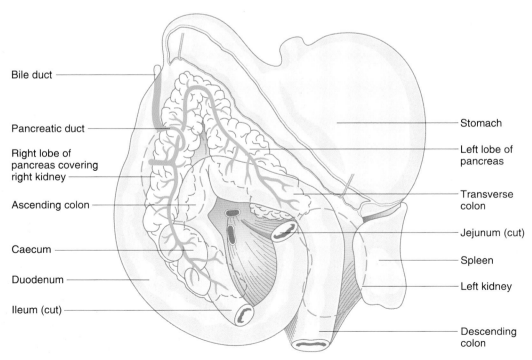

Figure 5.7 Abdominal viscera of the dog

Bile duct

Pancreatic duct

Right lobe of pancreas covering right kidney

Ascending colon

Caecum

Duodenum

Ileum (cut)

Stomach

Left lobe of pancreas

Transverse colon

Jejunum (cut)

Spleen

Left kidney

Descending colon

molecule is an enzyme). Small quantities of salivary amylase are also produced by the submandibular salivary glands. Salivary amylase starts the process of carbohydrate digestion in the oral cavity and continues its actions within the stomach for a short period. Complex carbohydrates are broken down into shorter-chain sugars known as polysaccharides. Only a small amount of salivary amylase is secreted in saliva and consequently the amount of carbohydrate digested at this stage is small. The further digestion of carbohydrates and polysaccharides is continued in the small intestine and will be discussed later in this section.

Gastric secretions

Gastric glands within the body and fundus of the stomach contain two types of cells. Oxyntic or parietal cells secrete hydrochloric acid and intrinsic factor while the chief or zymogen cells secrete an inactive pro-enzyme called pepsinogen. Together, these secretions are known as gastric juice. Hydrochloric acid lowers the pH of the stomach contents to approximately 1.5 to 2. The acidic environment kills most of the organisms that may be ingested, as well as denaturing any proteins (facilitating their digestion by gastric enzymes). It also breaks down any connective tissues and activates the pro-enzyme, pepsinogen, by changing it into pepsin. Pepsin is a proteolytic enzyme that breaks down proteins into shorter-chain polypeptides.

The enzyme rennin, also called chymosin, is also secreted by cells in the stomach wall. Rennin coagulates milk proteins. In the stomachs of un-weaned animals, an enzyme called gastric lipase is also produced, which initiates the digestion of the fats in the milk.

Pyloric glands, located in the pyloric region, produce the mucus that covers the lining of the stomach. Other cells known as 'G cells' within the pyloric area secrete a hormone called **gastrin** in response to the presence of food in the stomach. Gastrin is carried in the circulatory system to the parietal and chief cells, stimulating them to produce gastric juice and hydrochloric acid. It is also thought to stimulate contractions of the stomach wall which promote digestion.

After a period of time in the stomach, the semi-liquid substance leaving through the pyloric sphincter is a highly acidic mixture of digestive enzymes and partially digested food. This mixture is known as **chyme** and enters the proximal region of the small intestine.

Secretions into the small intestine

There are two main secretions into the small intestine from the pancreas and the gall bladder, as well as the secretions from cells in the wall of the small intestine itself. Secretions from the pancreas and gall bladder are discussed later in this chapter.

Secretory cells of the wall of the small intestine are stimulated by the presence of acidic chyme in the duodenum. Pockets of glandular tissue, known as **intestinal crypts** (or crypts of Lieberkuhn), are present at the base of the villi. Stem cells located at the base of the crypts divide constantly to produce new epithelial cells, to replace those of the lining of the small intestine as they are shed. As the older epithelial cells are shed into the intestine they release several enzymes (collectively known as brush-border enzymes) into the contents of the intestine. It is in this way that the enzyme **enterokinase** enters the small intestine. Although not directly involved with digestion, enterokinase is responsible for activating the pancreatic pro-enzyme, trypsinogen and will be discussed later in this section. In addition to the secretion of brush-border enzymes, the crypts also contain endocrine cells that secrete hormones such as cholecystokinin (CCK) and secretin that together control the activity and secretory activity of the gastro-intestinal tract.

The exocrine function of the pancreas

The watery, alkaline secretion produced by the pancreatic duct cells is regulated by the hormone secretin, which is secreted by the intestinal crypts

---

The pancreas is probably most renowned for its endocrine function in the regulation of blood sugar levels. However, it also has a significant exocrine input in the process of digestion through the secretion of pancreatic juice into the duodenum via the pancreatic duct. Pancreatic juice is a combination of secretions from both the acinar cells of the pancreas and the cells lining the pancreatic duct. It is alkaline and contains digestive enzymes (secreted by the acinar cells), water and ions, primarily bicarbonate (secreted by the cells lining the pancreatic duct).

(crypts of Lieberkuhn) in the duodenum, as discussed previously. The activity of the acinar cells, producing the enzyme component of pancreatic juice, is regulated by the hormone CCK. The enzymes secreted are as follows:

1. **Pancreatic amylase**

   Pancreatic amylase continues the digestion of complex carbohydrates that started initially in the mouth by the action of salivary amylase. Brush-border enzymes of the small intestine (maltase, sucrase, and lactase) facilitate the final conversion of disaccharides into simple sugars or monosaccharides, such as glucose, fructose, and galactose for absorption into the circulation via the villi.

2. **Nucleotidase** (or **nuclease**)

   Nucleotidase assists with the breakdown of nucleotides which form the genetic material (DNA and RNA) of animal and plant cells.

3. **Pro-enzymes**

   Many digestive enzymes are secreted in an inactive form to protect the secretory cells from their own digestive function (**autodigestion**). For example, trypsinogen is an inactive pro-enzyme contained in pancreatic juice which, when activated by enterokinase (a brush-border enzyme), is converted into trypsin. The function of trypsin is to continue the action of pepsin in the stomach, breaking down peptides into shorter chains and ultimately into single amino acids that can be absorbed into the circulation via the villi.

4. **Lipase**

   Lipase is the enzyme that digests lipids (or fats) into fatty acids and glycerol (or monoglyceride). Unlike the other products of digestion, such as amino acids and monosaccharides, fatty acids and glycerol are absorbed in the small intestine into small vessels called lacteals, which are part of the lymphatic system, rather than into the circulation. This will be discussed in more detail in Chapter 6.

In conclusion, we can see that pancreatic juice contributes significantly to the digestive process in the small intestine, with particular emphasis on continuing the digestion of carbohydrates, proteins, and lipids. There is a second secretion into the duodenum that also plays an important role particularly in the digestion of lipid and this is considered in the following section.

Bile

Bile is secreted into the small intestine from the gall bladder, through the bile duct which joins the pancreatic duct before entering the duodenum. Bile does not itself contain any digestive enzymes. It is composed of water, ions, bile pigments (bilirubin, derived from the breakdown of haemoglobin), cholesterol, and a range of lipids called bile salts. Bile salts assist in the break up of lipid droplets within the digestive tract into smaller droplets to increase the surface area on which the enzyme lipase can act. This process is known as emulsification and is rather similar to the action of some detergents. Washing-up liquids contain detergents that break up large volumes of fat into smaller droplets, making it easier for them to mix with water and consequently easier for us to clean the frying pan! Bile salts also aid the absorption of fatty acids and glycerol further along the small intestine.

Although the gall bladder is associated with the secretion of bile, its main function is to act as a storage organ for bile, although some concentration of the bile occurs during its storage. Bile is synthesized in the liver from where it is secreted continuously into the hepatic bile ducts and stored in the gall bladder. During storage, the gall bladder absorbs some of the water from the bile, effectively concentrating the bile pigments and salts. Bile is released from the gall bladder into the duodenum under the influence of CCK, which itself is secreted when chyme enters the duodenum.

Absorption of the products of digestion

Once the contents of the digestive tract have reached the more distal region of the jejunum, most of the digestive process is complete. Complex carbohydrates will have been broken down into disaccharides and then into monosaccharides through the action of both salivary and pancreatic amylase and brush-border enzymes. Proteins will have been digested into peptides and then into amino acids through the actions of pepsin and trypsin. Lipids will have been digested by lipase (with the assistance of the bile salts and emulsification) into fatty acids and glycerol. This is summarized in Figure 5.8.

These much simpler products of digestion are now small enough to be absorbed across the epithelium of the villi in the small intestine.

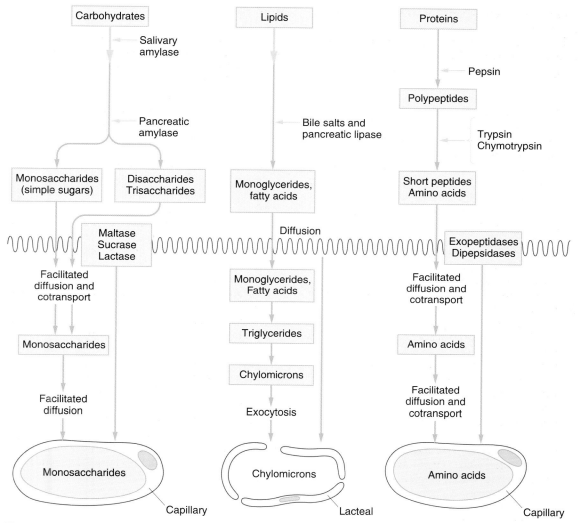

Figure 5.8 Summary of the chemical process of digestion

Monosaccharides and amino acids are absorbed into the epithelial cells. From here, they move first into the interstitial fluid and then into the capillary of the villi, thereby entering the circulation. They pass directly to the liver in the hepatic portal vein. However, fatty acids and glycerol, once absorbed into the epithelial cells, are used to synthesize new lipid molecules. These are then coated with protein to form a lipid/protein complex called a **chylomicron**. The chylomicrons are secreted by the epithelial cells into the interstitial fluid, but the protein coat prevents them from entering the capillary. The majority of chylomicrons are taken into the lacteal within the villus and pass into the

lymphatic system before finally entering the circulation at the subclavian vein.

Absorption of vitamins

Vitamins can be divided into fat-soluble and water-soluble forms. Water-soluble vitamins include vitamin C and the B group of vitamins. All the water-soluble vitamins are easily absorbed across the intestinal epithelium apart from vitamin B_{12} which needs to associate with intrinsic factor, secreted by parietal cells of the stomach, before it can be absorbed. The fat-soluble vitamins (A, D, E and K) remain associated with the lipid through their digestion and absorption. Vitamin K is produced by specific bacteria in the colon and is absorbed in this region.

Absorption of water and ions

Osmosis accounts for the movement of water across the epithelium of the intestine. Water is primarily absorbed in the small intestine and colon, depending upon osmotic gradients. The effects of ions, in particular Na^+, can also have effects upon the movement of water. The direct mechanism whereby specific ions are absorbed is uncertain. Final absorption of water takes place in the large intestine.

Defecation

The anus is the terminal opening of the digestive tract and is surrounded by an internal and external sphincter (circular ring of muscle). Faecal matter consists of food residues, cellular debris, secretions from the digestive tract, and bacteria from the large intestine. The colour of the faeces depends upon the content of the diet, in addition to the content of bile pigments. Observation of the faeces of an animal can give a good indication of its general health and can aid in the diagnosis of certain diseases. The consistency should be firm. Colour may vary from yellow to green and brown. Undigested blood appears red while digested blood appears black, with a tar-like consistency. This is known as **melaena**. There may also be other material present within the faecal matter, such as tapeworm segments, roundworms, bony segments, hair, fur, and other foreign bodies that the dog or cat has ingested. The presence of any of the latter may be a cause for concern.

Vomiting or emesis

Vomiting is initiated by a specific centre in the brain and results in the violent expulsion of the contents of the stomach through the mouth. This is caused by strong contractions of the muscles of the abdomen and diaphragm as the cardiac sphincter of the stomach relaxes. The cause of vomiting is irritation of the mucosa of the stomach which can be due to a number of factors including disease, toxins, or excessive stomach distension (perhaps due to an intestinal blockage). This should not be confused with regurgitation, which is expulsion of undigested food from the oesophagus rather than the stomach.

5.2 The liver

> Metabolism of the products of digestion
> The composition of blood

Introduction

The liver is the largest organ of the mammalian body excluding the skin, which some consider to be an organ. It appears as a firm, red/brown organ located in the anterior abdomen where it lies close to the diaphragm and is protected by the caudal ribs. Its functions are numerous, over 200 having been identified to date. It contributes to the metabolism of the products of digestion, storage of vitamins and minerals and recycling of hormones. It is also responsible for the synthesis of bile, and plays a key role in the production of heat in the regulation of body temperature. In the following sections we will examine some of the more important functions of the liver in more detail.

Metabolism of the products of digestion

Nearly all of the products of digestion pass directly from the small intestine into the circulation and are transported via the hepatic portal vein directly to the liver. The only exceptions to this are the products of fat digestion that pass into the lacteals of the lymphatic system, before returning to the circulation through the thoracic duct that drains into the left subclavian vein (see Chapter 6). The liver consequently has first access to the main products of digestion and regulates the composition of the blood by removing and storing excess nutrients whilst synthesizing or mobilizing those that are in deficit. It is also capable of removing toxins before they enter the bloodstream.

Amino acids are removed from the circulation and are either used in the synthesis of proteins or converted through a biochemical pathway into lipids or glucose that can be used for storage. Excess amino acids are converted by the liver into ammonia, then urea and uric acid, following which they are excreted by the kidneys. As proteins or amino acids cannot be explicitly stored by the body, a constant dietary intake is required in the healthy animal.

The metabolism of glucose, produced by the digestion of carbohydrates, is finely balanced to produce relatively constant blood glucose levels in the healthy animal. When in surplus, for example following eating, the liver removes excess glucose

> Although the products of lipid digestion (fatty acids and glycerol) bypass the liver initially, the liver has an important role to play in the breakdown of fatty acids for energy and regulation of blood lipids. It can release its own stored lipid when levels in the circulation are low and remove them from the circulation for storage when levels are high.

from the circulation, converting it into a storage product called **glycogen**, a process known as **glycogenesis**. Excess glucose may also be converted into lipid. When blood glucose levels fall the glycogen reserves are broken down to release glucose, a process known as **glycogenolysis** or **glucogenesis**. When glycogen reserves are exhausted, other carbohydrates or amino acids can be utilized to produce glucose. The regulation of blood glucose has already been discussed in Chapter 2.

In addition to the metabolism and regulation of the products of digestion, the liver also has an important role in the storage of certain vitamins and minerals. The fat-soluble vitamins A, D, E, and K, as well as vitamin B_{12}, are all stored in the liver. Iron is also stored as ferritin, for use when dietary intake is inadequate.

Synthesis of bile

Earlier in this chapter we examined the role of bile in the emulsification of dietary fat and its effects upon digestion. Bile salts and pigments are synthesized in the liver from where they are excreted and stored in the gall bladder prior to being secreted into the duodenum. The functions of bile were discussed above in more detail in the digestive system.

The composition of blood

The liver also has many effects upon the composition of blood. It synthesizes plasma proteins such as albumen, which is involved in the maintenance of osmotic pressure of plasma and blood clotting, e.g. fibrinogen and prothrombin. Specialized cells within the liver, known as Kupffer cells, are responsible for destroying old or damaged red blood cells, pathogens, and cellular debris by phagocytosis. Kupffer cells also play an important role in initiation of the activa-

tion of T-lymphocytes as part of the immune response (see Chapter 6).

The liver also inactivates some drugs by breaking them down into pharmacologically inactive molecules. Drugs that are broken down rapidly by the liver therefore need to be administered more frequently than those that remain within the circulation for a longer period of time. In addition to the removal of certain drugs, the liver is also responsible for the breakdown and removal of circulating hormones such as adrenaline, noradrenaline, and steroid hormones, as well as the removal and storage of toxins. Some toxins are broken down and excreted in bile whereas others are stored within lipid deposits in the liver itself, where they cannot affect cellular function.

Cholecalciferol (vitamin D_3), synthesized by the skin (integument) due to the effect of ultraviolet radiation (see Chapter 6). It is absorbed from the bloodstream by the liver, where it is converted into an intermediate compound that is then released back into the circulation for use by the kidneys in the synthesis of calcitriol (see Chapter 2).

5.3 The urinary system

> Structure of the urinary system
> Structure and function of the kidney
> The ureters, urinary bladder and urethra
> Neural control of urination
> Composition of urine

Introduction

The urinary system comprises the kidneys, ureters, urinary bladder, and urethra. The kidneys remove toxic nitrogenous compounds (e.g. urea and uric acid, produced by the liver) from the blood whilst excreting excess water and salts to assist with the long-term maintenance of blood concentration. In this section, we will examine the structure and function of the kidneys and associated structures of the urinary system.

Structure of the urinary system

The gross structure of the urinary system is illustrated in Figure 5.9. There are two kidneys (left and right) located behind the peritoneum of the abdominal cavity (described as a retroperitoneal location). They lie on either side of the vertebral column around the region of the first

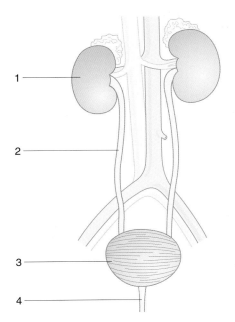

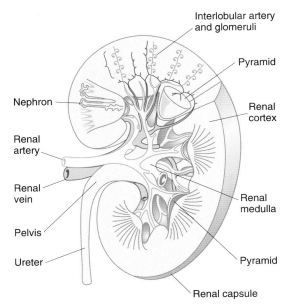

Figure 5.9 Structure of the mammalian urinary system. 1, Kidney (produces urine); 2, ureter (transports urine toward the urinary bladder); 3, urinary bladder (temporarily stores urine prior to elimination); 4, urethra (conducts urine to exterior)

Figure 5.10 Cross-section of the mammalian kidney

three lumbar vertebrae. The ureters connect the kidneys to the urinary bladder (a storage vessel) allowing the drainage of the urine they produce. The urethra connects the urinary bladder to the exterior and permits the passage of urine, a process known as urination or micturition.

Structure and function of the kidney

A cross-section of the kidney is illustrated in Figure 5.10. Two distinct zones can be identified, the outer, darker, **cortex** and the inner, paler, **medulla**. The renal pelvis appears as a white structure in the centre of the kidney and acts as a collecting space for the urine produced by the kidney before it passes down the ureter to the bladder.

On microscopic examination, it can be seen that the kidney consists of a collection of fine tubules with the specific function of filtering the plasma from toxic nitrogenous compounds. These tubules are called **nephrons**, and their structure is illustrated in Figure 5.11. The function of the nephrons is to filter toxic nitrogenous compounds from the plasma.

The blood supply to the kidney is via the renal artery. Following many subdivisions, the artery forms a network of capillaries, primarily in the cortex of the kidney, hence its darker appearance, which is due to the rich blood supply. Each network of capillaries forms an intertwining 'knot' of vessels called a **glomerulus**. The glomerulus sits in a 'cup' formed from simple squamous epithelial cells. This cup is known as the glomerular or Bowman's capsule and it is here that the blood is filtered. The afferent arteriole of the glomerulus has a much larger diameter than the efferent arteriole resulting in the blood within the glomerulus being under high pressure. Consequently, fluid from the plasma is filtered through the wall of the arteriole and into the capsule, rather similar to the way in which tissue fluid is formed. Larger proteins, such as plasma proteins and blood cells, are too large to pass through the capillary cell wall in the healthy kidney and consequently remain in the circulation. The fluid produced by this process (sometimes referred to as ultra-filtration) is called the **glomerular filtrate** and this travels along the rest of the nephron. The filtration pressure is defined as the difference in pressure

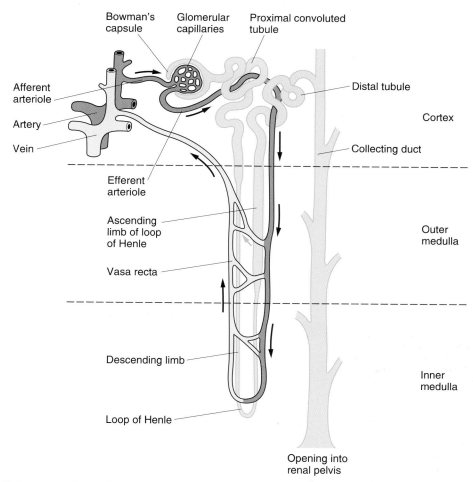

Figure 5.11 Structure of a nephron

between the blood in the capillary of the glomerulus and the pressure of the filtrate in the glomerular or Bowman's capsule. On entering the proximal convoluted tubule (PCT), the filtrate is in close association with a network of capillaries. It is here that the absorption of some water, salts, and glucose from the filtrate into the peritubular fluid (fluid surrounding the PCT) and ultimately the blood, takes place.

The loop of Henle

After leaving the PCT, the filtrate passes into the **loop of Henle** that travels from the cortex into the medulla and out again. Two regions can be identified in the loop of Henle, the ascending limb and the descending limb. The loop of Henle is responsible for further re-absorption of water from the filtrate, as well as sodium and chloride ions. The process of re-absorption occurs due to the effects of a counter-current exchange mechanism. This can be simply explained as follows: the counter-current exchange occurs due to the very close association of the ascending and descending limbs. In the ascending limb, which is impermeable to water and solutes, there is an active transport mechanism that moves sodium and chloride ions from the filtrate into the peritubular fluid. This results in an increased concentration of the fluid surrounding the descending limb. Consequently, water is drawn out of the descending limb into the peritubular fluid by osmosis, further concentrating the tubular fluid, and resulting in an increased movement of ions from the ascending limb. This

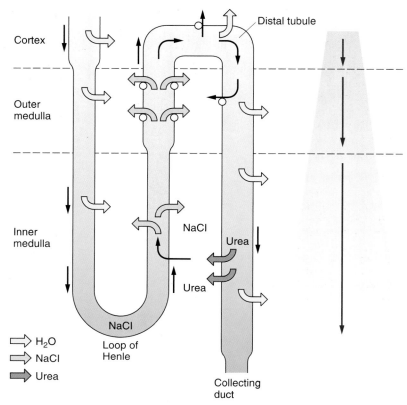

Figure 5.12 The counter-current exchange mechanism

positive feedback loop in the loop of Henle provides an extremely efficient way of re-absorbing water, sodium and chloride ions before the fluid reaches the distal convoluted tubule (DCT). This is illustrated in Figure 5.12.

The distal convoluted tubule and collecting duct

On leaving the loop of Henle, the tubular fluid has had the majority of some substances re-absorbed, e.g. glucose, water, and sodium and chloride ions. The remaining fluid contains a high percentage of urea and other organic waste products. The DCT carries out selective absorption and active secretion of certain compounds to adjust the composition of the tubular fluid. Remaining sodium and chloride ions are re-absorbed into the capillary network under the control of the hormone aldosterone. Secretion of aldosterone causes an increase in the amount of sodium ions re-absorbed and a consequent decrease in their excretion in urine.

Calcium ions are also re-absorbed under the regulation of the hormones calcitriol and parathyroid hormone. The movement of water into the peritubular fluid is associated with this movement of ions.

The DCT may also secrete certain substances, should their concentration become too high in the peritubular fluid. These include potassium and hydrogen ions, as well as some drugs, for example penicillin, atropine, and morphine. It is through the active secretion of hydrogen ions that the kidneys have a direct effect upon blood pH and the maintenance of homeostasis.

The filtrate from several nephrons passes into a collecting duct. It is here that the final adjustments to the composition and volume of urine take place. Aldosterone continues to have its effects on proximal regions of the collecting duct that lie within the renal cortex, while antidiuretic hormone (ADH) affects the permeability of the walls of both the DCT and the collecting duct to water. Secretion of ADH causes the walls to become permeable and consequently water moves from the tubule into the peritubular fluid. The resultant urine produced is concentrated (hypertonic). In the absence of ADH, the walls of the DCT and the collecting duct are impermeable to water and the urine produced remains dilute. Consequently, depending upon whether or not the animal needs to conserve water at any particular time, the secretion of ADH can be altered to regulate the volume of urine produced and the resultant amount of water lost.

Diabetes insipidus

> The inability to produce sufficient quantities of ADH results in the inability to concentrate urine effectively and the secretion of copious quantities of hypotonic urine. This condition is known as diabetes insipidus, and should not be confused with the other form of diabetes, diabetes mellitus, as discussed in Chapter 2.

The juxtaglomerular apparatus

Specialized cells of the DCT lie close to an unusual type of smooth muscle fibre in the wall of the afferent arteriole of the nephron (refer to Figure 5.11). Together, these form the juxtaglomerular apparatus (JGA) which is responsible for the secretion of the hormones erythropoietin and renin, discussed in Chapters 2 and 4, respectively. This mechanism is illustrated in Figure 5.13.

Maintenance of acid/base balance

In order that the pH of body fluids is maintained, it is essential that any changes in the pH or acid-base balance are detected so that appropriate action may be taken to maintain homeostasis. The kidneys have the ability to regulate pH through the effects of the cells of the DCT in secreting bicarbonate and hydrogen ions. In cases of acidosis, hydrogen ion secretion is increased in an attempt to decrease the acidity of the body fluid. The kidney also

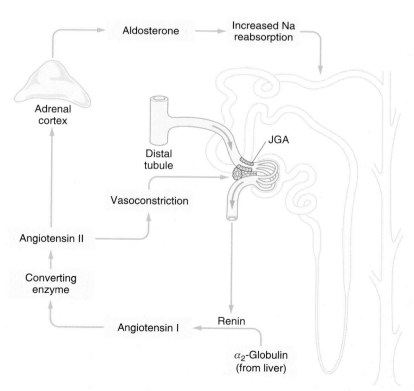

Figure 5.13 The renin–angiotensin feedback loop and the juxtaglomerular apparatus

secretes bicarbonate ions into the bloodstream; this helps to counteract any changes in pH through the buffering effects of these ions.

The ureters, urinary bladder and urethra

On leaving the kidney, the filtrate passes into the corresponding ureters (left or right). The ureters are relatively thick-walled, containing layers of smooth muscle that contract on stimulation from the autonomic nervous system to assist the flow of urine towards the urinary bladder. The ureters enter the bladder at an oblique (sloping) angle at the point of entry and this prevents the back-flow of urine into the ureters as the bladder fills. The bladder acts as a storage organ, and consists of a double layer of smooth muscle lined with transitional epithelial cells that are able to stretch as the bladder fills, so that it is capable of considerable distension.

The urethra leaves the bladder and carries urine to the external orifice. It passes through the internal sphincter, which is under involuntary control, as well as the external urethral sphincter which is under voluntary control. The external urethral sphincter must be voluntarily relaxed in adult animals to allow urination to occur. In the male animal the urethra is common to both the urinary and reproductive systems.

Neural control of urination

The wall of the bladder contains stretch receptors that are stimulated as the bladder fills with urine. The receptors trigger the sensation of a full bladder as the urine volume increases. Activity in the sensory fibres carries this information to the spinal cord where it is relayed to the thalamus of the brain and cerebral cortex and the animal becomes aware of a full bladder. Efferent fibres are also stimulated, due to increased activity in the sensory fibres, and muscle surrounding the bladder contracts. However urination does not occur until both the internal and external urethral sphincters relax. Relaxation of the external sphincter is under voluntary control and if urination is suppressed, eventually the urinary bladder relaxes for a period of time. The cycle continues until the bladder exceeds a certain volume, upon which the internal sphincter is forced open, causing a reflexive relaxation of the external sphincter and urination occurs involuntarily. Although puppies lack voluntary control over urination, they develop voluntary control of urination with age, in response to an appropriate stimulus to which they have been trained, e.g. newspaper, a command, or being placed on an area of grass.

Composition of urine

Approximately 85–99% of the glomerular filtrate is re-absorbed along the length of the nephron in a normal, healthy dog and the resultant urine consists of approximately 96% water and 4% solids. The solid fraction includes urea, urates, and uric acid (the end-products of protein metabolism), in addition to chlorides, phosphates, sulphates and creatinine (a by-product of the metabolism of muscle cells). The average dog or cat will pass 20 ml urine per kg body weight each day, although this is extremely variable, being dependent upon factors such as temperature, activity of the animal, diet, etc. Being primarily carnivorous, the pH of canine and feline urine is between five and seven, i.e. slightly acidic. Herbivorous species such as the rabbit usually have alkaline urine. The specific gravity of urine (i.e. compared to water) is usually 1.015–1.045 (range 1.001–1.065) in the healthy dog and 1.035–1.060 (range 1.001–1.080) in the normal cat. Due to the variable nature of these normal ranges, different texts may quote slightly different values.

Various abnormal constituents may also be evident in a sample of urine. The presence of fresh blood may be due to trauma of the urinary tract, e.g. from recent catheterization or may indicate cystitis. Alternatively, it may be a contaminant if taken from a female animal in season. Glucose in the urine may indicate diabetes mellitus, although a small quantity may be detected if the animal has recently been fed. The presence of ketones may also indicate diabetes mellitus, as the animal starts to utilize its fat reserves for cellular energy production. Proteins in the urine may be an indicator of damage to the urinary tract, as in the case of chronic renal failure, while bile may indicate some form of liver disease or a blockage of the bile duct. Deposits such as cells from the urinary tract, casts, or crystals, may also be evident. The examination of urine as a diagnostic aid to the veterinary surgeon can be a valuable tool. However, it must be remembered that conclusions should not be drawn from these results alone.

5.4 The respiratory system

Basic principles of respiration
Composition of inspired and expired air
Structure of the respiratory system
The mechanism of respiration
Control of respiration

Introduction

The respiratory system is the mechanism whereby the body supplies oxygen to each cell for the process of aerobic respiration to produce the energy required for all cellular processes. It must also be able to remove the waste products of the respiratory process, namely carbon dioxide. It is essential to have a system specifically devoted to this process, as the multicellular nature of the animal means that cells cannot conduct the process on an individual basis. Consequently, a transport mechanism is required to distribute the oxygen and carbon dioxide. This is the cardiovascular system, discussed in detail in Chapter 4. In this chapter we examine the structure and function of the mammalian respiratory system and the process by which oxygen is supplied to the cells of the body and carbon dioxide is removed.

We can divide the respiratory process into two parts which take place in different areas: **external respiration** describes the process of inspiration and the diffusion of oxygen from the air sacs (alveoli of the lungs) into the blood and carbon dioxide from the blood into the air sacs/alveoli. **Internal** or **tissue respiration** represents the diffusion of gases between the blood and tissues of the body. These are illustrated in Figure 5.14.

Basic principles of respiration

The process of respiration can be represented in a very basic way by the following equation:

Respiration → energy + carbon dioxide + water vapour

Oxygen is required for this process to occur and the respiratory process follows a complex cycle known as the Krebs cycle or the Citric Acid cycle. This will not be discussed in detail in this text. Interested readers should refer to Purves and Orions, 1987 (see References and Further reading) for more information. In these cycles, energy is produced in the form of adenosine triphosphate

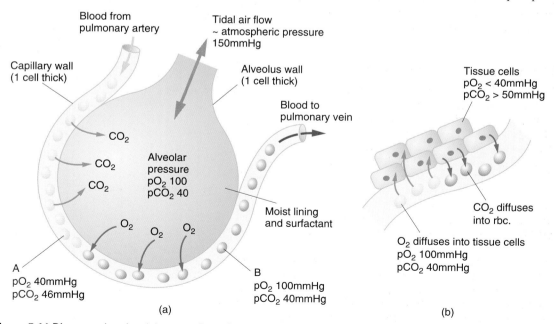

Figure 5.14 Diagram showing (a) external respiration and (b) internal or tissue respiration. A, red cells low in oxygen, haemoglobin is purple/red (deoxygenated). The air in the alveolus is high in oxygen, therefore O_2 diffuses from alveolus → blood; B, red cells rich in oxygen, oxyhaemoglobin is bright red (oxygenated). Goes to body cells/tissues via pulmonary vein and left side of the heart. pO_2 and pCO_2 refers to the partial pressures of oxygen and carbon dioxide

(ATP); this molecule can be broken down to release energy by cells in the body whenever energy is required.

Figure 5.14 shows that the movement of gases is dependent upon the difference in their partial pressures measured in mm Mercury (mmHg), gases diffusing from areas of high partial pressure to low partial pressure, until the pressures across either side of the membranes are equal.

Composition of inspired and expired air

The composition of inspired and expired air is illustrated in Table 5.1. It should be noted that nitrogen is not utilized during the respiratory process. Only approximately 5% of the oxygen breathed in is actually utilized by the animal, the remaining 16% being expired. This explains how mouth-to-mouth resuscitation can still be effective.

Table 5.1 Composition of inspired and expired air

	Inspired air (%)	Expired air (%)
Nitrogen	79	79
Oxygen	21	16
Carbon dioxide	0.04	4.5
Water vapour	varies	saturated
Other gases	trace	trace

Structure of the respiratory system

A basic outline of the structure of the respiratory system of the dog is illustrated in Figure 5.15. From the diagram it can be seen that the respiratory system comprises the nose and nasal chambers, the pharynx, the larynx, the trachea, two bronchi, many bronchioles, alveolar ducts and alveoli. We shall consider the function of each of these areas in the following sections.

Nose and nasal chambers

The nose and nasal chambers provide the entrance to the entire respiratory system. Air enters the nasal cavity through the nostrils or external nares. The alar fold forms a bulbous enlargement that attaches to the wing of the nostril. Its function is to cause turbulence of the air entering the nasal chamber, the reasons for which will be discussed later in this section. The nostrils lead to the internal nares of the nasal chamber that is divided into two by the cartilaginous nasal septum. The turbinate bones inside the nasal chamber are highly vascular and are lined with ciliated mucous epithelial tissue. These act to increase the surface area with which the inspired air comes into contact. The vascularity of the nasal chamber permits the warming of inspired air whilst the ciliated mucous epithelium acts to moisten the air and to trap any large dust particles that may be inhaled, thereby protecting the delicate lung tissue. Turbulence caused by the alar fold ensures that these effects are maximized and air is warmed, moistened, and filtered prior to entering the rest of the respiratory tract.

Pharynx

The pharynx is located towards the caudal aspect of the oral and nasal chambers and is common to both the respiratory and digestive systems. It can be considered in three regions: the **nasopharynx**, the **oropharynx** and most caudally, the **laryngopharynx**.

The **nasopharyngeal region** continues from the nasal chambers and is lined with ciliated, mucous epithelium. It is here that the Eustachian tube from the middle ear opens, to permit the equilibration of the pressure on either side of the tympanic membrane (see Chapter 2). It is separated from the rest of the pharynx by the soft palate.

The **oropharynx** lies towards the back of the mouth, below the soft palate. It contains folds of lymphoid tissue known as the tonsils and is lined with stratified epithelial tissue to resist the effects of friction caused during swallowing. The soft palate normally moves upwards during swallowing to prevent food entering the respiratory tract.

The **laryngopharynx** forms the caudal part of the pharynx and leads to the larynx.

Larynx

The **larynx** is composed of muscle and fibro-cartilage. It lies at the cranial end of the trachea and its functions are to permit vocalization and to act as a valve via the action of the epiglottis, preventing the inspiration of foreign bodies. The structure of the larynx is illustrated in Figure 5.16.

The larynx is supported by the hyoid apparatus, a series of many small bones that articulate with the temporal bone of the skull. The joints between the bones of the hyoid apparatus are termed synchondroses.

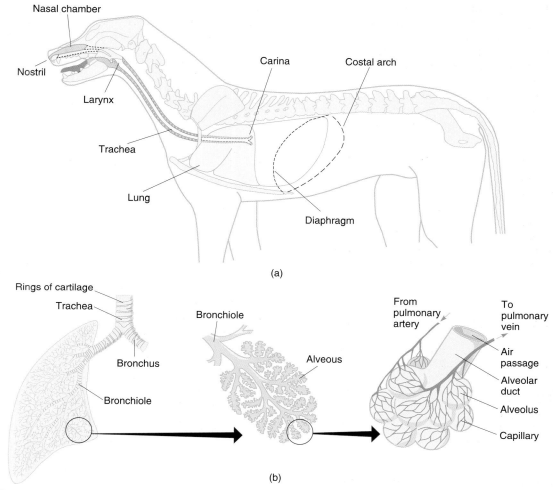

(a)

(b)

Figure 5.15 (a) Outline of the structure of the respiratory system of the dog; (b) air passages in the lungs

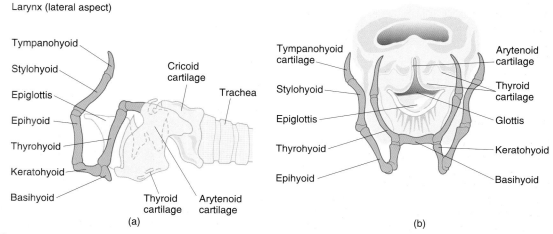

Larynx (lateral aspect)

(a)

(b)

Figure 5.16 Structure of the (a) larynx (lateral aspect) and (b) the hyoid apparatus

The vocal cords are folds that form a narrow passageway into the larynx and are responsible for vocalization as they vibrate. Should a foreign body touch the vocal folds, they quickly come together producing an involuntary reflex expiration that pushes them apart, resulting in a forceful gust of air that blows the foreign object away. This is known as coughing.

Trachea

The **trachea** is a long tube composed of smooth muscle and fibrous tissue. It extends from the larynx to the point at which it divides into two bronchi that supply the left and right lungs. Along its length there are incomplete, 'C'-shaped rings of hyaline cartilage which act to give strength and support. The space in the ring lies at the point where the oesophagus lies and permits the expansion of the oesophagus during swallowing. Ciliated mucous epithelium lines the trachea to further trap particles present in the inspired air. The cilia move the mucus toward the pharynx where it is swallowed.

The bronchi and bronchioles

In the area of the mediastinum, the trachea divides into two bronchi that supply the right and left lungs. The point of division is marked by a ridge known as the carina. At this point, the bronchi also have strengthening 'C'-shaped rings of cartilage but when they begin to divide repeatedly into smaller bronchioles, the rings become less significant until they are no longer apparent. The walls of the bronchioles are composed of smooth muscle and are capable of dilation and constriction under the innervation from the autonomic nervous system. This provides a controlling mechanism for the flow of air into the respiratory system. Bronchodilation, caused by increased activity in the sympathetic part of the autonomic nervous system, increases the amount of air available, preparing the animal for situations such as fight or flight. Bronchoconstriction reduces the diameter of the airways as a result of activity in the parasympathetic nervous system. This may occur in some allergic reactions, such as anaphylaxis caused by a bee sting.

Alveolar ducts and alveoli

Fine bronchioles terminate at alveolar ducts. These connect the alveolar sacs, each containing many alveoli. This structure gives the lungs a spongy appearance. The alveoli lie in close association with an extensive capillary network to permit gaseous exchange. Elastic fibres help to keep the structures in place, in addition to helping with the recoil of the lungs, pushing air out during expiration. Each alveolus is formed from a single layer of simple squamous epithelium that permits the rapid diffusion of gases. Septal cells (or Type II cells) secrete a fluid known as a surfactant. This phospholipid-based fluid covers the entire alveolar surface where it reduces the surface tension within these extremely small structures, preventing their collapse and keeping them open.

Gaseous exchange occurs across the epithelia of the alveoli and the endothelial cells of capillaries. This distance is exceeding small and consequently diffusion in this area is a very rapid process.

The lungs and pleural membranes

There are two lungs that lie within the thoracic cavity on either side of the mediastinum. They are extremely delicate and are protected by the ribs and intercostal muscles. On examination they can be seen to be divided into lobes, the left lung with three and the right lung with four.

The serous membrane that covers the lungs is known as **pulmonary pleura** (sometimes referred to as visceral pleura in other texts) whereas those that line the thoracic cavity are termed the parietal pleura. These are illustrated in Figure 5.17. It can be seen that each lung lies within a sac formed by the pulmonary pleura. This is termed the pleural cavity. Both serous membranes secrete a thin, watery, fluid (pleural fluid) that acts as a lubricant, preventing friction between the membranes as the lungs inflate and deflate. The maintenance of an air-tight pleural cavity is critical in the mechanical process of respiration and is discussed in the following section.

The mechanism of respiration

The process of respiration can be considered in two consecutive phases, inspiration (or inhalation) and expiration (or exhalation).

1. **Inspiration**
   During inspiration, the circular muscles of the diaphragm contract, pulling it from its relaxed,

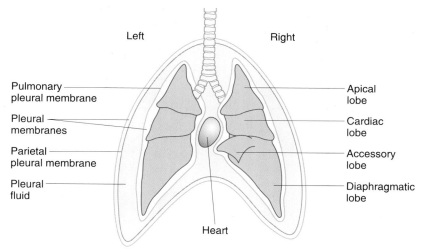

Figure 5.17 Illustration of the lungs and pleural membranes

domed position into one that is more flattened. This acts to increase the length of the thoracic cavity. Simultaneously, the external intercostal muscles contract, pulling the ribs upwards and outwards. This also acts to increase the volume of the thoracic cavity and decreases intra-thoracic pressure. As the thorax of the animal is air-tight, apart from the opening into the trachea, air is drawn into the lungs via the trachea to accommodate the reduced pressure in the thorax. Figure 5.18 illustrates the mechanisms involved.

2. **Expiration**
Following inspiration, the muscles of the diaphragm relax and the diaphragm returns to its resting dome-shaped position. The external intercostal muscles relax and the ribs move downwards and inwards. Both these movements act to decrease the volume of the thorax, thereby increasing intrathoracic pressure. The lungs recoil and air is driven out through the trachea. This process is primarily passive during quiet breathing, requiring very little effort, however, in laboured breathing, the internal intercostal muscles may also contract to aid the lowering of the rib cage. Figure 5.18 illustrates the mechanisms involved.

Lung capacity

The volume of air held in the lungs during the respiratory process can be measured using a spirometer. This can be used to establish the relationships between respiratory volume and lung capacity, which can aid the diagnosis of problems with pulmonary ventilation. Although this technique is not used on the dog and cat, it does have its uses in evaluating the performance and lung function of race horses and humans. A tracing obtained from the spirometer is illustrated in Figure 5.19.

- The tidal volume (TV) is the volume of air breathed in or out during respiration at rest.
- The expiratory reserve volume (ERV) is the total volume of air that can be voluntarily expired following normal breathing, i.e. without taking a deep breath in beforehand.
- The residual volume (RV) is the volume of air remaining in the lungs following maximum exhalation.
- The inspiratory reserve volume (IRV) is the volume of air that can be inhaled, above the tidal volume.
- The inspiratory capacity is TV+IRV, i.e. the volume of air that can be inhaled following quiet respiration.
- The functional residual capacity (FRC) is ERV +residual volume, i.e. the volume of air in the lungs after completion of a cycle of quite respiration.
- The vital capacity is the maximum volume of air that can be inhaled and exhaled, i.e. ERV+IRV +tidal volume.
- The total lung capacity is the total volume of the lungs, i.e. vital capacity+residual volume.

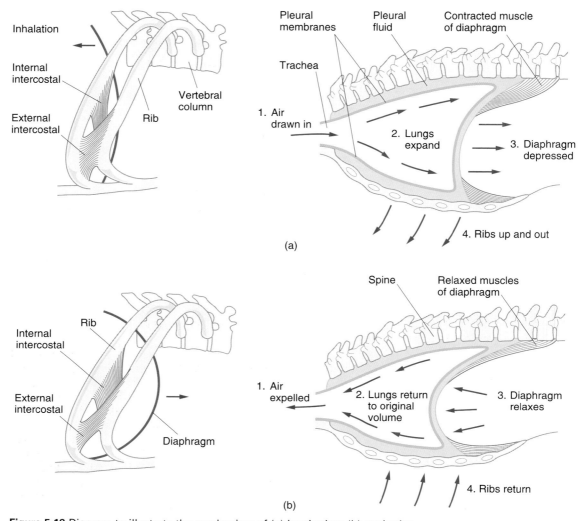

Figure 5.18 Diagram to illustrate the mechanism of (a) inspiration; (b) expiration

Factors affecting lung function

Lung function in the dog and cat can be affected by several conditions. Pneumothorax, or air in the pleural cavity, results in the lung being unable to inflate. Pyothorax, or pus in the pleural cavity, and haemothorax, blood in the pleural cavity, may also prevent expansion of the lungs during inspiration, as can a tumour either within the lungs themselves or within the mediastinum. A ruptured diaphragm will also prevent lung inflation as the diaphragm will be unable to flatten to increase the volume of the thoracic cavity. Pulmonary congestion and pulmonary oedema associated with heart disease

are frequently associated with an enlarged heart, and can also affect functioning of the lungs. There are many more conditions that can affect lung function; those mentioned above are probably the most commonly seen pulmonary conditions in general practice.

Control of respiration

The respiratory rate varies depending upon the size of the animal. Larger individuals have a rate that is at the lower end of the scale for their species. The respiratory centre in the medulla oblongata and pons of the hindbrain is responsible for the

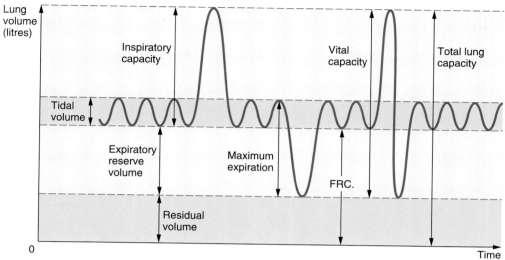

Figure 5.19 Spirometer tracing demonstrating the relationship between lung capacity and respiratory volume

---

The normal respiratory rate of the dog and cat is:

Dog   10–30 breaths per minute
Cat   20–30 breaths per minute

---

underlying, unconscious, event of respiration which is under the control of both neural and chemical feedback.

Neural control of respiration

Specialized receptor cells in the walls of the bronchioles of the lungs detect the degree to which the walls are stretched or distended. Impulses from these stretch receptors inhibit inspiration when the lungs are stretched and stimulate inspiration when the lungs are deflated. This is known as the Hering-Breuer reflex. Impulses from the stretch receptors travel to the respiratory centre in the brain via the vagus nerve.

Baroreceptors within the carotid and aortic sinuses monitor the degree of stretch of the vessels as an indicator of blood pressure. Stimulation of the receptors also affects the respiratory centre of the brain. When blood pressure rises, the respiratory rate falls and when blood pressure falls the respiratory rate increases.

Pain, fever, or impulses from exercising limbs all cause an increase in the rate and depth of respiration.

Chemical control of respiration

pH is detected by specialized receptors called chemoreceptors. Central chemoreceptors are situated on the surface of the medulla oblongata. They are stimulated by a lowering of pH (due to an increase in the levels of dissolved CO_2) in the CSF around the brain and spinal cord. This directly reflects any change in blood pH. An increase in the level of dissolved CO_2 will cause a lowering of the pH of the CSF that will stimulate the chemoreceptors. This results in an increase in both the rate and depth of respiration, the effect of which will be to eliminate any excess CO_2.

Peripheral chemoreceptors are located in the aortic arch and carotid body, close to the carotid artery. These receptors are stimulated by a fall in the oxygen content of the blood and stimulate the respiratory centre to increase the depth and rate of respiration. If CO_2 levels are also increased, the sensitivity of these receptors to a fall in oxygen, is increased. It is interesting to note that a fall in the oxygen content of the blood on its own is not a very effective stimulus to increase respiration. A rise in dissolved CO_2 content is a much more powerful stimulus. Animals that are subjected to breathing air low in oxygen content show no sense of suffocation and will very often collapse from oxygen deprivation before an increase in respiratory effort due to rising levels of dissolved CO_2 is observed.

Review questions

1. Which of the following is the first site at which fat digestion occurs in the alimentary tract?
   (a) mouth
   (b) stomach
   (c) duodenum
   (d) jejunum

2. Which of the following is not a region of the stomach?
   (a) fundus
   (b) pylorus
   (c) cardus
   (d) cardia

3. In young animals, where is the enzyme rennin secreted?
   (a) stomach
   (b) mouth
   (c) duodenum
   (d) jejunum

4. What is the name given to the milky white secretion leaving the stomach?
   (a) gastric juice
   (b) chyle
   (c) gastrin
   (d) chyme

5. Which of the following statements is correct?
   (a) the ileum is the terminal section of the small intestine
   (b) the bile duct enters the small intestine at the jejunum
   (c) the function of the duodenum is absorption of the products of digestion
   (d) the function of the ileum is digestion

6. Which of the following muscle types forms the wall of the small intestine?
   (a) skeletal muscle
   (b) striated muscle
   (c) smooth muscle
   (d) cardiac muscle

7. In which part of the small intestine would you find villi?
   (a) stomach
   (b) duodenum
   (c) ileum
   (d) colon

8. Fats that are digested and absorbed into lacteals are then carried almost directly into the
   (a) cisterna chyli
   (b) hepatic vein
   (c) portal vein
   (d) right azygous vein

9. The stomach of the dog produces hydrochloric acid, mucus and
   (a) amylase
   (b) bile salts
   (c) pepsin
   (d) trypsin

10. The process by which rabbits appear to eat their own faeces is called:
    (a) hind gut fermentation
    (b) caecal recycling
    (c) coprophagia
    (d) faecal nutrition

11. Name the two main processes involved with digestion.

12. What is the dentition of an adult dog?

13. Name the four pairs of salivary glands.

14. Describe peristalsis.

15. Name the end products of digestion of the following:
    (a) fats
    (b) proteins
    (c) carbohydrates

16. Describe the role of enterokinase during digestion.

17. Describe the function of bile in the digestive process.

18. Describe the fate of excess glucose on reaching the liver.

19. List the gastric secretions and briefly describe their functions.

20. State what is secreted by the Crypts of Lieberkhun.

21. The glomerular filtrate consists of:
    (a) water and waste products from the circulation
    (b) plasma without the larger plasma proteins
    (c) blood without cells or plasma proteins
    (d) none of the above

22. The filtration pressure is:
    (a) equal to the systolic blood pressure
    (b) equal to the diastolic blood pressure
    (c) the pressure of the fluid in the Bowman's capsule
    (d) the difference in pressure between that of the blood in the glomerulus and the fluid in the first part of the nephron

23. Water absorption along the nephron is controlled by:
    (a) anti-diuretic hormone
    (b) aldosterone
    (c) renin
    (d) angiotensin

24. Glucose is only seen in urine:
    (a) if the animal is suffering from diabetes insipidus
    (b) in conjunction with ketones
    (c) when the body's glycogen reserves are complete
    (d) when the renal threshold for glucose is exceeded
25. In which part of the nephron does selective reabsorption occur:
    (a) glomerulus
    (b) Bowman's capsule
    (c) proximal convoluted tubule
    (d) collecting duct
26. In which part of the nephron is there a counter current multiplier effect?
    (a) loop of Henle
    (b) distal convoluted tubule
    (c) proximal convoluted tubule
    (d) collecting duct
27. Where is the Juxtaglomerular Apparatus located?
    (a) the glomerulus
    (b) the proximal convoluted tubule
    (c) the distal convoluted tubule
    (d) the collecting duct
28. Which part of the nephron is associated with acid/base balance?
    (a) the glomerulus
    (b) the proximal convoluted tubule
    (c) the distal convoluted tubule
    (d) the collecting duct
29. Approximately what percentage of glomerular filtrate is reabsorbed along the nephron?
    (a) 50%
    (b) 70%
    (c) 80%
    (d) 90%
30. Which of the following structures lies predominantly within the medulla?
    (a) loop of Henle
    (b) distal convoluted tubule
    (c) proximal convoluted tubule
    (d) glomerulus
31. Explain the cause of diabetes insipidus.
32. Explain the function of the distal convoluted tubule.
33. Describe the role of ADH in the conservation of water within the body.
34. Name the two hormones secreted by the Juxtaglomerular Apparatus (JGA).
35. Name the hormone that exerts its effects on the JGA.

36. Draw a diagram to illustrate the structure of a nephron.
37. Explain the difference between the urethra and the ureter.
38. Explain the process occurring at the proximal convoluted tubule.
39. Name the type of transport occurring when sodium and chloride ions are moved against the concentration gradient from the filtrate into the peritubular fluid of the loop of Henle.
40. Which of the following statements is correct? During inspiration:
    (a) the muscles of the diaphragm relax
    (b) the diaphragm becomes flattened and lowered
    (c) there is an increase in intrathoracic pressure
    (d) the external intercostal muscles relax
41. Which of the following is not produced by the respiratory process?
    (a) nutrients
    (b) energy
    (c) carbon dioxide
    (d) water
42. Oxygen comprises approximately what percentage of expired air?
    (a) 3%
    (b) 12%
    (c) 16%
    (d) 20%
43. Which of the following represents the passage of air through the respiratory tract?
    (a) trachea, bronchi, bronchioles, alveoli
    (b) trachea, bronchioles, bronchi, alveoli
    (c) trachea, bronchi, alveoli, bronchioles
    (d) trachea, alveoli, bronchi, bronchioles
44. What is the normal respiratory rate of the cat?
    (a) 5–10 breaths per minute
    (b) 10–20 breaths per minute
    (c) 20–30 breaths per minute
    (d) 30–40 breaths per minute
45. Specialized stretch receptors in the walls of the bronchioles detect the degree of distension and inhibit inspiration when the lungs are stretched and stimulate inspiration when the lungs are deflated. This process is known as:
    (a) the respiratory reflex
    (b) the inspiratory reflex
    (c) the Herring Breuer reflex
    (d) the Messiner's reflex

46. Baroreceptors that detect changes in blood pressure are located:
    (a) within the walls of the lungs
    (b) within the capillaries of the alveoli
    (c) within the medulla of the brain
    (d) within the aortic and carotid sinuses
47. Chemoreceptors are located:
    (a) within the walls of the lungs
    (b) within the medulla of the brain
    (c) within the aortic arch and carotid body
    (d) b and c
48. The 'C' shaped rings of the trachea are formed from:
    (a) hyaline cartilage
    (b) smooth muscle
    (c) fibrocartilage
    (d) bone
49. The vocal cords are located in the:
    (a) pharynx
    (b) larynx
    (c) epiglottis
    (d) trachea
50. Bronchodilation is caused by activity in the:
    (a) parasympathetic nervous system
    (b) sympathetic nervous system
    (c) somatic nervous system
    (d) all of the above
51. Draw a diagram to illustrate the process of external respiration.
52. Explain the reasons for the nasal chamber being highly vascular with a lining of mucous epithelium.
53. Describe the function of the soft palate.
54. Explain the purpose of surfactant.
55. Draw a diagram to illustrate the lungs and pleural membranes.
56. Name the term used to describe the amount of air breathed in or out at rest.
57. List four conditions that may reduce lung function.
58. Explain the role of chemoreceptors in the control of respiration.
59. Describe the movements of the diaphragm during inspiration and expiration.
60. Name the two areas of the brain that are associated with the control of respiration.

Survival, development and defence

6.1 The integument

Structure of the integument/skin
Specialization of the integument
Hair
Specialized glands

Introduction

An animal is under constant attack from invading organisms that can threaten its health, such as bacteria, viruses, and fungi, as well as environmental toxins. It is critical for the survival of the individual that these invaders can be fought off without serious damage to the health of the animal. In the following chapter we will consider the mechanisms on which the animal can draw to defend itself against invasion.

Structure of the integument/skin

Skin is composed of three layers of tissue: the outer **epidermis**, the middle **dermis** and the inner **hypodermis** or **subcutaneous layer** (see Figure 6.1).

The outer epidermis is formed from stratified squamous epithelial tissue and can itself be considered in four layers. The lower layer is called the **stratum germinativum** or **stratum basale** as it is in this layer that the cells divide rapidly to replace those that are shed from the surface. Moving outwards from the stratum germinativum or basale, the cells become flatter and are interwoven with strands of the structural protein, keratin, that gives the skin strength and some

Probably the most logical of defence barriers is the integument, or skin, to which it is more commonly referred. In its protective function it can be considered as a non-specific defence mechanism. It provides a physical barrier that prevents the entry of many pathogens (organisms that cause disease). It has many other functions and is an extremely complex organ. These functions will be discussed in the following chapter.

waterproof properties. This layer is known as the **stratum granulosum**. The adjacent layer is the **stratum lucidum** and it is here that the cells can be seen to lose their nuclei before entering the most external layer, the **stratum corneum** where the cells are completely flattened and keratinization is complete. It is this layer that is sloughed off during the lifetime of the animal and is constantly replaced by the rapidly dividing cells of the stratum germinativum or basale. The entire epidermal layer is avascular.

The dermis forms the middle of the three layers and is comprised of dense connective tissue that is vascular. It is this layer that contains the nerve fibres, nerve endings and elastic fibres in addition to the hair follicles, and the sweat and sebaceous glands that grow down from the epidermis.

The hypodermis or subcutaneous layer lies beneath the dermis and consists of loose connective tissue. It is this layer that contains the subcutaneous fat stores.

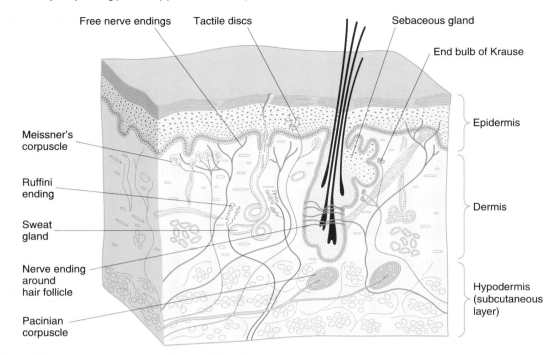

Figure 6.1 Structure and nerve endings of the skin

Functions of the integument

Functions of the integument are many and varied. Some are more apparent than others as will become clear in the following section.

1. **Barrier protection**

   One of the main functions of the skin is to provide a barrier between the animal and its environment. Epidermal cells prevent the entry of many pathogens, while accessory structures such as hair protect against mechanical abrasion and prevent some hazardous substances or insects coming into contact with the skin. Specialized secretions such as those from the sebaceous and sweat glands flush the surface, washing away pathogens. They may also contain **bacteriocidal** enzymes (**lysozymes**) and **antibodies**. Mucus on many epithelial surfaces (e.g. in the respiratory tract and digestive tract) traps foreign bodies, while in the stomach hydrochloric acid destroys many potential pathogens. There are many epithelial and glandular secretions that help to protect the body from invasion.

2. **Maintenance of homeostasis**

   The skin maintains homeostasis via two principal mechanisms. Firstly it acts to conserve water within the body. This is particularly evident in species such as reptiles where the skin is covered with scales, further reducing water loss in warmer climates. Its second homeostatic function is in the maintenance of body temperature. Heat loss can be controlled from the surface of the skin by the dilation or constriction of blood vessels close to the surface. The production of sweat also allows heat to be lost as it evaporates from the surface of the skin. The presence of hair can also be utilized to trap an insulating layer of air close to the skin in cold conditions, thereby reducing heat lost. This partly explains why the majority of breeds of dog that have evolved in colder climates have a thick, dense fur. In some animals the presence of a subcutaneous layer of fat can also act as insulation.

3. **Excretion**

   The skin acts as an organ of excretion through the presence of two types of exocrine glands. Sebaceous glands (see Figure 6.1) produce an oily secretion called sebum, which is secreted into the hair follicles and onto the surface of the skin. Sebum is a mixture of triglycerides, cholesterol, proteins, and electrolytes. Its prime function is to lubricate the hair and skin whilst helping to prevent the growth of some bacteria. It also acts to waterproof the hair and skin.

Sweat glands are the major excretory glands of the skin, although when compared to the entire excretory capacity of the animal, they contribute very little. Apocrine sweat glands are coiled and can be associated with the hair follicles (refer to Figure 6.1). They produce a secretion that has a distinctive odour, containing pheromones, and is thought to be associated with recognition of a mate and marking territory. Eccrine sweat glands (also referred to as merocrine sweat glands) produce sweat which is composed of water, sodium chloride, urea, lactic acid, and potassium ions. Sweat is produced as a means of regulating heat loss. Eccrine glands are present in the skin of the nose and footpads of the cat and dog.

In the female mammal during pregnancy, mammary gland tissue develops and the production of milk occurs following parturition. This will be discussed later in this chapter.

Ceruminous glands are modified sweat glands that are located in the external ear canal. The secretion, known as cerumen (ear wax), helps to protect the tympanic membrane by trapping dust and foreign bodies that enter the canal. Excessive production in some cats and dogs can cause problems leading to ear infections and irritation.

4. **Synthesis of vitamin D$_3$**
   The cells of the epidermis, when exposed to ultraviolet (UV) light can convert a vitamin D precursor into vitamin D$_3$ or cholecalciferol. This is converted by the liver into an intermediate compound which is used by the kidneys to synthesize the hormone calcitriol. Calcitriol is an important hormone that is necessary for the absorption of dietary calcium and phosphorus from the intestine. In cases where an animal is not allowed exposure to the correct UV wavelengths of light, e.g. rabbits kept permanently in dark hutches and reptiles kept without UV lights, the animal is at risk of developing hypovitaminosis D (deficiency of vitamin D) or rickets to which it is sometimes referred. Bone growth and maintenance is impaired due to the inability to absorb dietary calcium and phosphorus and this may lead to malformations and fractures.

5. **Storage**
   In healthy animals a subcutaneous layer of fat is stored within the adipose tissue of the hypodermis. This can become excessive if the animal is obese or depleted if the animal is undernourished. As well as acting as an energy reserve the subcutaneous fat layer also contributes towards a degree of mechanical protection in addition to providing an insulating layer, preventing heat loss in cold climates.

6. **Sensation**
   The integument is often described as the largest sensory organ of the body and contains specialized receptor cells within the dermis that can detect chemical, mechanical or thermal stimuli (see Chapter 2). It was originally thought that each receptor could detect only one stimulus, although it would now appear that receptors can respond to more than one type of stimulus. Their purpose is to protect the animal against injury and damage.

7. **Pigmentation**
   Specialized cells called melanocytes are located at the junction of the dermis and epidermis. They produce a pigment, melanin, which protects the animal from the damaging effects of UV light, in addition to having a camouflage function in most animals. The distribution and structure of melanin determines the colour of the coat of an animal. Animals that lack the genetic material required to produce melanin are called albinos and are at risk from the damaging effects of UV light due to their lack of protection. Sun-tan creams with a high UV-protection factor can help prevent this damage if applied to the extremities, e.g. ear tips and nose, during the summer months.

8. **Accessory structures**
   Certain accessory structures, such as hair, feathers, claws, and beaks, are associated with the integument of certain species. Those relating to the dog and cat will be discussed in the following section.

Specialization of the integument

In certain areas of the cat and dog the integument is slightly different from the generalized structure described above.

The footpads

The foot of the cat and dog has four toes, each with a claw and a digital footpad. There is also a central pad known as the metatarsal or metacarpal pad on the hind limb or fore limb, respectively. The fore limb also possesses a carpal pad. A dew claw (digit 1) with a digital pad may also be present, if it has not been removed. Very occasionally, a dew claw may be present on the hind limbs, although these are frequently removed as they are at great risk of being torn. Figure 6.2 illustrates the palmar aspect of the fore limb.

The epidermis of the skin of the footpads is thickened and hairless. There is a collection of adipose tissue in the dermal region that forms the digital cushion and the dermis itself is thick and vascular. The structure of the epithelium differs between the dog and the cat. Dogs have an epithelial layer that is arranged in conical papillae, giving a rough feel. These can wear down if the dog is routinely exercised on hard surfaces. The pads of cats have a much smoother epithelial surface. Whilst sweat glands are absent in the haired skin of the cat and the dog, they are present in the hairless foot pads, consequently the feet are capable of considerable heat loss and in animals at risk from hypothermia they should be covered, to prevent unnecessary loss of heat.

Skin of the nose

Nasal skin (rhinarium) is also hairless and contains a high proportion of keratin, giving additional toughness. It is also heavily pigmented in the majority of animals, to protect the tissue from UV radiation. It should be moist in the healthy animal and contains numerous sweat glands, indicating that this area also contributes to heat loss. Animals that live in cold climates often sleep with their noses covered by their paws. This helps to warm the air before entering the nasal cavity in addition to preventing heat loss.

The scrotum

The skin of the scrotum has a thin layer of epithelium and a sparse distribution of hair. There is very little subcutaneous adipose tissue as the testes should be kept comparatively cool to facilitate sperm production. Their position within the body also keeps the temperature below that of the body.

Claws

Claws have several functions in the dog and cat. They can be used during attack and defence, during hunting (particularly so in the cat), for climbing, to aid grip on rough terrain, and also to mark territory through the scratching of soil or trees.

The hard outer part of the claw grows from a specialized part of the epidermis called the coronary band. This is illustrated in Figure 6.3.

The coronary band grows in two sheets that form the wall of the claw and cover the ungual process of the third phalanx. A softer type of epidermis forms the sole of the claw that lies between the two walls. The vascular dermis lies

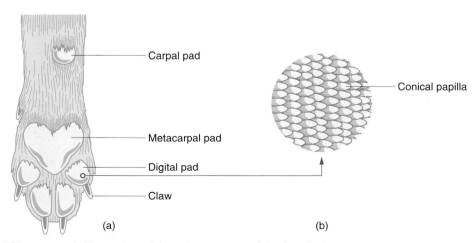

Carpal pad

Metacarpal pad

Digital pad

Claw

Conical papilla

(a)   (b)

Figure 6.2 Diagrammatic illustration of the palmar aspect of the fore limb

There are five major differences in the structure of the claw between the dog and cat.

1. Claws of the dog are tubular whereas those of the cat are laterally flattened.
2. Cat's claws are brittle and easily shed whereas those of the dog are not.
3. Cats can retract their claws when not in use; those of the dog are not retractable.
4. Cat's claws are less pigmented than those of the dog.
5. Claws of the cat are sharper than those of the dog.

between the horn of the claw and the bone of the third phalanx. Considerable care must be taken, particularly in animals with heavily pigmented claws, that this region is not cut whilst trimming the claw. Growth of claws can be rapid and, if not naturally worn down or trimmed, they can grow round into the footpad. This is particularly common with dew claws. Cats should be provided with and trained to use, a scratching post, as this facilitates the maintenance of healthy claws and protects furniture and carpets!

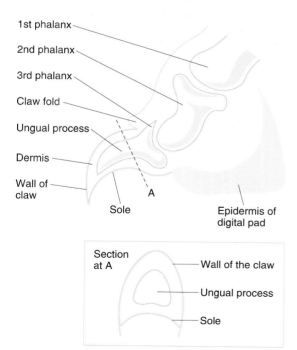

1st phalanx
2nd phalanx
3rd phalanx
Claw fold
Ungual process
Dermis
Wall of claw
Sole
A
Epidermis of digital pad

Section at A
Wall of the claw
Ungual process
Sole

Figure 6.3 Anatomy of the canine digit and claw

Hair

Hair covers most of the surface of the skin in the dog and cat. It has several functions that contribute to protection and survival.

Through pilo-erection (the raising of the hair) a layer of air can be trapped close to the skin that acts as insulation in cold weather. This aids temperature regulation to some degree. In certain species the hair is pigmented at the extremities, e.g. the tips of ears, nose and feet of a Siamese cat. The darker colour reduces heat loss from these areas. Some owners may request that their Siamese cat is spayed via a ventral midline incision rather than the more usual flank incision. This is due to the fact that the hair may grow back darker than the rest as it has been at a lower temperature (due to the site being clipped). This is far less obvious if a ventral midline incision has been used.

Different hair types can be identified, each with a role to play in the protection of the animal. Outer **guard hairs** form the long top coat. Sebum, secreted by the sebaceous glands, coats the hair shaft, protecting it and conditioning the skin whilst conferring some waterproofing properties. In addition, each guard hair is attached to an arrector pili muscle that can raise the hair for insulation. Guard hairs grow from primary follicles, each follicle producing only one hair. The undercoat is formed from **wool hairs** that are shorter and more dense. Their primary role is one of insulation and their numbers increase during autumn in preparation for the colder winter months. Breeds that have evolved to live in cooler climates usually have thick undercoats. Wool hairs grow from secondary follicles and there are several hairs produced by each follicle. **Vibrissae** are the third hair type and form the thick whiskers. Their function is tactile, as at their root they have nerve endings that respond to movement of the hair. Their distribution is specialized, being primarily located around the upper lips, eyes, and cheek regions.

Often overlooked, hair also has a role in communication between individual animals. Raised hackles indicate that the dog is fearful and/or likely to be aggressive, as does a 'bottle brush' tail in the cat. This has evolved from the principle that making oneself appear larger is more likely to frighten an adversary. Whether this works or not remains open to debate.

Finally, we should not overlook the role that man's influence has had upon the selection of breeds for their individual appearance. Many toy breeds that were selected purely for companionship have long coats that will have increased their appeal as companions.

Specialized glands

In addition to the ceruminous and mammary glands discussed earlier, there are two other areas of specialized sebaceous glands.

The **tail glands** are located on the dorsal surface of the tail around the fifth to seventh coccygeal vertebrae in the dog, while in the cat they run along the entire length of the tail. Hair in this region may be coarser than normal and the skin may appear more yellow due to the glandular secretion. It is thought that the secretion may aid species recognition by olfaction (smell). This area may become particularly prominent in middle aged/elderly dogs when the hair can become sparse and the cells become hyperplastic (abnormally enlarged).

Anal sacs are located between the internal and external sphincters of the anus. They consist of numerous sebaceous glands that secrete a brown, oil-like secretion with a distinctive odour. It is thought that this secretion assists in individual recognition in dogs. In the healthy dog, defecation results in the emptying of the sacs. It is not uncommon, however, for these sacs to become inflamed and infected, requiring manual expression and sometimes surgical removal if the case is severe and does not respond to more conservative treatment.

6.2 The defence function

> Non-specific defences
> Specific defences: immunity

Introduction

In the section above we considered the many functions of the integument, although from a defence perspective, the skin can be described as having a non-specific defence function. In this section, we discuss other non-specific defences relating to the body.

Non-specific defences

Phagocytic cells

These cells respond in the first instance to invasion by pathogens and include neutrophils and eosinophils (discussed in more detail in Chapter 4 dealing with the transport of blood). These polymorphonuclear leucocytes enter tissue when there is injury and/or infection. Neutrophils phagocytize damaged cells and invading bacteria whereas eosinophils ingest pathogens that have been coated with antibodies.

Macrophages (sometimes referred to as **histiocytes**) are derived from monocytes. These are present in every tissue in the body and these collections are sometimes termed the **reticuloendothelial system**. Macrophages are capable of a varied response to an invading pathogen. They may engulf the pathogen and destroy it with lysosomal enzymes, they may bind to the pathogen and remove it from the circulation (but are unable to destroy it without the assistance of other cells), or they may destroy the pathogen by the release of toxic chemicals.

Immunological surveillance

Natural killer cells (NK cells) recognize and destroy any of the body's own cells that are abnormal. They are responsible for monitoring the cells of the body, a process called immunological surveillance. NK cells detect the abnormal antigens that are present on the surface of abnormal or foreign cells, following which they bind to the cells and release a substance that attacks the membrane. This results in the abnormal cell being unable to maintain its own internal environment and causes cellular destruction.

Interferons

Interferons are small proteins which are released by macrophages, lymphocytes, and cells infected by viruses. They bind to the membranes of healthy cells, triggering the production of antiviral proteins in neighbouring cells. Should these cells be invaded by a virus, the antiviral proteins prevent viral replication within the cells.

Complement

Plasma contains complement proteins that assist with and enhance the action of antibodies. The systems involved are complex and are not within the scope of this text. They can, however, contribute towards the inflammatory response through the attraction of phagocytes to an injured area, the enhancement of phagocytosis, and the destruction of cell membranes. For more details about complement activation (Reeves, 1987).

Inflammatory response

Inflammation is a local response of tissue to injury, which can be caused by a variety of stimuli. Damaged cells and tissues stimulate mast cells, basophils, and platelets, to release histamine. Mast cells also release serotonin and heparin with injured cells releasing kinins and prostaglandins. These chemicals act to increase the permeability of the capillaries in the injured area which allows an increased number of white blood cells (e.g. neutrophils and macrophages) to migrate to the injured site. This helps to protect against infection and removes damaged cells from the area. Vasodilation also causes a local increase of temperature which is thought to help with defence by increasing the activity of certain antimicrobial enzymes. Eosinophils are also supplied in increased numbers to the site of an injury, where they are involved with the immune response (see below).

Fever or pyrexia

Certain pathogens can act as, or cause the release of, pyrogens, small proteins that reset the body's temperature-control thermostat in the hypothalamus of the brain. If this occurs, the body temperature increases and fever or pyrexia can occur, i.e. the body temperature is maintained at above 38.7°C (101.7°F). It is thought that, in some cases, pyrexia may have a beneficial effect by inhibiting the replication of some viruses and bacteria. However, it should be noted that the most probable benefit is that of raising metabolism, so that cellular reactions occur at a faster rate, which may help to combat the effects of disease.

Specific defence: immunity

Specific defences protect the animal against specific antigens, in contrast to the non-specific defences discussed in the previous section. For example, the animal may be resistant to infection by one particular strain of kennel cough, although it may be susceptible to a slightly different strain.

The majority of specific defences are acquired after the birth of the animal, following accidental or deliberate exposure to the particular pathogen. Acquired immunity can be **active**, for example, when the immunity is as a consequence of direct exposure to an antigen. In other cases, immunity is **passive**, for example, when the antibodies are transferred from one animal to another via the **placenta** or milk as in the case of a mother and her offspring. Some specific defences, however, are innate, i.e. present when the animal is born, irrespective of whether it has been exposed to the disease, and a consequence of the genetic make-up of the animal. An example is that dogs are not susceptible to feline leukaemia virus.

The cells primarily involved in the immune response are lymphocytes. There are two forms of lymphocytes, B-lymphocytes and T-lymphocytes. T-lymphocytes are formed from bone marrow tissue in the embryo and migrate to the thymus. During development of the foetus they become associated with the **lymphatic** tissue of the spleen, liver, and gut-associated-lymphoid-tissue or GALT (see the section on the lymphatic system below). B-lymphocytes are also formed from cells in the embryonic bone marrow and again, migrate to the lymphoid tissues. Together these two cells allow the animal to respond to specific antigens. T-lymphocytes attach themselves to antigens (e.g. viruses, parasites and fungi) and destroy them by the secretion of cytotoxic substances, lysosymes, or interferon (see above). This mode of action is often referred to as **cell-mediated** or **cellular immunity**. In contrast, B-lymphocytes produce antibodies that are specific to the invading antigen. These lymphocytes are responsible for the **antibody-related** or **humoral immunity**.

Antibodies

Antibodies are very large proteins called gamma globulins or immunoglobulins, that are present within the circulation as well as on the surface of T- and B-lymphocytes. The structure of an antibody is such that it can recognize a particular antigen (a substance that the body recognizes as being foreign, such as invading bacteria) and attach itself to it. On binding with the antigen, the antibody changes shape which results in its inactivation. Antibodies are only activated by specific antigens and the relationship between the two molecules is so specific that it is often referred to as a lock and key mechanism. Formation of an antibody–antigen complex causes the antigen to become inactive, e.g. through lysis, neutralization, or precipitation, allowing its subsequent destruction by phagocytic cells.

Other antibodies attach to the surface of certain invasive bacteria and prevent them adhering to mucous membranes, thus preventing their penetration into the tissues. When an antibody on a B-lymphocyte binds with an antigen, the B-lymphocyte is stimulated to replicate, to produce memory cells and plasma cells. The plasma cells produce immunoglobulins or antibodies, which appear in the bloodstream. Plasma cells have a relatively short lifespan while the memory cells are longer lived and continue to circulate once the original antigen has been destroyed. It is these cells that are capable of rapid proliferation should the animal be exposed to the same antigen again in the future. We have been able to exploit this to our advantage through the development of vaccines for many potentially fatal pathogens.

T-lymphocytes react in a slightly different way to B-lymphocytes. When an antigen binds to the surface antibody, they produce killer T cells and memory cells. Killer T cells attach themselves to cells containing the antigen and damage the cell membrane leading to its destruction. They are short-lived. Memory cells are also produced in larger numbers. These remain within the circulation and if the antigen is encountered again, they can differentiate very quickly into killer T cells. Helper T cells are also produced by T-lymphocytes when exposed to antigens. These helper cells are thought to contribute to the activation of B-lymphocytes by enhancing their replication and production of plasma cells and antibodies.

Immunological competence

This is the term given to the ability of an animal to produce an immune response on exposure to an antigen. During pregnancy, maternal antibodies are transferred across the placenta to the developing foetus. This is continued post-partum through the transfer of antibodies in colostrum in the first few days of lactation. Ideally, the newborn kitten or puppy should receive adequate colostrum within the first 24 hours of birth, as after this time the morphology of the intestinal mucosa changes,

preventing the absorption of large protein molecules such as antibodies. During the 8 weeks after birth, the levels of maternal antibodies in the circulation of puppies and kittens slowly decline and at 8 weeks they are very susceptible to pathogens, although they are able to produce their own antibodies when exposed to antigens. It is at about this age that many vaccines for the cat and dog are ideally administered (the exact age varies, depending upon the type of vaccine and manufacturer). Vaccines are designed to trigger the formation of antibodies to particular antigens, without causing the disease itself. This is achieved either by using synthetic vaccines that mimic the live pathogen very closely, by using killed antigens, or by using a live form of the antigen at a very low dose (often referred to as an attenuated vaccine).

Allergy

An allergic reaction is defined as an inappropriate or excessive response to an **antigen** or **allergen** (a substance which causes an allergic response). Allergies can manifest themselves in many ways. Some animals have an allergy to certain food products, commonly wheat and certain types of animal protein. Others may exhibit an allergic response to flea bites, the house dust mite, or synthetic materials, or to inhaled allergens such as pollen. The list is varied and growing continuously as the field of veterinary science expands its knowledge in this area. During the sensitization phase, on first exposure to the allergen, the animal does not usually exhibit an allergic response. The specific antibodies produced by this initial exposure are unusual in that they bind to mast cells and basophils. When the animal next encounters the allergen, the mast cells and basophils release histamine and prostaglandins into the surrounding tissue. This causes a massive inflammatory and allergic response that can be very severe in certain individual animals and in some cases, life-threatening.

Anaphylaxis

This is a specific type of severe allergic response where exposure to the allergen affects the mast cells within the body, producing a very rapid allergic reaction. Symptoms include swelling and oedema in the dermis of the skin, caused by changes in capillary permeability, and contraction of smooth muscle lining the respiratory system, resulting in bronchospasm or difficulty in breathing. A severe response can result in peripheral vasodilation which can cause a dramatic fall in blood pressure that may lead to circulatory collapse. Hence the name to which this is commonly referred, **anaphylactic shock**.

6.3 The lymphatic system

Circulation of tissue fluid
Structure of the lymphatic system
Lymphatic tissue

Introduction

As blood passes through the capillaries of the circulatory system, gaseous exchange occurs between the cells of the tissue and the blood, as discussed in Chapter 5. Gases such as oxygen and carbon dioxide are carried in the blood dissolved in solution. For gaseous exchange to occur (along with the exchange of nutrients and waste products) fluid and dissolved gases pass out of the capillaries and circulate around the tissue cells forming interstitial fluid (or tissue fluid). As this is a continuous process, there has to be a mechanism for the draining away of interstitial fluid from the tissues, other than by return at the venous end of capillary beds (see Figure 6.4), as it constantly leaks out of the capillaries. The lymphatic system acts as a drain for this interstitial fluid, in addition

to having other important functions that will be discussed within this chapter.

Circulation of tissue fluid

The diagram in Figure 6.4 illustrates the circulation of tissue fluid within the animal. Fluid from the blood arriving at the tissue moves through the permeable capillary membranes into the spaces surrounding the cells of the tissue due to a difference in hydrostatic pressure between the blood and tissue fluid. Large molecules such as plasma proteins (e.g. albumin and globulin) and corpuscles remain within the circulatory system, as they are normally unable to pass through the capillary cell walls. Consequently, interstitial fluid is clear, watery, and similar in composition to plasma, except that it does not contain plasma proteins and corpuscles. As the fluid moves from the circulatory system it carries dissolved gases, nutrients and water to the cells. Waste products from cellular metabolism such as carbon dioxide and urea diffuse out of the cells and into the interstitial fluid.

Not all of the fluid can return directly to the circulatory system as the difference in hydrostatic pressure is not large enough at the venous end of the capillary bed. The fluid which is unable to return via this route is collected and returned to the circulatory system by another set of vessels which form the lymphatic system. Lymphatic vessels permeate throughout most body tissues and are blind-ended, being a one-way transport system. Fluid within these vessels is termed **lymph**.

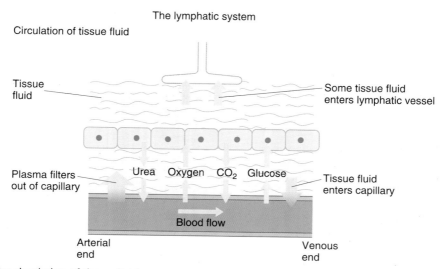

Figure 6.4 The circulation of tissue fluid

The lymphatic system has vessels within every tissue of the body except those of the central nervous system. These vessels are similar in structure to veins, having thin walls, although they are far more numerous. They also possess valves along their length (again, similar to veins) in order to prevent backward lymph flowing. Periodically, the vessels pass through collections of lymphatic tissue known as lymph nodes.

The structure of the lymphatic system

Lymph nodes

Lymph nodes vary in size and are distributed throughout the body (see Figure 6.5). They are comprised of cells similar to lymphocytes, held together by layers of connective tissue, known as trabeculae. The lymph passes through the nodes where it is filtered to remove bacteria and debris. When an area of tissue is infected, the lymph nodes within that region swell and become tender (lymphadenopathy), as the infected lymph is filtered by the node and the bacteria are destroyed. If the bacteria within the lymph are not destroyed they are at risk of entering the bloodstream when the animal may develop septicaemia. Enlarged superficial lymph nodes may be palpated and used as an aid in diagnosis. The lymph nodes also produce fresh lymphocytes which enter the circulatory system.

In addition to acting as a filter, the lymph nodes also contain macrophages, whose function is to aid in the recognition of antigens so that they can be destroyed by B-lymphocytes produced within the lymph node. The macrophages are also thought to contribute to the removal of dead cells and bacteria by phagocytosis. The lymph nodes contain cells that produce T-lymphocytes (see Specific defence: immunity, above).

Lymphatic ducts

After passing through the lymph nodes, the lymphatic vessels drain into larger lymphatic ducts. There are three major lymphatic ducts within the cat and dog, the thoracic duct, the tracheal duct and the right lymphatic duct. These are illustrated in Figure 6.5.

The thoracic duct is the largest duct of the lymphatic system, starting in a small pouch called the cisterna chyli located in the dorsal abdomen. Vessels from the hind limbs, pelvic and abdominal organs empty into this duct. As it travels cranially, other lymphatic vessels join it including the tracheal duct. It drains into the cranial vena cava, returning the lymph to the main circulatory system. The right lymphatic duct is smaller than the tracheal and thoracic ducts, and drains the lymphatic vessels from the right side of the head,

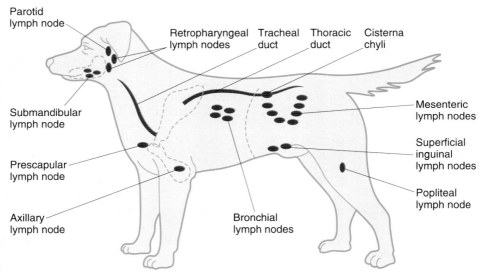

Figure 6.5 The main lymph nodes and lymphatic ducts of the dog

thorax and right fore limb. It empties into the right subclavian vein. Within the larger ducts the flow of lymph is facilitated by the presence of valves, contraction of the body muscles, and negative pressure in the larger ducts close to the heart, the heart creating suction in the ducts as it relaxes following contraction.

Lacteals

As discussed in Chapter 5, fatty acids and glycerol from the digestion of dietary fats are converted into chylomicrons by the addition of a protein coat. These chylomicrons enter the lacteals of the lymphatic system within the villus of the digestive epithelium and pass further along the lymphatic system before finally entering the circulation through the subclavian vein.

Lymphatic tissue

In addition to the lymph nodes, other collections of lymphatic tissue are located within the body of the dog and cat.

The thymus

The thymus is found in the mediastinum and is thought to be an important site of lymphocyte production in young animals. It decreases in size as the animal ages and the lymphatic tissue is replaced with fat. It is thought to be an important contributor to the resistance of young animals to certain diseases and infection through the production of T-lymphocytes (see Specific defence: immunity). It also produces hormones known as thymosins that are involved in the maturation of the thymus and other lymphoid tissue.

The spleen

The spleen is a purple/red organ located in the left cranial abdomen. It consists of splenic pulp, containing cells of various types, contained within a capsule of fibrous tissue. It is involved with the production of lymphocytes, the initiation of the immune response, the breakdown of red blood cells and storage of iron, and the removal of abnormal blood cells and other components in the blood through phagocytosis. It is not uncommon for the spleen to be damaged, either through direct physical injury, e.g. when an animal is involved in a road traffic accident, or through infection, inflammation or the proliferation of cancer cells. Treatment may involve the complete removal of the spleen (a splenectomy). Fortunately, the animal is able to survive without its spleen as other areas within the body are capable of taking over the organ's functions.

Galt and Peyer's patches

Gut-associated lymphoid tissue (GALT) is a collection of lymphoid tissue associated with the digestive system and Peyer's patches are collections of lymphoid tissue specifically located in the wall of the small intestine. These tissues assist with the battle against invading antigens from their location within the intestinal mucosa. Other areas of lymphoid tissue are located within other areas of mucosa, such as the tonsils (located in the pharynx). In some texts these types of tissue are collectively referred to as MALT (mucosa-associated lymphoid tissue).

6.4 Reproduction

> The male reproductive system
> The female reproductive system
> Mating and pregnancy
> Parturition
> Lactation

Introduction

Without the ability to reproduce, species would become extinct. Reproduction can be sexual, involving the combination of genes from both the male and female, or asexual, when the genes of the offspring are from one parent only. Asexual reproduction does not occur in mammals, being more common in certain species of plants. It produces offspring that are genetically identical to their parents in every way. Mammals reproduce by sexual reproduction, the offspring being a result of the random combination of the genes of two parents. As a result, the offspring are genetically different from either parent. They can be said to exhibit genetic variation.

For the survival of the bloodline of a successful individual at least one copy of its genes must be passed on to the next generation. Reproductive strategies for dealing with this have evolved two very different approaches. The first approach involves the production of larger numbers of female and male **gametes** (reproductive cells, e.g. eggs and sperm), often thousands, which are released into the environment at the same time (**external reproduction**). It is left to chance as to whether or not they meet, develop, and survive into adulthood. Neither parent is involved in protecting the offspring and consequently the survival rate is poor. However, a few individuals usually survive into adulthood and consequently the reproductive strategy is a success. This method of reproduction is commonly seen in many species of fish and amphibians. Mammals and other terrestrial species adopt a far less random approach and have evolved to allow the release of the male gametes into the female animal, thereby greatly increasing the chance of fertilization. This is known as **internal fertilization**. This mechanism, together with the increased parental care of the developing offspring, both before and after birth, which has evolved among mammalian species, has greatly increased the chance of survival of individual mammalian offspring.

The male reproductive system

The male reproductive system is adapted for the production, storage, and nutrition of the male gamete or **spermatozoon** (pl = **spermatozoa** or sperm), its transport into the reproductive tract of

the female and the production of male reproductive hormones called androgens, e.g. testosterone. The major parts of the reproductive tract of the dog and tom cat are illustrated in Figures 6.6 and 6.7.

The testes

There are two testes, sometimes referred to as the male **gonads** or **testicles** (sing = testis). During gestation, they descend from the abdomen, through the inguinal ring in the wall of the abdomen to lie in the scrotal region. In the dog this area lies between the hind legs whereas in the tom cat it is located on the perineum below the anus. In some individuals, the testes fail to descend into the scrotum and remain within the abdomen or within the inguinal region. This is termed cryptorchidism. When one testis fails to descend the animal is said to be monorchid. It is necessary for the testes to be outside the body cavity, 2–3°C lower than body temperature, for the viable production of spermatozoa. The retained testes of monorchid and cryptorchid animals are unlikely to be productive. There is also an increased risk of the retained testis becoming cancerous and consequently they should be removed. In a monorchid animal it is also recommended that the descended testis be removed

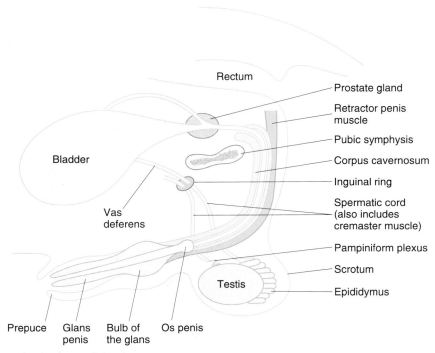

Figure 6.6 Reproductive tract of the dog

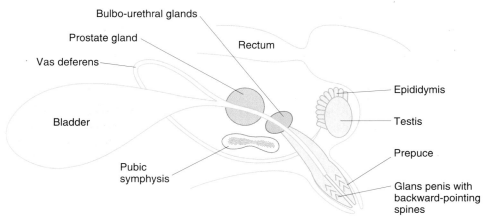

Figure 6.7 Reproductive tract of the tom cat

to prevent the animal siring offspring, as the condition is thought to be hereditary. In an entire male animal the cremaster muscle, originating from the internal abdominal oblique muscle of the abdominal wall, allows the raising and lowering of the testes within the scrotum, dependent on the external temperature.

The formation and development of spermatozoa

At puberty there is a surge in the production of testosterone in the male animal. This stimulates the production of luteinizing hormone (LH), sometimes called interstitial-cell-stimulating hormone (ICSH) in some texts when referring to the male animal. LH has a positive feedback effect, stimulating further testosterone production that in turn stimulates the production of spermatozoa within the seminiferous tubules of the testis. The semi-

niferous tubules form the internal structure of the testis, along with supportive connective tissue. Three different cell types can be identified and are illustrated in Figure 6.8.

1. **Spermatogenic cells**
   These cells produce the male gametes, spermatozoa. The spermatozoa have undergone a meiosis, resulting in cells that contain half the number of the parent cell, i.e. are haploid (see Chapter 1).
2. **Sertoli cells**
   Sertoli cells provide support for the development and maturation of spermatozoa. They are stimulated by follicle-stimulating hormone (FSH) from the anterior pituitary gland and produce inhibin, a hormone that has a negative feedback on the production of FSH. In this way, the faster the rate of sperm production (due to increase FSH secretion) the more inhibin is produced to slow the production of FSH. They therefore act as regulators of spermatogenesis through this negative feedback effect. In addition, they control the release of spermatozoa into the lumen of the tubules.
3. **Interstitial cells of Leydig**
   These cells lie in the spaces between the seminiferous tubules, within the supportive connective tissue. They produce the male hormones, androgens, e.g. testosterone.

The epididymis

Spermatozoa pass from the seminiferous tubules of the testis via the efferent ducts (or vasa efferentia)

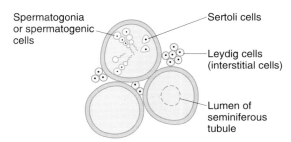

Seminiferous tubules of testis

Figure 6.8 Diagrammatic illustration of the three different cell types in seminiferous tubules

to the epididymis, a large, coiled tube that lies along the testis. It acts as a storage area for the spermatozoa as they mature.

The vas deferens

The **vas deferens** (pl = **vasa deferentia**), or deferent duct, lies within the spermatic cord and carries the sperm during ejaculation from the epididymis to the urethra, via the accessory glands (discussed below). The wall of the vas deferens is comprised of a largely smooth muscle that helps to propel the ejaculate along its length by peristalsis.

Accessory glands

There are two accessory glands in the tom cat and only one in the dog. The prostate gland is common to both species and is a relatively large, walnut-shaped gland that secretes a thin, milky, alkaline secretion known as seminal fluid. This forms the bulk of the ejaculate and aids the survival of the spermatozoa within the acidic environment of the female reproductive tract. It also contains certain enzymes that are necessary for sperm motility. The second set of accessory glands, present only in the tom cat, are called the bulbo-urethral glands. They lie caudal to the prostate gland along the urethra and secrete a thick mucous substance that forms part of the seminal fluid in the cat.

The urethra, penis and prepuce

The urethra is common to both the urinary and reproductive systems, and runs from the bladder to the tip of the penis, carrying both urine and semen to the exterior. The penis is a tubular organ and consists of the root, the body, and the glans. When not erect, it is covered entirely by the prepuce, a fold of skin that extends from the skin of the wall of the abdomen. The penis is a complex organ and in a simplified form can be considered to consist of the **urethra**, the **os penis**, the **corpus cavernosum**, the **corpus spongiosum**, and the **retractor penis muscle**.

The urethra has already been discussed in relation to the urinary system in Chapter 5. The os penis is a small bone that develops unattached and is separate from the remainder of the skeleton and as such is sometimes referred to as the splanchnic skeleton. It lies almost entirely within the glans of the penis and has a groove along its length in which the urethra is located. The os penis lies dorsal to the urethra in the dog (the cat does not have an os penis). The tip of the os penis is composed of fibrocartilage. The corpus cavernosum consists of two strips of erectile tissue that run through the body of the penis to the os penis whereas the corpus spongiosum lies underneath the corpus cavernosum, expanding to encircle the urethra in the bulb of the penis at the root and distally into the glans. Following erection of the penis, primarily by increased flow of blood to the corpus cavernosum and corpus spongiosum, the retractor penis muscle returns the penis into the prepuce, as the penis returns to its non-erectile state. Further detail can be found in Evans and Cristensen (1993).

The female reproductive system

The female reproductive system is adapted for the production of the female gamete or ovum (pl = ova), its fertilization by the male gamete, and transport of the fertilized egg to the uterine horns where the embryo can implant and develop until parturition. It is also responsible for the preparation of the female animal during pregnancy for the process of parturition and the resultant care of the neonate, including lactation. The major parts of the reproductive tract of the bitch are illustrated in Figure 6.9.

The ovaries

The ovaries are also referred to as the female gonads as they develop from the same embryonic tissue as the male testes. They are paired and are located in the abdomen, caudal to the kidneys. Each ovary is attached to the suspensory ligament, the broad ligament, and the proper or ovarian ligament, which all secure it within the abdomen.

The ovaries lie within a fold of mesentery called the mesovarium attracting them to the peritoneum of the body wall. The mesovarium has a small opening known as the ovarian bursa from which the ovum can escape at ovulation. The functions of the ovaries are two-fold. Not only do they produce the ova via a process known as oogenesis, but they also secrete the female steroid hormones, oestrogen and progesterone.

The formation and development of ova

Figure 6.10 shows the maturation of oocytes and ovulation. Only one follicle is shown, but it must be remembered that in multiparous species such as

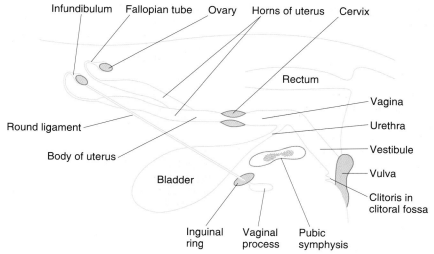

Figure 6.9 Reproductive tract of the bitch

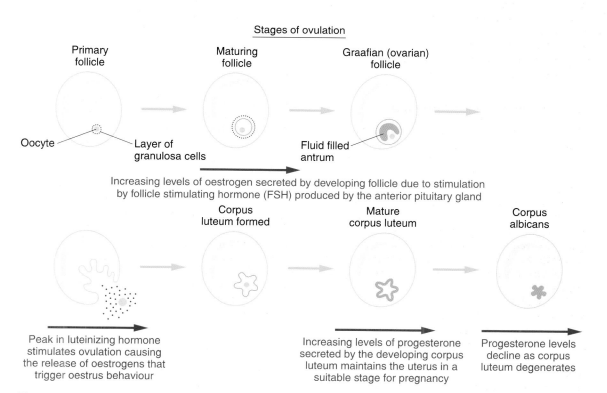

Figure 6.10 The stages of ovulation

the dog and cat, many follicles will develop simultaneously.

The oviducts (fallopian or uterine tubes)

At ovulation, the ova are 'caught' by the fimbriae (finger-like processes) of the infundibulum and the ova travel through the oviducts to the uterus, aided by peristaltic contractions of the smooth muscle within the oviduct walls. In the majority of cases, when mating has occurred, fertilization also occurs in the oviduct rather than the uterus itself.

The uterus

This structure is a hollow, muscular 'Y'-shaped organ comprising a neck or cervix, a body, and two uterine horns in the dog and cat. The horns of the uterus are attached to the ovaries by the proper and broad ligaments. The round ligament attaches the ovary to the tip of the horn and runs through the inguinal ring to the vaginal process, a pad of fatty tissue. All these ligaments contain some smooth muscle that permits stretching as the uterus expands during pregnancy. Depending upon the reproductive status of the bitch or queen, the uterus can vary in size. The wall of the uterus is formed from layers of smooth muscle known as the myometrium with an inner layer of mucous epithelial cells called the endometrium.

The vagina, vestibule and vulva

The vagina extends from the cervix to the external urethral orifice, where the urinary and reproductive systems join and share a common link with the exterior. At this point there is a sharp bend of the tract marking the point of the vestibule, which is common to both systems, as shown in Figure 6.9. The vestibule is extremely muscular and is thought by some to contribute towards the tie seen in dogs during mating, discussed later in this chapter. The term vulva is considered by some to include the vestibule, labia and clitoris, although others make a distinction between the three anatomical areas. The labia, or lips, form the external boundary of the reproductive tract and is visible in most bitches, being particularly swollen when the bitch is in oestrus. The clitoris is analogous to the male penis, although it consists of fatty rather than erectile tissue. Its location is illustrated in Figure 6.9.

Mating and pregnancy

Now that we have familiarized ourselves with the reproductive anatomy of both the male and female dog and cat, in addition to the formation and development of ova and spermatozoa, we can examine the anatomical and physiological aspects of mating and pregnancy. However, before we consider these we must have some appreciation of the factors to take into account when selecting individual animals for breeding.

Reproductive cycles

Most species of animal have particular breeding seasons which depend upon the time of year. These are usually timed to exploit optimal conditions for survival such as warmer temperatures and increased food supply. Many grazing animals time their reproductive cycles to ensure that offspring are born when the grass quality is at its best, the aim being to support the increased nutritional demands of lactation. This is usually in the spring months of April or May in the UK, the time we associate with the appearance of lambs in the fields. Similarly, predators may time their cycles to coincide with an abundance of prey species. Due to this dependence on seasonal effects, the triggers for reproduction are usually changes in temperature, day-length (or photoperiod) or rainfall. In some pack species the reproductive cycle may be triggered by the presence of another female in their reproductive cycle (season or heat). It is thought that this effect is due to olfactory cues from pheromones released by the cycling female.

Within a breeding season, the number of cycles a female animal has is dependent upon the species. Some are receptive to the male animal only once during the breeding season. These can be described as **monoestrus** species, of which the bitch is an example. Although the bitch has, on average, two breeding seasons per year, she is only receptive to the male during one stage of each season. Other species have no clearly defined breeding season and cycle throughout the year. These are termed **polyoestrus**, and the domestic Guinea Pig is an example of a polyoestrus species. Species such as the cat and rabbit have a long breeding season during the spring and summer months, during which they cycle repetitively until mated. During the autumn and winter months the majority do not come into season. This type of reproductive pattern can be described as **seasonally polyoestrus**. In the rabbit and the cat, the onset of the reproductive phase is triggered by increasing photoperiod and temperature.

Therefore, when dealing with different species and planning a breeding programme, it is important to be aware of the variation in reproductive cycles and seasons.

The oestrus cycle

Classically, the mammalian reproductive or oestrus cycle can be split into five stages. These are listed in Table 6.1, along with the events that occur at each stage. However, there is considerable species variation in the classical stages illustrated in Table 6.1, and Tables 6.2 and 6.3 illustrate the similarities and differences between the oestrus cycles of the bitch and queen. In contrast to the bitch, which ovulates irrespective of whether mating occurs, i.e. she is a spontaneous ovulator, ovulation of the queen is stimulated by the act of mating. This is described as reflex ovulation. Other species that are reflex ovulators include the rabbit and ferret.

Selection of breeding stock

Many factors should be considered before planning a breeding programme with any species of animal. In this section we will give consideration to both the dog and cat, although the same principles apply to all species.

Table 6.1 Stages of the oestrus cycle

Stage of cycle	Events
Pro-oestrus	The period during which the follicles of the ovaries enlarge and mature
Oestrus	The ovarian follicles rupture (ovulation) and ova are released
Metoestrus	A corpus luteum is formed at the site of each ruptured follicle
Dioestrus	Corpora lutea become established or, if the ova are fertilized, pregnancy is established
Anoestrus	No ovarian activity

It remains a popular myth with many dog and cat owners that a female animal must have the opportunity to have a litter. Many believe that it will 'settle the animal down', making her more loyal, obedient and 'loving'. This is not the case and it should be emphasized to owners that there are no medical grounds for a bitch or queen to have a litter, nor will it make her a 'better' pet. Owners should be encouraged to think about their own reasons for wanting to breed from their bitch or queen, before a mating is planned.

Pet owners should consider the following points:

- **Do they have potential homes for the puppies/kittens?**
  Some breeds of dog, in particular, have very large litters. It is not uncommon for a labrador retriever to produce litters in excess of 10 pups.
- **Do they have the time and space for the puppies until they are homed?**
  For example, a litter of 10 Rottweiler puppies that are 8 weeks old will demand a great deal of time, energy and space.
- **Have they considered the potential costs of rearing a litter?**
  The bitch or queen may experience difficulties during parturition and require a caesarean section. This is likely to be out of normal surgery hours and may prove expensive. In addition, the bitch/queen will require good quality food during pregnancy and lactation and the puppies/kittens will also require good nutrition when weaned. Should any of the puppies/kittens become ill, they will require veterinary attention.

Support, information and advice will also be needed for the new owners of the puppies/kittens. Some breeders like to produce an information pack for each new owner containing information sheets and a few basic essentials such as a few days supply of food, a puppy collar and lead, and a suitable puppy toy. Whilst this is excellent practice, when repeated for 10 puppies it can be a considerable cost, both in time and money.

Table 6.2 Stages of the oestrus cycle of the bitch

Stage of oestrus cycle	Duration	Notes	Physiology
Pro-oestrus	9–10 days	Swelling of the vulva will be seen due to rising levels of oestrogens. A blood-stained mucous (serosanginous) discharge is evident in most bitches and the endometrium thickens. The bitch may urinate more frequently and male dogs may be attracted to her.	FSH secretion stimulates maturation of the follicles and both oestrogen and LH levels start to increase as follicles mature. The oestrogen released by the ovarian follicles stimulates an increase in LH production from the anterior pituitary gland.
Oestrus	7–10 days (variable)	The vulva softens due to a peak in the release of LH. The discharge is less bloody as the follicles rupture. The female accepts the male's advances and he is attracted to her due to the high levels of oestrogen. She exhibits inviting behaviours such as tail flagging and lordosis. When the male mounts her she stands rigid (often termed standing oestrus).	A pre-ovulatory surge of LH stimulates ovulation and the ovarian follicles rupture. The surge of LH also helps to promote development of the corpora lutea.
Metoestrus	5–15 days	The period of pregnancy if mating has occurred. Metoestrus and dioestrus are often considered together in the reproductive cycle of the bitch. If not mated most bitches will show some signs of false pregnancy as the hormones at this time are similar to those of a pregnant bitch. One of the more important hormones causing false pregnancy is thought to be prolactin (see later section).	Corpora lutea are formed and become established during dioestrus (the late luteal phase). Progesterone levels increase as the corpora lutea mature. Progesterone helps in the maintenance of pregnancy.
Dioestrus	6–7 weeks		
Anoestrus	Approx 5 months	No signs of sexual behaviour.	

Total duration of the oestrus cycle of the bitch is approximately 21 days, although this is variable depending upon the individual animal.

● **Can they provide a clean, healthy environment for mother and offspring?**

It is essential that both mother and offspring are kept in conditions that promote good health. A place should be available that can be routinely cleaned and disinfected as required. It may be necessary to restrict the access of other household pets whilst the offspring are still young.

● **Are they able to provide socialization opportunities for the puppies/kittens before they are sold?**

This is one of the most critical aspects of rearing young animals that is often over-

looked. Under the Sale of Goods Act the owner has both a moral and legal responsibility to ensure that the offspring are healthy with a sound temperament. This can only be achieved through adequate socialization that should be started as soon as the puppies are a few days old. They should be accustomed to touch from a very early age and once their ears and eyes open they should be exposed to as many strange stimuli as possible; the vacuum cleaner, the television, travel in the car, the sight of traffic, other healthy vaccinated animals, young children and adults. The list is

Table 6.3 Stages of the oestrus cycle of the queen

Stage of oestrus cycle	Duration	Notes	Physiology
Pro-oestrus	3–10 days	Pro-oestrus and oestrus are difficult to distinguish in the queen as no significant signs are visible during the pro-oestrus stage, although some queens may 'call' for a male.	When the queen will accept mating by the male, follicles are well-developed, secreting maximum levels of oestrogens.
Oestrus		When in oestrus the queen will exhibit lordosis and trample her hind feet in the presence of a male. She will rub against inanimate objects.	
Interoestrus	10–14 days	In the absence of mating the queen will return in season following a 'quiet' period with no obvious signs. Some queens will show a continuous season as the waves of growth of the follicles overlap.	Preparation in ovary for next round of follicular development. The queen is a reflex ovulator. She will only ovulate if mated. If not, she will continue returning to oestrus.
Pregnancy	64 days	Weight gain observed. Foetuses palpable at 3–4 weeks post mating.	Corpora lutea develop in response to the LH surge triggered by ovulation. Progesterone levels increase as corpora lutea mature.
Metoestrus (pseudo-pregnancy)	25–40 days	If ovulation occurs but fertilization does not, then short period of pseudopregnancy occurs. Queen then returns to interoestrus before commencing with oestrus again, providing that it is still within the breeding season. If not, she will return to anoestrus.	Corpora lutea develop and produce progesterone for short period.
Anoestrus	Autumn–Spring	No reproductive activity.	No ovarian activity.

endless. If exposed to many different experiences, it is more likely that the puppies/kittens will make well-adjusted pets.

Potential breeders should also pay consideration to the suitability of their bitch/queen for breeding:

- **Is she of a suitable age?**
  Recommended age for breeding is 1.5 to 2 years for a bitch (although this may vary depending upon the individual animal and breed) and 12 months for a queen. The Kennel Club will not register any offspring from a bitch over 7 years old unless special permission is obtained prior to mating.

- **Is her temperament good?**
  No animal should be used for breeding unless their temperament is suitable.
- **Is she in good condition/health?**
  The bitch/queen should be on a good quality diet and have no known health problems. She should not be over or under weight. She should also be up to date with worming and vaccination prior to mating.
- **Does she (or any of her close relations) have any hereditary defects?**
  This can be a particular problem in certain breeds, e.g. congenital cardiac disease in some Cavalier King Charles Spaniels, hip dysplasia in large breeds of dog, and progressive retinal atrophy and Collie Eye Anomaly in Border Collies.

- **If she is a pedigree, is she a good example of the breed and what is her breeding?**

  Reference to the breed standard should identify any weaknesses of a particular female and a male animal can be identified that will improve on these. It is important that the pedigrees of the sire and dam be considered to avoid inbreeding.

In this way, the mating can be planned to produce offspring that have the best chance of survival and are free from hereditary defects. Consideration should also be given to the above points when identifying an appropriate male animal for use as a stud. It is usual for the owner of the bitch/queen to approach the owner of the stud and request to use their dog/tom cat. The owner of the stud has a responsibility to:

- **Present the stud in good health**

  Similar consideration should be given to those of the bitch/queen.
- **Offer a free return should the bitch/queen fail to conceive**

  If the stud is unproven (i.e. has not yet sired a litter) then it is usual for no fee to be charged until the bitch/queen is confirmed to be in whelp/kitten. Should a mating with a proven stud fail to result in conception, then it is usual for the owner to allow a mating on the second season at no charge.
- **Offer a second mating if the first fails to result in a tie**

  Some stud owners recommend that a bitch is mated twice during a season (2–3 days apart) to maximize the chance of conception. Should a tie not occur then it is usual to try the mating again in 2–3 days. This is not necessary in the cat as the queen is a reflex ovulator and the tie does not occur during mating.

Mating

Now that we are aware of the reproductive cycles of both the cat and the dog, and also issues that should be given consideration in the selection of appropriate breeding stock, we can consider mating. It is important to remember that mating will only be successful if the female animal is presented to the male during the oestrus stage of the reproductive cycle. It will be necessary for the owner of the female to determine the optimum time for mating, in order to maximize the chances of success. This is less important in the queen than

the bitch as the queen will ovulate after mating, being a reflex ovulator. However, as the bitch is a spontaneous ovulator, the optimum time is more difficult to detect and can be easily missed. There are several techniques that are available that will be discussed briefly below. Further details can be found in Simpson et al. (1998).

1. **Clinical observation**

   Unfortunately clinical indicators do not correlate well with physiological events. Most texts state that the average bitch ovulates 12 days after the start of pro-oestrus and should be mated at day 14 after the first sign of bleeding. However, some bitches may ovulate as early as 8 days or as late as 26 days. If the latter bitch were presented to the male on day 14 as recommended, it is unlikely that he would be interested in mating as she would not be in the oestrus phase of the cycle. Some authors have suggested that vaginal softening gives an accurate indicator of the LH surge that occurs 2 days prior to ovulation.
2. **Levels of plasma progesterone**

   Measurement of the levels of plasma progesterone are possible using a simple test kit. Progesterone levels increase at the time of the LH surge, as the corpora lutea develop at the time of ovulation. This provides an extremely reliable indicator that ovulation has occurred, providing that routine blood sampling is possible near the predicted time of ovulation.
3. **Vaginal cytology**

   Examination of the cells of the vagina under the microscope can, to the experienced eye, indicate the most suitable time for mating. During the oestrus cycle, the vaginal cytology changes under the influence of the reproductive hormones. Cells appear larger during the oestrus period, keratin can be seen within the cytoplasm and the cells have no nucleus (anuclear). When the percentage of anuclear cells is maximal, at around 80% or above, this coincides with the fertile period following ovulation. This technique is a reliable indicator of the optimum time for mating, providing it is performed by someone experienced in the technique. It also requires the bitch to be available for routine vaginal smears.

Irrespective of the method used to determine the optimum time for mating, an experienced stud dog will often let the owner know whether the bitch is in oestrus or not by his response when she is presented to him. If she is receptive the bitch will also exhibit specific responses to attention from the male. She may exhibit lordosis, arching the spine downwards in order to draw the dog's attention to the vulval region. She will hold her tail to one side, a process known as flagging, and will stand very still (this is why she is often said to be in standing oestrus). As the dog's interest increases she will allow him to mount and enter the vulva. Full erection of the penis is achieved after entry and swelling of the bulbus glands locks the penis within the female's reproductive tract.

The ejaculate is comprised of three components. The first portion is released during initial erection and contains prostatic fluid only. The second portion is the sperm-rich fraction and is released after full erection, usually once thrusting has stopped. Following this stage, the dog will try to rotate himself so that he is tail-to-tail with the bitch. Some dogs may not turn fully and prefer to be parallel to the bitch or rest on her back. This penultimate phase is termed the tie and during this phase the third portion of ejaculate, primarily prostatic fluid, is released. The duration of the tie can vary from 10 minutes to over one hour and is not an indication of successful fertilization. One theory is that the bitch also contributes towards the tie by contraction of the vestibular muscles. Eventually the tie breaks due to a reduction of the swelling of the bulbus and the dog and bitch part. A more detailed account of the mating process is given by Simpson et al. (1998). Figure 6.11 illustrates the key stages in the mating process.

The mating of the cat is much less complex. The male is drawn to the female by her behaviour, smell, and vocalization. He grasps her by the scruff of the neck and mounts her, treading on her back to stimulate her further. Intromission is quicker than in the dog, only taking a few seconds and as he withdraws the female cries due to the discomfort caused by the spines on the penis that stimulate ovulation. Some females will turn on the male and try to swipe at him, following which they roll intensely and lick their genitals. Females will usually allow remounting within 10 minutes although it may take up to one hour and it is recommended that the male is allowed to remain with the female until at least four matings have occurred to ensure that ovulation has been stimulated.

Control of reproduction

Consideration of methods for controlling the reproduction of the dog and cat is essential as it is undesirable for the majority of animals kept as pets to breed, either from the owner's point of view or from the point of view of population control. There are several methods available for controlling the reproduction of the cat and the dog. These can be broadly categorized into surgical methods and hormonal manipulation.

Surgical methods

These are probably the most common forms of controlling reproduction in the cat and dog.

In the female, ovariohysterectomy involves the removal of both ovaries and the uterus, to the level of the cervix. A more commonly used term is 'spaying' although this technically means the removal of only the ovaries (this technique is more commonly practised in some European countries). The advantages of this procedure are not only that it eliminates the possibility of unwanted offspring, but also that it reduces the incidence of mammary tumours, and eliminates

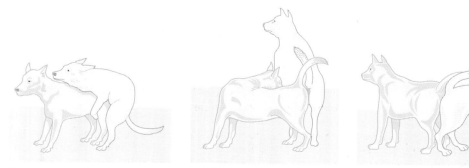

Figure 6.11 Key stages in the mating of the dog and bitch

the risk of pseudopregnancy and pyometra. There may be disadvantages in that it is thought to cause urinary incontinence in some bitches, it may lead to a change in coat texture, and it may lead to increased weight gain (but only if the owner continues to provide the same diet as before and does not adjust it to take account of changed metabolic rate and activity). Some studies indicate that it may also lead to increased aggressive tendencies in some bitches, although this area is still under study.

Castration involves the removal of the testicles in the male animal. The advantages of this technique are not only that it prevents the male from siring unwanted offspring, but also that it prevents benign enlargement of the prostate gland as well as tumours of the prostate, anal adenomas and perineal hernias. It may also decrease the incidence of some undesirable male sexual behaviour, e.g. scent marking in tom cats, roaming and some inter-male aggression in dogs. Disadvantages are that it may cause a change in coat texture and may lead to an increase in weight, if the owner continues to feed as before.

Vasectomy is the third method of surgical control of reproduction but it is rarely performed in the dog or cat, being more commonly performed in the ferret. It involves the cutting of the vas deferens preventing the passage of spermatozoa from the epididymis of the testis. As the testes are retained, they still continue to produce spermatozoa and associated hormones, in particular testosterone. The female ferret (the jill) has a similar pattern of oestrus to that of the queen, commencing cyclical activity as the days lengthen with a period of anoestrus during the winter months. If she is not mated she will continue to cycle and is at risk of developing pseudopregnancy. This may cause anaemia and bone marrow suppression due to the high circulating levels of oestrogen and these can prove life-threatening. If the female is mated she will cease cycling and consequently her health is not at risk. Use of a vasectomized male means that the female can be mated but that offspring are not produced. If the female is not required for breeding she should have an ovariohysterectomy.

Hormonal manipulation

In addition to the methods of surgical control of reproduction, it is also possible to administer synthetic hormones that mimic the effects of the naturally occurring reproductive hormones.

The oestrus cycle can be prevented by the administration of a progestogen (a progesterone or progesterone-like compound). These are usually administered as a depot injection (long-acting, slow-release) or as tablets towards the end of anoestrus, and they prevent the occurrence of oestrus. Delmadinone acetate (Tardak®), megestrol acetate (Ovarid®) or proligesterone (Delvosterone®) can all be administered to prevent oestrus. Normal oestrus usually occurs 4–6 months following administration.

Megestrol acetate (Ovarid®) can also be administered during pro-oestrus and oestrus to suppress the signs of oestrus. Manufacturers recommend that these products should not be used in animals intended for breeding and that contact with other females in oestrus may cause a failure in contraception. Side-effects of the progestogens used for oestrus prevention and suppression may cause increased appetite and weight gain, lethargy, mammary enlargement, and changes in coat and temperament as well as an increased risk of pyometra.

It is sometimes necessary, following an unwanted mating or misalliance, to prevent pregnancy. If the female is not required for breeding then an ovariohysterectomy should be performed during metoestrus. If this is not considered possible, then oral oestrogens (e.g. oestradiol benzoate) can be administered at a high dose within five days of mating. This usually prolongs oestrus and can increase the risk of the development of pyometra (an accumulation of pus in the uterine cavity). There are also products available that can be administered in late pregnancy that lower blood progesterone. This induces resorption or abortion. Their use is not common in the UK.

Oral oestrogens can also be administered in low doses followed by equine chorionic gonadotropin to induce oestrus in bitches that either have long periods of anoestrus, are slow to reach puberty, or do not show behavioural signs of oestrus. This technique varies in its success.

Progestogens, e.g. delmadinone acetate (Tardak®), can also be used to suppress testosterone production in the male animal and consequently may lead to a reduction in certain male sexual behaviours such as libido, inter-male aggression, roaming and territory marking. It should be remembered that these drugs do not cause infertility and at present there is no single drug that is available as a male contraceptive. The most common use for progestogens in the male animal is as a means of preventing some behavioural problems; however, this should always be combined with appropriate behavioural modification for desired long-term effects.

Pregnancy

Following a successful mating, pregnancy can be diagnosed by several methods. Clinical signs such as an increase in body weight and abdominal enlargement may be observed in both the bitch and the queen, although they are not a very reliable indicator in the bitch, as they may also be seen in animals with pseudopregnancy. Other clinical signs that may be observed in the bitch include enlargement of the mammary glands from day 40 after mating, production of milk from day 40–55 onwards, and behavioural changes such as nest building. However, it is important to note that these can all be observed in cases of pseudo-pregnancy and do not therefore provide a reliable diagnosis on their own.

Other methods that can be used include abdominal palpation, identification of fetal heartbeat, radiography, detection of plasma hormones, detection of plasma proteins, and ultrasound. These will be discussed briefly in the following section. For further information the reader is referred to Simpson et al. (1998).

1. **Abdominal palpation**
   This is one of the more commonly used methods of diagnosis by many Veterinary Surgeons. In the bitch the foetuses can be felt as a swelling at approximately 4–6 weeks after mating (days 21–30 following mating in the queen). This method is usually accurate, although it can be difficult in nervous or obese animals. It becomes more difficult to palpate the foetuses after 35 days following mating.
2. **Presence of foetal heartbeat**
   This can be detected using a stethoscope or by ECG, although it is only detectable during late pregnancy.
3. **Radiography**
   Enlargement of the uterus can be observed by radiography from 30 days following mating, however it may also be enlarged due to a pyometra. The foetal skeletons are visible as they become mineralized, about 45 days following mating. This method of diagnosis presents some risk to the dam and foetuses, however, as sedation or anaesthesia is usually required. If conducted during late pregnancy it allows the number of foetuses to be determined.
4. **Plasma hormones**
   Detection of plasma progesterone is of no diagnostic reliability as levels in the pseudo-pregnant animal are also elevated. Test kits are now available that detect the hormone relaxin and these provide a more reliable indicator of pregnancy in the bitch.
5. **Plasma proteins**
   An increase in certain plasma proteins occurs from day 20 onward in the bitch and is used as a reliable indicator of pregnancy, forming the basis of some commercial test kits. False positives can occur in inflammatory conditions such as pyometra that also causes elevated plasma protein levels.
6. **Ultrasound**
   This is one of the more commonly used methods of diagnosis due to its non-invasive nature. Using B-mode ultrasound it is possible to diagnose pregnancy as early as day 16 after mating in the bitch, although the technique is easier if left until day 28 when fluid around the foetus is easily visible. In the queen, pregnancy can be diagnosed as early as day 12. This technique also allows an estimation of number of foetuses present and their viability, as heart-beats can be detected.

The duration of pregnancy can be taken as 64–66 days from the LH surge in the bitch or 56–72 days from the time of mating. The variability is due to the bitch being a spontaneous ovulator, consequently when mated she may not yet have ovulated, resulting in an apparently longer gestation, or she may have ovulated before mating, resulting in an apparently shorter gestation period. As the queen is a reflex ovulator the variation in duration of gestation is minimal, the majority taking 65 days (with a range of 64–68 days).

Pseudopregnancy (pseudocyesis or false pregnancy)

It is now thought that most bitches that come into season and are not mated suffer to some degree from pseudopregnancy approximately weeks 6–14 after oestrus. Some bitches may show few overt clinical signs and the owner may be unaware that there is any difference in behaviour. Others may show a marked change, however, becoming more aggressive, withdrawn, protective over toys, and even producing milk. It has traditionally been the view that rising levels of progesterone in the non-pregnant bitch (similar to those in the pregnant bitch) were responsible for the signs of false pregnancy. More recent opinion identifies the cause as being due to either excessive levels of the hormone prolactin or an increased sensitivity of the bitch to this hormone. Prolactin levels increase in both the pregnant and non-pregnant bitch around day 30 of metoestrus, preparing the mammary glands for lactation and maintaining the corpora lutea. In pack animals it would be advantageous to have some subordinate females able to suckle the offspring of the dominant female, in order to reduce the demands on the dominant bitch. Pseudopregnancy can therefore be seen to have evolutionary advantages in the ancestors of the domestic dog, perhaps explaining why so many entire bitches are seen today in practice with varying severities of the condition. Simpson et al. (1998) discuss the various treatment options in greater detail. Anti-prolactin drugs, e.g. cabergoline (Galastop®) is now available in the UK and has a high success rate in the treatment of most cases of pseudopregnancy.

Parturition

During the last few weeks of pregnancy, the bitch or queen will start to make a nest and should be encouraged to select an appropriate area. The requirements for such an area are discussed in detail by Evans and White (1994). Pre-partum hypothermia (a fall in rectal temperature by 2°C) will be observed 24–26 hours before parturition due to the sudden fall in plasma progesterone, indicating the start of parturition. It is possible that the fall in progesterone is triggered by a hormone produced by an, as yet, unidentified hormone produced by the foetuses. This is thought to be a stress response, as a consequence of competition for space and restricted nutrients within the uterine horns. This can be identified as the first stage (the stage of preparation) of the five stages of parturition listed below.

1. **Stage of preparation**
   This commences with the onset of pre-partum hypothermia, discussed above. The tissues of the vagina and the perineum relax; other than this there are no obvious signs.
2. **First stage parturition**
   Uterine contractions begin at this stage. Milk may become apparent within the mammary glands and the dam may show general signs of discomfort, restlessness, panting and nesting behaviour. She may try to seek seclusion and

may shiver and/or vomit. The uterine contractions are a result of the release of oxytocin from the posterior pituitary gland that will cause the cervix to dilate in preparation for the passage of the foetus. Relaxin, a hormone produced by the placenta, causes relaxation of the pubic symphysis, again to facilitate the passage of the foetus. The allantochorion (formed during development of the embryo by the fusion of the allantois and chorion, two of the foetal membranes) may rupture at this stage and allantoic fluid may be seen at the vulva.

3. **Second stage parturition**
   During this stage there is an increase in the frequency and strength of contractions of the uterus as the foetus is pushed through the cervix into the vagina. Strong abdominal straining is observed as the foetus is presented (usually feet and head first) and delivered. The foetus may remain contained within the amnion, which the dam will normally tear as she licks the foetus vigorously. If this does not occur it may be necessary to intervene and break the sac to help the neonate (newborn) breathe. The placenta usually follows the foetus within 20 minutes. The dam normally breaks the umbilical cord but again, intervention may be required. Should the second foetus not follow within 60 minutes then **dystocia** (difficulty during parturition) may be indicated and assistance of a veterinary surgeon should be sought.
4. **Third stage parturition**
   This coincides with the passage of the placenta. In the bitch and queen, this occurs in the second stage so cannot be strictly defined as a separate period. A dark-coloured discharge may be seen (green in bitches and brown in queens) from the marginal haematomas of the placentae (localized collections of blood clots around the edges of each placenta). This is considered normal.
5. **Puerperium**
   This is the period during which the reproductive tract returns to its normal state. The time for the uterus to return to normal can take 4–6 weeks, during which it is not abnormal to observe a mucoid discharge.

Following parturition, the loss of the placenta coupled with a decline in oestrogen and progesterone results in the removal of the inhibition of the secretion of prolactin. Once this inhibition is removed, prolactin is released and stimulates the production of milk, or lactation, which will be discussed in the following section.

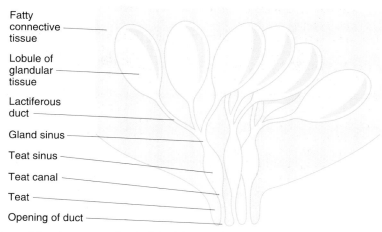

Fatty connective tissue

Lobule of glandular tissue

Lactiferous duct

Gland sinus

Teat sinus

Teat canal

Teat

Opening of duct

Figure 6.12 Structure of the mammary gland of the bitch

Lactation

During pregnancy, under the influence of various hormones, mammary tissue develops in preparation for the requirements of the neonates. Mammary glands are modified sweat glands; bitches usually have five pairs and queens four. The males of most species have rudimentary teats. The structure of a mammary gland is illustrated in Figure 6.12.

During pregnancy, the mammary tissue becomes active and develops secretory ducts and alveoli. As a consequence the mammary glands enlarge. This is primarily due to the production of a hormone, lactogen, by the placenta, but also to the effects of oestrogen and progesterone. The hormonal control of mammary gland development is illustrated in Figure 6.13.

Milk may be produced towards the end of pregnancy in some animals, but the most important stimulus for the production of milk occurs when the inhibition of prolactin ceases, due to expulsion of the placenta at parturition. The first milk to be produced is thicker in consistency than normal, with a yellowish tinge. This is called colostrum and carries maternal antibodies, important for conferring passive immunity to the neonate for its first few weeks of life. It is also more energy-rich than normal milk, again to give the neonate a 'head start'. It is important that the colostrum is consumed as soon as possible, ideally within the first 24 hours following parturition. After this time the morphology of the intestine of the neonate changes to prevent the absorption of the large maternal antibodies. It is possible for young animals to survive if they do not receive maternal colostrum. However, their chances of survival are reduced and they are particularly prone to infection, e.g. parvovirus, distemper, etc. as they have no resistance to disease. Commercial colostrum and milk substitutes are available, but, wherever possible, maternal milk is preferable. Fresh milk from other species should not be used due to the difference in nutritional composition, as illustrated in Table 6.4. If maternal milk is unavailable it is preferable to use a commercial milk replacement.

Hormonal control of lactation

Following development of the mammary tissue during pregnancy, as outlined in Figure 6.13, a variety of hormones are associated with the process of lactation following parturition. The act of suckling by the neonate causes the release of prolactin from the anterior pituitary gland and

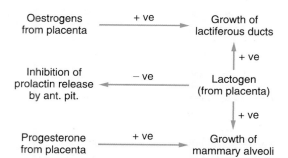

Oestrogens from placenta → + ve → Growth of lactiferous ducts

Inhibition of prolactin release by ant. pit. ← – ve ← Lactogen (from placenta)

Progesterone from placenta → + ve → Growth of mammary alveoli

+ ve

+ ve

Figure 6.13 Hormonal control of mammary gland development during pregnancy

Table 6.4 Nutritional content of the milk from various species

Content (%)	Bitch	Queen	Cow	Goat
Moisture	77.2	81.5	87.6	87.0
Dry matter	22.8	18.5	12.4	13.0
Protein	8.1	8.1	3.3	3.3
Fat	9.8	5.1	3.8	4.5
Ash, e.g. vitamins	4.9	3.5	5.3	6.2
Lactose	3.5	6.9	4.7	4.0
Calcium	0.28	0.04	0.12	0.13
Phosphorus	0.22	0.07	0.10	0.11
Energy (kcal/100 g)	135	106	66	70

oxytocin from the posterior pituitary gland. Prolactin stimulates secretion of milk from the glandular tissue of the mammary gland and oxytocin stimulates the ejection of the milk, a process known as milk 'let down'. Consequently, once suckling commences, there is a positive feedback of the action of suckling upon the secretion and let down of milk. Suckling is also thought to have an inhibitory effect upon the production of FSH and LH from the anterior pituitary gland, preventing the development of ovarian follicles whilst the animal is suckling. This lack of ovarian activity is termed lactational anoestrus and prevents species such as the cat, in particular, returning to the reproductive cycle whilst suckling young. The hormones associated with lactation are illustrated in Figure 6.14.

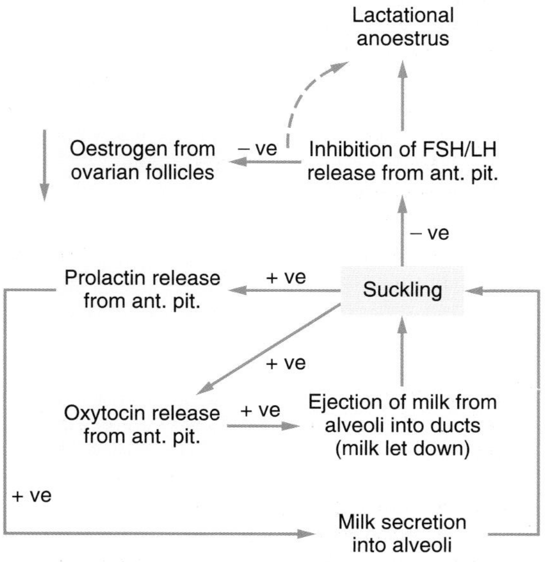

Review questions

1. How many pads does a dog have on one front leg, assuming the dew claw is present?
   (a) 4
   (b) 5
   (c) 6
   (d) 7
2. In what order are the layers of the epidermis, starting with the most superficial?
   (a) stratum corneum, stratum lucidum, stratum granulosum, stratum germinativium
   (b) stratum germinativum, stratum granulosum, stratum lucidum, stratum corneum
   (c) stratum granulosum, stratum germinativum, stratum lucidum, stratum corneum
   (d) stratum lucidum, stratum corneum, stratum granulosum, stratum germinativum
3. Which one of the following is not an epidermal structure?
   (a) arrector pili muscles
   (b) melanocytes
   (c) sebaceous glands
   (d) sweat glands
4. Which one of the following is not a function of sebum?
   (a) lubrication of hair
   (b) production of pheremones
   (c) stimulation of further growth of hair
   (d) waterproofing of hair

Figure 6.14 Hormonal control of lactation

5. The production of which vitamin by the skin is stimulated by ultraviolet light?
   (a) Vitamin A
   (b) Vitamin B_{12}
   (c) Vitamin C
   (d) Vitamin D_3

6. Which cells are involved with the immune response?
   (a) eosinophils
   (b) neutrophils
   (c) monocytes
   (d) lymphocytes

7. An allergic response is characterized by the release of:
   (a) histamine
   (b) anti-histamine
   (c) pyrogens
   (d) T-lymphocytes

8. Anaphylaxis is a result of activation of which cell types in the body?
   (a) neutrophils
   (b) B-lymphocytes
   (c) T-lymphocytes
   (d) mast cells

9. The use of vaccines against disease can be described as what type of immunity?
   (a) innate
   (b) passive
   (c) active
   (d) maternal

10. Another term for macrophage is:
    (a) histiocyte
    (b) lymphocyte
    (c) monocyte
    (d) neutrophil

11. Explain why animals deprived of natural sunlight may develop brittle bones.

12. Outline the purpose of sweat production.

13. Describe interferons.

14. Describe the role of the subcutaneous fat deposit.

15. State why the skin of the scrotum have little subcutaneous fat.

16. List the five differences between the claws of a dog and cat.

17. Describe what happens during inflammation.

18. Outline the role of fever in defending the body against pathogens.

19. State the type of immunity conferred by colostrums on the neonate.

20. Describe what occurs during anaphylaxis.

21. Fats that are digested and absorbed into lacteals are then carried almost directly into the
    (a) cisterna chyli
    (b) hepatic vein
    (c) portal vein
    (d) right azygous vein

22. Tissue of the lymph nodes produce which type of white blood cell?
    (a) monocytes
    (b) neutrophils
    (c) lymphocytes
    (d) eosinophils

23. Which of the following is the name given to lymphoid tissue associated with the intestine?
    (a) thymus
    (b) Peyer's patches
    (c) tonsils
    (d) cisterna chyli

24. Fertilization of the ova by the spermatozoa occurs in the:
    (a) uterine or Fallopian tubes
    (b) uterus
    (c) vagina
    (d) vestibule

25. During the oestrus cycle of the bitch, dioestrus is followed by:
    (a) anoestrus
    (b) metoestrus
    (c) oestrus
    (d) pro-oestrus

26. Another name for interstitial cells of the testis is:
    (a) accessory cells
    (b) Leydig cells
    (c) seminiferous cells
    (d) Sertoli cells

27. The main hormone secreted by the corpus luteum of the ovary is:
    (a) oxytocin
    (b) follicle-stimulating hormone
    (c) oestrogen
    (d) progesterone

28. Which one of the following is not part of the female reproductive tract?
    (a) oviduct
    (b) vas deferens
    (c) urethra
    (d) vestibule

29. Which of the following is not a function of the ovaries?
    (a) secretion of luteinizing hormone
    (b) secretion of progesterone
    (c) secretion of oestrogen
    (d) formation, development and release of ova

30. Which hormone is responsible for milk 'let down'?
    (a) oxytocin
    (b) oestrogen
    (c) prolactin
    (d) progesterone
31. Describe the formation of lymph.
32. Explain how dietary fats are absorbed following digestion.
33. State the three different cell types of the seminiferous tubules and outline their role.
34. Describe the stages of ovulation and the hormones involved.
35. Describe the oestrus cycle of the bitch, including significant hormonal events.
36. Explain when a bitch should be mated.
37. State which hormone is now thought to be the major contributor to pseudopregnancy in the bitch.
38. Describe the stages of parturition and the significant events occurring at each stage.
39. Name the hormones that are involved in the growth of mammary tissue during pregnancy.
40. State which hormones are released during the act of suckling, thus stimulating milk secretion and let down.

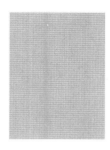

References

Blood DC and Studdert VP (1999) *Saunders Comprehensive Veterinary Dictionary,* 2nd edn. Harcourt Brace and Company Limited

Budras K, Fricke W and McCarthy PH (1994) *Anatomy of the Dog. An Illustrated Text,* 3rd edn. Mosby-Wolfe

Clancy J and McVicar A (1995) *Physiology and Anatomy: A Homeostatic Approach.* Edward Arnold

Ebbing D (1987) *General Chemistry,* 2nd edn. Houghton Mifflin Company

Eckert R, Randall D and Augustine G (1988) *Animal Physiology: Mechanisms and Adaptations,* 3rd edn. Cambridge University Press

Evans HE and Cristensen GC (1993) *Miller's Anatomy of the Dog,* 3rd edn. WB Saunders Company

Evans M and White K (1994) *Book of the Bitch.* Henston

Keele CA, Neil E and Joels N (1982) *Samson Wright's Applied Physiology,* 13th edn. Oxford University Press.

Green NPO, Stout GW, Taylor DJ and Soper R (1985) Biological Science 1: Organisms, Energy and Environment. Cambridge University Press

Hutchinson M (1990) *Manual of Endocrinology.* BSAVA

Lane DR and Cooper B (1999) *Veterinary Nursing,* 2nd edn. Butterworth Heinemann/ BSAVA

Purves WK and Orians GH (1987) *Life: The Science of Biology,* 2nd edn. Sinauer Associates Inc

Reeves G (1987) *Lecture Notes on Immunology.* Blackwell Scientific Publications

Simpson G, England G and Harvey M (1998) *Manual of Small Animal Reproduction and Neonatology.* BSAVA

Wheater PR, Burkitt HG and Daniels VG (1988) *Functional Histology,* 2nd edn. Churchill Livingstone

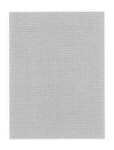

Further reading

Blood DC and Studdert VP (1999) Saunders Comprehensive Veterinary Dictionary (2nd edn). Harcourt Brace and Company Limited
An excellent, comprehensive veterinary dictionary that no-one should be without.

Eckert R, Randall D and Augustine G (1988) Animal Physiology: Mechanisms and Adaptations (3rd edn). Cambridge University Press
A clear, concise text that explains the basic physiological principles with some clear illustrations. This text covers a wide range of species from reptiles, through to birds and fish. The dog and cat take a bit of a back seat!

Evans M and White K (1994) Book of the Bitch. Henston
Aimed essentially at the dog owner, this book provides a good guide to the care of the bitch during mating, pregnancy, whelping and lactation. Although the physiology is kept to a minimum, it is a good book for those wanting a deeper appreciation of the factors involved in breeding a litter.

Green NPO, Stout GW, Taylor DJ and Soper R (1985) Biological Science 1: Organisms, Energy and Environment. Cambridge University Press
A general text that covers a wide range of biological principles relating to both plants and animals. Excellent, detailed chapter on the structure of the mammalian cell.

Lane DR and Cooper B (1999) Veterinary Nursing (2nd edn). Butterworth Heinemann/BSAVA
A comprehensive book covering all aspects of veterinary nursing for first and second year students, as well as qualified nurses wishing to keep up to date or refresh their memory. The chapter on anatomy and physiology provides a concise summary of the most important biological systems of the cat and dog.

The College of Animal Welfare (2000) Multiple Choice Questions in Anatomy and Physiology. Butterworth Heinemann
A popular text with first year students preparing to take their examination. It includes 300 multiple choice questions relating to anatomy and physiology that will assess your comprehension of the principles in this book

Evans HE and Cristensen GC (1993) Miller's Anatomy of the Dog (3rd edn). WB Saunders Company
An in-depth guide to the anatomy of the dog. For those who want to know more about anatomy in detail.

Clancy J and McVicar A (1995) Physiology and Anatomy: A Homeostatic Approach. Edward Arnold.
A human text that, if used with caution, helps to explain some of the basic physiological principles of the major body systems. The reader does need to remember that it is a human text and so some principles do not apply to the cat and dog.

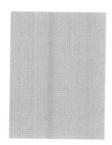

Answers

Chapter 1

1. c, Electrons. Protons and neutrons are located in the nucleus. Electrovalents are not nuclear particles.
2. a, Ionic. Covalent bonding is associated with the sharing of electrons as in the formation of a water molecule. Hydrogen bonding is used to represent the weak forces of attraction that exist between two molecules of water due to their polarity.
3. d. Salt is the solute, water the solvent and an ionic solution is formed. The solute dissolves in the solvent to form an ionic solution.
4. b, Iso-osmotic. 0.9% saline has the same osmotic pressure as body fluids.
5. b. Water molecules will move into the blood cell. This occurs as the water moves from weak solution (outside the cell) to strong solution (inside the cell) according to the principles of osmosis. The cell will swell and eventually burst (haemolyse).
6. a, 1. pH 1 is strongly acidic, 7 is neutral and 12 is strongly alkaline.
7. a. 1×10^4. The decimal place after the 1 has to move four places to the right to give 10,000. Alternatively, remember that the power 10 is equal to the number of 0s.
8. b, Protons and electrons. In an atom (which always carries a neutral charge) the number of positive particles (protons) always equals the number of negative particles (electrons).
9. d. Osmosis is always associated with a semi-permeable membrane and the movement of water from weak to strong solution.
10. a. Mercury. Although it is a metal, mercury is liquid at room temperature and atmospheric pressure (think about the clinical thermometer).
11. Points to include: Consists of three sub-atomic particles, protons, electrons and neutrons; Protons carry a positive charge, electrons carry a negative charge and neutrons are neutral; Protons and neutrons are contained within the nucleus, whereas the electrons orbit around the nucleus like planets orbiting the sun.
12. An isotope is a chemical element with the same atomic number as another (i.e. the same number of protons and electrons) but has different mass number (i.e. a different number of neutrons).
13. Two hydrogen atoms combine with an oxygen atom, each sharing an electron with the oxygen in a single covalent bond. Refer to Figure 1.5.
14. Refer to Figure 1.6 and explanatory text.
15. A buffer is a substance which in solution, resists changes in pH by either 'mopping up' excess protons if the environment becomes too acidic or by releasing protons should the environment become too alkaline. They allow the maintenance of a stable pH in biological systems.
16. Refer to Figure 1.8 and explanatory text.
17. 2.5×10^4. The number before the power 10 should be expressed as a number between 1 and 9.
18. As there are 2.2 lbs in 1 kg, 30 lbs = 30×2.2 = 66 kg.

19. Using the equation: $\dfrac{(F-32)\times 5}{9} = \,^{\circ}C$

$$\dfrac{(101-32)\times 5}{9} = 69 \times 5$$

$$\dfrac{345}{9} = 38.33°C \text{ (to 2 decimal places)}$$

20. Using the equation: $\dfrac{(C \times 9)}{5} + 32 = \,^{\circ}F$, i.e. multiply by 9, divide by 5 and add 32.

$$0\,\dfrac{(40 \times 9)}{5} + 32 = \dfrac{360}{5} + 32 =$$
$$72 + 32 = 104°C$$

21. a, Mitochondria. These organelles generate ATP that acts as an energy store and can be broken down to ADP releasing energy.
22. b, Golgi body. Ribosomes on the rough ER synthesize proteins that then pass to the Golgi body for modification and secretion. These include enzymes.
23. b, Nucleus. The nucleus contains the DNA (genetic information) of the cell.
24. b. A phospholipid bilayer. See Figure 1.10.
25. b. See answer to question 11.
26. a. This is the only structure that is visible with a light microscope due to its large size.
27. a, Phacocytosis. Pinocytosis describes the ingestion of liquids.
28. c, 65%. This is the average for a healthy adult animal. In older animals the percentage is less and in younger animals the percentage is greater than average.
29. a, Collagen. A structural protein of connective tissue that gives strength to the tissue.
30. c, Synovial joints. Hyaline cartilage or articular cartilage to which it is sometimes referred provides a smooth, durable surface facilitating movement of the joint whilst acting to absorb some of the forces within the joint.
31. Epithelial tissue, connective tissue, nervous tissue, muscular tissue.
32. Simple epithelia, compound or stratified epithelia and glandular epithelia. Refer to Figures 1.13, 1.14 and 1.15.
33. (1) **Simple epithelia** – Associated with covering and lining surfaces of the body. It is located in areas of the body where diffusion,

absorption, secretion or filtration occur; for example, the respiratory surfaces of the lungs, internal surfaces of blood and lymph vessels and lining major body cavities. (2) **Compound/stratified epithelia** – The tissue is resistant to wear and tear as the surface cells are replaced by those underneath; consequently they are located in areas that are subject to some degree of friction. Stratified squamous epithelial tissues line the skin, oral cavity, oesophagus, vagina and anus. Transitional epithelial tissue lines the bladder and urinary tract. (3) **Glandular epithelia** – This type of epithelial tissue is comprised of glandular cells that produce and secrete/excrete materials, for example milk, sweat, sebum, cerumen, hormones and enzymes. **Exocrine** glands such as sweat glands, sebaceous glands, gland of the pancreas and mammary glands secrete the glandular products onto the surface of a cavity or skin. **Endocrine** glands secrete their products into the blood supply for distribution to target organs. Examples of endocrine glands include the adrenal glands, thyroid gland, ovary and testis.

34. Skin is cornified or keratinized stratified squamous epithelium.
35. Transitional epithelium lines the bladder.
36. See question 33.
37. A sweat gland is an example of a simple coiled gland.
38. A salivary gland is an example of a compound alveolar/acinar gland.
39. Refer to pages 14 and 15 for the events during mitosis.
40. Meiosis is similar to mitosis. However, it has two stages of cellular division rather than one. In Meiosis the cell nucleus divides to produce **four daughter nuclei, each with half the number of chromosomes of the parent cell**. It can also be referred to as reduction division as it reduces the number of chromosomes from diploid ($2n$, two sets of each chromosome) to haploid (n, one set of each chromosome). Compare this to mitosis whereby the nucleus divides to produce two daughter nuclei containing identical sets and numbers of **chromosomes** to the parent cell (i.e. is diploid, $2n$).
41. c. Plasma contains the bigger plasma proteins such as albumen and fibrinogen that are too large to pass through the spaces between the epithelial cells of the capillaries into the interstitial spaces.

42. c. The pericardial cavity contains the heart. The pleural cavity contains the lungs. The peritoneum is the serous membrane lining the walls of the abdominal and pelvic cavities. The cardium is a fictitious term.

43. a. Dorsal means towards, or on the back of, an animal. Ventral means towards the belly, cranial means towards the head and caudal means towards the tail.

44. b. Chloride. In this question there were only two possible answers as both potassium and sodium exist as cations (positively charged ions).

45. d, Sodium. Again there were only two possible options as both chloride and bicarbonate are anions (negatively charged ions).

46. c, Potassium. See comments for 45.

47. d, Pleura. The mediastinum is a cavity in the thorax that contains the heart. The peritoneum is the serous membrane lining the walls of the abdominal and pelvic cavities. The perineum is the region between the tail and ischiatic arch of the pelvis, especially the region between the anus and genital organs.

48. b, Thorax. See comments above.

49. d. CSF is classified as Transcellular fluid as it is secreted by specialized cells within the brain in an area called the choroid plexus.

50. d. 60% of the total body fluid is intracellular fluid.

51. A serous membrane lines body cavities. It is smooth and shiny and is comprised of serous endothelial cells that secrete a watery fluid that acts as a lubricant between surfaces.

52. Each pleural cavity is lined by serous membranes called pleura. The pleural layer lining the lungs is called the visceral pleura and that opposite the parietal pleura.

53. Homeostasis is the ability of an animal to maintain a stable internal environment whilst continually adjusting to varying external conditions.

54. Interstitial fluid is the fluid in the spaces between the cells, whereas intracellular fluid is the fluid within the cells themselves.

55. Younger animals have a greater percentage of their body weight as water; therefore a puppy would have a larger percentage of body water than an adult dog.

56. The three types of extracellular fluid are interstitial fluid, plasma and transcellular fluid.

57. Distal means towards the extremities of the limbs (the toes) or further away from.

58. Medial means 'towards the middle of'.

59. Lateral is the opposite of medial.

60. Superficial means situated on or near the surface.

Chapter 2

1. b. The parasympathetic nervous system is under involuntary control and supplies smooth and cardiac muscle and glands of the body.

2. a. Both the autonomic and parasympathetic nervous systems are under involuntary control. The visceral motor system supplies the internal organs. The somatic motor neurones carry information from the CNS to skeletal muscle.

3. b. The autonomic system controls the activity of the heart and smooth muscle. See above for further explanation.

4. b. Myelination acts as an 'insulator', preventing the leaking of the electrical impulse thereby increasing its speed of transmission, whereas a, c and d would all decrease the speed of nervous transmission.

5. c. Myelin is produced by Schwann cells.

6. d. Astrocytes are thought to contribute towards the maintenance of the blood–brain barrier.

7. b. The sodium/potassium pump uses a carrier protein located within the membrane to exchange sodium and potassium ions. This process requires energy and is therefore defined as active transport.

8. a. Anaxonic neurones are found in the CNS.

9. d. Visceral sensory neurones carry information from the organs of the animal to the CNS.

10. b. Sodium and potassium are the ions responsible for the generation of an action potential.

11. The four classifications of neurones according to structure are anaxonic, unipolar, bipolar and multipolar.

12. The four glial cells of the CNS are astrocytes, oligodendrocytes, microglia and ependymal cells.

13. The two glial cells of the PNS are satellite cells and Schwann cells.

14. The transmembrane or resting potential occurs due to an overall excess of negative charge on the inner surface of the membrane when compared to the outer surface, resulting in a difference in electrical charge of inner and outer surfaces of the membrane.

15. An electrochemical gradient occurs when both an electrical and chemical gradient exist across a cell membrane. This can be due to the difference in distribution of sodium and potassium ions across the membrane as a consequence of the different concentrations and their electrical charge. The electrochemical gradient that exists across the cell membrane acts as a store of energy.

16. An action potential is generated when a part of the membrane becomes depolarized, i.e. when the inside of the cell becomes positively charged and the outside negatively charged for a momentary period (remember that with the resting potential the inside of the cell is negatively charged whereas the outside has a positive charge).

17. Saltatory conduction is when an action potential 'jumps' from one Node of Ranvier to another in myelinated fibres (*saltare* – Latin – to leap). This type of nervous transmission occurs much quicker than that in non-myelinated axons as the action potential can 'leap' across lengths of the myelinated axon from node to node.

18. A synapse is the region where one nervous impulse transfers from one neurone to the next.

19. The all-or-none principle refers to the generation of action potentials within neurones. They either occur or not. A graded response is not possible. The magnitude and duration of the action potential is constant, once the initial threshold has been overcome.

20. During the generation of an action potential sodium ions move very quickly out of the axon (at the point of the stimulus) into the extracellular fluid. This causes a local change in the electric potential that triggers a movement of an electrical current to the next segment of the axon. This further causes a depolarization that, when it reaches the threshold, causes the generation of another action potential. In such a way, successive action potentials are triggered along the length of the axon and the impulse travels away from the point of stimulus.

21. c. The sub mater is not one of the meninges.

22. b. CSF can be sampled from the sub-arachniod space, below the arachnoid mater.

23. a. The cerebrum is part of the forebrain, divided into the left and right cerebral hemispheres.

24. b. The cauda equina is the terminal part of the spinal cord resembling a mare's tail.

25. b, Cranial nerve II. The optic nerve carries the impulses associated with sight.

26. c. The parasympathetic nervous system predominates when the animal is relaxed; therefore when digestion would be a priority. Answers a, b and d are all associated with activity of the sympathetic nervous system.

27. c. See above.

28. c. Visceral motor fibres predominate carrying impulses to the organs, cardiac and smooth muscle. There will also be some visceral sensory neurones providing feedback to the CNS.

29. d. Nociceptors are triggered by stimuli causing tissue damage or injury.

30. a. The Vagus nerve (X) carries the majority of the impulses associated with the parasympathetic nervous system.

31. The limbic system is an area of the brain that includes a large number of the structures of the forebrain that are interconnected. It is associated with emotional response and is thought to be associated with certain aspects of emotional behaviour.

32. The somatic nervous system can be subdivided into two sections, cranial nerves and spinal nerves.

33. A plexus is a complex network of nerve fibres that innervate a particular region of the body such as the brachial plexus that innervates the forelimb.

34. When a dog stands on a piece of glass the pain receptors will trigger a stimulus that passes along the sensory afferent neurone to the spinal cord. An interneurone carries the impulse to the motor efferent neurone that causes muscular contractions that remove the limb away from the sharp object. This is known as a reflex response.

35. Adaptation can occur in some receptors that are continually exposed to a stimulus and results in a decline in response. It prevents the unnecessary wasting of energy by preventing the animal responding to a stimulus that is insignificant.

36. The sympathetic portion of the nervous system helps to prepare the body for activity, in particular to meet emergencies (often called the fight or flight response). Activity of the sympathetic nervous system causes dilation of smooth muscle (hence dilation of the pupils, blood vessels to the skin, dilation of the bronchus) increase in metabolic rate, and increased respiration rate.

37. A neurotransmitter is a chemical substance that is released at the synapse. Its function is to diffuse across the gap and interact with the post-synaptic neurone causing either depolarization of the neurone, stimulating the generation of an action potential or hyperpolarization of the neurone, reducing the chance of the generation of an action potential. Neurotransmitters can therefore have either an excitatory or inhibitory response.

38. The neurotransmitter, released by the pre-synaptic neurone, diffuses across the synapse and reacts with the receptor sites of the postsynaptic neurone, causing depolarization and the generation of an action potential.

39. A neuromuscular blocking agent acts at the neuromuscular junction preventing the transmission of the nervous impulse to the muscle hence inhibiting muscular contraction. Drugs such as tubocurarine and pancuronium act by competing with acetylcholine for receptor sites on the muscle cell.

40. A conditioned reflex is achieved by training the animal to exhibit a reflex reaction in response to a conditioned stimulus (i.e. one that would not normally be associated with the reflex response). The classic example is the training of dogs by the Russian scientist, Pavlov, to salivate in response to the ringing of a bell. This involved training (or conditioning) the dogs to associate the ringing of the bell with food. Subsequently, when the bell rang in the absence of food the dogs salivated as they had been conditioned to associate the bell with feeding.

41. a. The pathway of light is cornea, aqueous humour, lens, vitreous humour and retina.

42. d. The tapetum is the reflective surface. The sclera is the outer surface (white of the eye), the retina is the inner surface that contains the receptor cells and rods are one of the two types of receptor cells.

43. d. The cornea is associated with refraction (the bending of light). Other areas where refraction occurs include the lens, aqueous humour and vitreous humour.

44. c. The third eyelid in the dog can be seen at the medial canthus (towards the nose).

45. d. The iris controls the amount of light entering the eye by dilation (in dim light) or constriction (in bright light).

46. a. The white of the eye is called the sclera.

47. d. The retina is the light sensitive layer that contains the photoreceptor cells (rods and cones).

48. b. The semicircular canals are positioned in three planes and movement of the fluid within the canals stimulates receptor cells that relay information to the brain regarding rotational movement of the head.

49. d. The eustachian tube connects to the middle ear that is filled with air. It permits the equalization of air pressure on either side of the tympanic membrane.

50. d. The malleus is the first of the ear ossicles and is consequently attached to the tympanic membrane.

51. Light passes first through the cornea and aqueous humour, where a slight degree of refraction occurs. It then passes through the lens, which changes its shape to focus the light, a process known as accommodation. After passing through the lens the light rays travel through the aqueous humour and are incident upon the retina, ideally in the area of the fovea where visual acuity is at its greatest. The retina contains the photoreceptor cells that are stimulated by the light and send impulses via the optic nerve to the brain.

52. Accommodation is the process whereby the lens changes its shape to focus light coming from either close or distant objects. If light is from a distant object, the ciliary muscles relax, tightening the suspensory ligaments and the lens is pulled into a thin shape so that light can be focused. If light is from a close object then the ciliary muscles contract, relaxing the suspensory ligaments so that the lens is more spherical in shape.

53. The lacrimal apparatus is the term given to the glands and associated structures associated with the dispersal of tears. It includes the lacrimal gland, the tarsal or meibomian gland, the mambrana nictitans gland, the nictitating membrane, goblet cells, the punctae, lacrimal canaliculi, lacrimal sac and naso-lacrimal duct.

54. The tapetum is the reflective layer on the caudal surface of the choroid. It acts to improve vision in dim light by reflecting light back into the eye, acting like a mirror.

55. The nictitating membrane serves to protect the eye being composed of cartilage. It covers the eye inside the eyelids when closed. In cats when they are ill, it sometimes fails to retract completely when the eye is open and is visible towards the medial aspect of the eye.

56. Sound waves enter the ear funnelled by the pinna and travel down the external auditory

canal. They cause the tympanic membrane to vibrate which in turn vibrates the ossicles of the middle ear (the malleus, the incus and the stapes). The stapes vibrates against the oval window that in turn causes vibration of the fluid (perilymph) within the inner ear. Movement of the perilymph causes the distortion of sensory cells that triggers a nervous impulse along the auditory nerve to the brain.

57. The eustachian tube connects the air filled middle ear to the pharynx. It allows the pressure within the middle ear to equilibrate with the pressure on the outside, thereby preventing rupture of the tympanic membrane.

58. The sensation of balance is as a result of feedback from the receptor cells of the semicircular canals, utricle and saccule of the inner ear. The semicircular canals detect rotation of the head via the movement of fluid (endolymph) that stimulates sensory hair cells that generate a nervous impulse. Both the utricle and saccule detect position of the head via sensory hair cells that are tipped with calcium carbonate crystals (otoliths) that 'bend' the hair cells as the head tilts due to the effects of gravity or linear acceleration. The bending of the hair cells generates a nervous impulse that is transmitted to the brain via the auditory nerve. Information from all three areas contribute towards the sensation of balance.

59. As discussed in 58, the semicircular canals detect motion of the head via the movement of fluid within the canals. As the canals are arranged in three perpendicular planes, movement of the head can be detected in any direction.

60. The Jacobson's organ is a structure that is present in the roof of the mouth of most animals and is associated with an enhanced ability to detect certain smells. It is particularly well-developed in the snake and is thought to be associated with both taste and smell. As the snake flicks its tongue in and out it draws it over the Jacobson's organ allowing it to taste/smell the surrounding air.

61. d. ADH or vasopressin is released by the posterior pituitary gland along with oxytocin. The remaining pituitary hormones are all released from the anterior pituitary gland.

62. b. PTH causes bone demineralisation; therefore calcium ion concentrations in extracellular fluid increase. Calcitonin has the opposite effects, causing mineralization of bone and hence a fall in blood calicium levels.

63. a. Glucagon is secreted by alpha cells, insulin be beta cells and somatostatin by delta cells.

64. b. See 63.

65. d. The adrenal medulla secretes adrenaline and nor-adrenaline (or epinephrine and nor-epinephrine).

66. c. Luteinizing hormone is produced by the anterior pituitary gland. Both ADH and oxytocin are produced by the posterior pituitary gland and calcitonin is produced by the thyroid gland.

67. a. The follicle stimulating hormone and luteinizing hormone have a direct effect on the ovary. Progesterone is produced by the corpus luteum of the ovary itself, as is oestrogen.

68. d. Posterior pituitary.

69. b. Anterior pituitary.

70. a. Kidneys.

71. The hormones produced by the anterior pituitary gland are: thyroid stimulating hormone, adrenocorticotrophic hormone, follicle stimulating hormone, luteinizing hormone, prolactin, growth hormone (somatotropin), and melanocyte stimulating hormone.

72. The parathyroid hormone is secreted when the calcium ion concentration in blood falls below the ideal level. It stimulates the increase in circulating blood calcium by stimulating the activity of osteoclasts and consequently the demineralization of bone. It inhibits the activity of osteoblasts, reduces the urinary excretion of calcium ions, and stimulates the secretion of calcitriol by the kidneys (this improves the efficiency of calcium absorption from the digestive tract). The latter three also help to retain calcium within the circulation, thereby preventing any further losses until the balance is restored.

73. Hyperparathyroidism can occur in one of three ways. Neoplasia of the gland can cause overproduction of PTH. This causes bone demineralization which become weak and susceptible to fractures. Chronic renal failure can cause secondary indirect hyperparathyroidism as the kidneys are unable to regulate the excretion of calcium ions. Excess PTH is secreted to try and compensate for the loss. This results in demineralization of bones, usually the mandible and maxilla, producing a condition known as 'rubber jaw'. Secondary nutritional hyperparathyroidism may also be seen in young animals fed butcher's meat (particularly low in calcium). The growth of bone is affected as calcium is preferentially

used to sustain circulating levels within normal limits.

74. Calcitonin is secreted by the thyroid gland in response to an increase in blood calcium ion concentration above the threshold level. It has the opposite effects of PTH, stimulating activity of osteoblasts increasing the mineralization of bone. It also increases the urinary excretion of calcium ions via effects on the kidneys.

75. The steroid hormones secreted by the adrenal cortex include mineralocorticoids, e.g. aldosterone; glucocorticoids, e.g. adrenaline; and adrenal sex steroids, e.g. testosterone.

76. The adrenal medulla secretes adrenaline (epinephrine) and noradrenaline (norepinephrine).

77. All three hormones secreted by the pancreatic islets are associated with the regulation of blood glucose levels. Insulin is secreted in response to an increase in blood glucose and promotes the uptake of glucose by the cells of the body for use during cellular metabolism, thereby removing it from the circulation. Glucagon has the opposite effect, being secreted when blood glucose levels are low. It triggers the breakdown of glucose stores (glycogen) within the muscle and liver in an attempt to sustain blood glucose levels within an ideal range. Somatostatin is the third pancreatic hormone and is secreted in response to dramatic peaks of insulin or glucagons, thereby preventing swings in blood glucose levels.

78. **Diabetes mellitus** is caused by an inability to synthesize sufficient or effective insulin. The patient is unable to regulate its blood glucose levels which are usually very high as the blood remains within the circulation being unable to be utilized by the body's cells for cellular metabolism. Blood glucose levels can exceed the renal threshold for the reabsorption of glucose, in which case glucose appears in the urine – which is copious and has a high specific gravity due to the presence of glucose. Being unable to use glucose for metabolism, lipid (fats) are used and consequently the animal can appear very thin and the breath/urine may smell of pear drops, characteristic of ketones produced as a by-product of fat metabolism. **Diabetes insipidus** is due to the inability to produce adequate or effective amounts of ADH. The animal is therefore unable to regulate the concentration of its urine, producing copious quantities of dilute urine. No glucose is present in the urine of an animal with diabetes insipidus.

79. Inhibin has a negative feedback effect upon the production of follicle stimulating hormone, thereby preventing the development of ovarian follicles in the female and the production of sperm in the male.

80. Hormones produced by the ovary include oestrogens (prior to ovulation) and progesterone (following ovulation). The corpus luteum of the ovary also produces a hormone called relaxin in preparation for parturition.

Chapter 3

1. c. The femur is a long bone and therefore develops by endochondral ossification. Intramembranous ossification relates to the development of bone by replacement of connective tissue, hence c is correct; a and b are incorrect.

2. d. Growth occurs at the epiphyseal or growth plate.

3. a. The calcaneus forms the point of the hock and is also known as the os calcis.

4. a. Long bone.

5. d. Flat bone.

6. b. The primary centre of ossification develops in the diaphysis, followed by secondary centres in each epiphysis once the growth plates are evident.

7. a. See above.

8. b. Blood vessels within bone are located in the haversian systems (or osteons).

9. c. Scapula.

10. c. The acetabulum is found in the pelvis and the obturator foramen is the hole at the base of the skull.

11. The five functions of the skeleton are: (a) to provide a framework and support for soft tissues; (b) to permit movement via articulations between bones at joints and the action of muscles; (c) to protect delicate organs, e.g. brain, heart and lungs; (d) to form blood cells in the marrow of long bones; (e) to act as a storage site for minerals, e.g. calcium and phosphorus.

12. The three parts of the skeleton are the axial skeleton, the appendicular skeleton and the splanchnic skeleton.

13. The two types of bone are cancellous (spongy) bone and compact bone.

14. Osteoblasts form new bone matrix whilst osteoclasts break down bone to release the stored minerals (calcium and phosphorus).

15. Bones are classified as follows: (a) long bones, e.g. femur and humerus; (b) flat bones, e.g. ribs and scapula; (c) irregular bones, e.g. vertebrae and maxilla; (d) short bones, e.g. carpal and tarsal bones; (e) sesamoid bones, e.g. patella and fabellae.

16. A foramen is a small hole in a bone where blood vessels or nerves pass through.

17. A condyle is a rounded enlargement at the end of a bone, usually covered with cartilage and involved with a joint.

18. Refer to Figure 3.6.

19. Refer to the answer for question 73, Chapter 2.

20. When a fracture occurs there is localized bleeding at the fractured site and osteocytes die around the area due to the disrupted blood supply. The endosteum and periosteum produce cells that move into the area forming an area of cartilage at the site of the fracture. The cartilage is then replaced by bone as osteoblasts become active at the site. This area is palpable as a callus. Over time activity of both osteoblasts and osteoclasts remodels the bone at the fractured site, replacing spongy bone with compact bone.

21. b. Anaerobic means without oxygen.

22. a. The epimysium is the outer layer. The prefix 'epi' usually infers 'outer'.

23. d. Intestinal muscle is smooth muscle.

24. d. Smooth muscle lines the walls of the blood vessels. It is under involuntary control.

25. b. Glycogen.

26. c. Hypertrophy. The prefix 'hyper' usually means 'larger/bigger than'.

27. d. Lactic acid.

28. a. Fibrous joint.

29. b. Vertebral bodies. Both a and c are examples of fibrous joints and d is a synovial joint.

30. c.

31. The three types of muscle are smooth, striated and cardiac.

32. The two proteins involved with muscle contraction are actin and myosin.

33. Acetylcholine is the neurotransmitter released at the neuromuscular junction.

34. Isometric contraction causes an increase in tension within the muscle, the length of the muscle remaining constant. Isotonic muscle contraction causes a shortening in length of the muscle with the tension within the muscle remaining constant.

35. The *triceps brachii* acts as an extensor of the elbow.

36. A muscle that is an adductor moves a limb towards the body when it contracts, whereas contraction of an abductor muscle moves the limb away from the body (remember: abduct = to remove/move away from).

37. Sesamoid bones redirect the pull of tendons so that they can function more efficiently whilst acting to protect them.

38. The two types of cartilaginous joint are hyaline cartilage (e.g. the costochondral junction of the rib) and fibrous cartilage (e.g. joints of the mandibular and pelvic symphysis).

39. See Figure 3.10.

40. A tendon is formed from fibrous connective tissue and usually connects muscle to bone. Ligaments are also formed from fibrous connective tissue; however, they connect bones or cartilage within joints, giving the joint stability.

Chapter 4

1. b. The number of eosinophils can be increased with a nematode infection.

2. a, Leucocytosis. Leucopaenia would be a decrease in the number of white blood cells.

3. d. In the healthy animal, the neutrophil is the most numerous.

4. c, Sodium ions. Prothrombin is converted into thrombin that then converts fibrinogen into fibrin. Calcium ions are required during the cascade reaction (for the formation of tissue thromboplastin, see Figure 4.6).

5. d. Platelets are associated with haemostasis (blood clotting).

6. a. Erythropoetin stimulates the production of erythrocytes.

7. d. An eosinophil is a granulocytes.

8. a. The most numerous blood cell is the erythrocye (compare this question to question 3).

9. d. Red blood cells are formed in the red bone marrow of calcellous (spony) bone that is found in the ribs, cranial bones, irregular bones and epiphyses of long bones.

10. d. The erythrocyte is not phagocytic whereas a, b and c are.

11. Haemostasis is a process that relies on a cascade of reactions that trigger a blood clot. Tissue damage causes localized constriction of the blood vessels in an immediate attempt to

reduce blood loss and platelets adhere to the site. If the tissue damage is minor, this may be all that is required to prevent further blood loss. As the platelets adhere they release various factors that cause further aggregation. The damaged tissue also releases tissue factor that combines with calcium ions and a clotting factor in the blood to produce tissue thromboplastin. A second source of thromboplastin is from the activation of the substances released by the platelets. When thromboplastin enters the plasma it forms an enzyme known as prothrombinase. This enzyme converts prothrombin into thrombin. Thrombin converts fibrinogen into insoluble threads of fibrin that form a mesh across the wounded site. Blood cells become trapped in the mesh and a clot is formed.

12. An erythrocyte is the only cell that loses its nucleus as it develops and matures. This is so that there is as much space as possible for carrying oxygen.

13. Lymphocytes are produced in the lymph nodes and lymphatic tissue of the spleen, liver and other organs.

14. The average lifespan of a circulating red blood cell is 120 days.

15. The blood cells that are involved with the specific immune response are B-lymphocytes and T-lymphocytes.

16. Plasma is a straw coloured, clear fluid that contains 90% water. The remainder is comprized of mineral salts, plasma proteins, dissolved gasses, waste products and nutrients. It also contains variable amounts of antibodies, hormones and enzymes depending upon the individual animal.

17. Serum is the same as plasma except that the clotting factors have been removed due to a clot being formed.

18. Erythropoiesis occurs in the red bone marrow of cancellous (spongy) bone, e.g. marrow of the ribs, cranial bones, vertebrae and the epiphyses of long bones.

19. The three protective functions of blood are: (a) haemostasis, preventing blood loss (platelets); (b) prevention against infection (white blood cells); (c) immunity (antibodies).

20. Erythropoeisis is the production of erythrocytes.

21. d. Blood returns to the heart from the lungs in the pulmonary veins.

22. a. Not to be confused with the atrio-ventricular node in the septum.

23. b. Also called the bicuspid valve.

24. b.

25. b. Blood leaving the pulmonary vein has just been to the lungs and is therefore oxygenated.

26. c. Closing of the mitral and bicuspid valves (atrioventricular valves) produce the first heart sound and closing of the semi-lunar valves produces the second.

27. a. The left ventricle has the thickest myocardium as it had to contract with greater strength to pump blood into the aorta to supply the systemic circulation.

28. d. The visceral pericardium (or epicardium) lines the surface of the heart.

29. a. Systole is contraction and diastole is relaxation.

30. c. The QRS complex represents the action potential passing down the bindle of His, along the Purkinje fibres and depolarization of the ventricles as they contract.

31. There are four valves in the heart. The atrioventricular valves, the bicuspid and tricuspid valves are located between the left and right atria and ventricles respectively. Their function is to close when the ventricles contract, preventing backflow of blood back into the atria. The two semi-lunar valves, the aortic and pulmonary, are located between the left ventricle and the aorta and the right ventricle and the pulmonary artery. Their function is to close following ventricular systole, preventing the backflow of blood into the ventricles as they relax.

32. Initial stimulus for the heartbeat arises spontaneously in the sino-atrial node within the wall of the right atrium. The wave of depolarization generated spreads across the atria causing the cardiac muscle to contract and the atria empty into the ventricles. The wave of depolarization reaches the atrio-ventricular node in the septum and this triggers another wave that spreads along the bundle of His and the Purkinje fibres. This causes the ventricles to contract as they empty their contacts into the pulmonary and systemic circuits.

33. The left atrium receives blood from the pulmonary circulation (via the pulmonary vein) and the left ventricle pumps blood into the systemic circulation (via the aorta). The right atrium receives blood form the systemic circulation (via the vana cavae) whereas the right ventricle pumps blood to the pulmonary circulation (via the pulmonary artery).

34. There are three types of blood vessels, arteries, veins and capillaries. Arteries conduct blood away from the heart. As the blood is under high pressure they are thick-walled and robust (they have a thick tunica media with increased amounts of smooth muscle and elastic fibres) when compared to the other vessels. Veins conduct blood back towards the heart. Blood in these vessels is under lower pressure than the arteries, consequently they are more flaccid in structure with less smooth muscle and elastic fibres. Most veins contain valves along their length that help to facilitate the circulation of blood by preventing the blood flowing in the wrong direction due to the effects of gravity. Capillaries are the smallest of the blood vessels and form a network between the arteries and veins. They are thin-walled and it is here that the exchange of interstitial fluid can occur. Capillaries have a smooth muscle sphincter that can contract or relax regulate the amount of blood flow through the capillary network.

35. The range of heart beat for a dog is 60–180 beats per minute, depending upon the size of the animal.

36. The following arteries can be used to monitor pulse in the conscious animal: femoral artery, brachial artery, carotid artery, coccygeal artery and ulnar artery. Some are more easily accessible than others.

37. Baroreceptors are located within the carotid and aortic sinuses and detect the degree of stretch of the vessel wall that gives an indication of the pressure of the circulating blood. If blood pressure increases the baroreceptors send impulses to the cardiovascular centre of the brain, which then takes action to cause a decrease in cardiac output and vasodilation, thereby reducing blood pressure.

38. Renin triggers a cascade reaction, stimulating the conversion if Angiotensinogen into Angiotensin I. Angiotensin converting enzymes then convert this into Angiotensin II. Angiotensin II is a powerful vasoconstrictor, reducing blood flow to the peripheral tissues, thereby ensuring blood flow to vital organs is maintained. It also stimulates the secretion of aldosterone from the adrenal cortex which promotes the retention of water via retention of sodium ions. Secretion of ADH is stimulated which also increases the retention of water and Angiotensin II also stimulates thirst so that the animal seeks water. By these mechanisms, blood pressure and circulating blood volume should increase.

39. ACE is secreted by the lungs.

40. Signs of circulatory shock include: pale mucous membranes and slow capillary refill time, cold extremities and a rapid, weak pulse. The animal may appear depressed.

Chapter 5

1. b. Lipase is secreted by the stomach of unweaned animals. In the adult the bulk of fat digestion occurs in the duodenum.

2. c. The cardia, fundus and pylorus are all parts of the stomach.

3. a. Rennin is secreted in the stomach and clots the milk diet of young animals to facilitate fat digestion.

4. d. Chyme is associated with the digestive tract whereas chyle is the fatty liquid found in the lacteals of the lymphatic system.

5. a. The dile duct enters at the duodenum, the duodenum is associated with digestion not absorption and the function of the ileum is absorption.

6. c.

7. c. Villi are located where absorption occurs.

8. a.

9. c. Pepsin is produces as an inactive form, pepsinogen. HCl within the stomach activates it into pepsin.

10. c.

11. The two stages during the digestive process are mechanical (the mastication of food and churning by the stomach) and chemical (the use of chemicals and enzymes to break down food).

12. The dentition of an adult dog is I3/3, C1/1, P4/4, M2/3.

13. The four pairs of salivary glands are the parotid, submandibular, sublingual and zygomatic.

14. Peristalsis is the name used to describe the waves of contraction of the smooth muscle of the intestine that propel food along the digestive tract.

15. The end products of digestion are: (a) fats are digested into fatty acids and glycerol; (b) proteins are digested into amino acids; (c) carbohydrates are digested into monosaccharides.

16. Enterokinase is a brush-border enzyme that is released into the small intestine. It activates

the pro-enzyme trypsinogen converting it into the active form, trypsin.

17. Bile is synthesized in the liver and stored in the gall bladder from where it is released into the duodenum. It does not contain any digestive enzymes and is associated with the emulsification of lipid (breakdown of fat into small droplets). Emulsification of the lipid makes it easier for lipase to digest any dietary fat. Bile salts also aid the absorption of fatty acids and glycerol further along the small intestine.

18. Excess glucose is converted into a storage product called glycogen by a process called glycogenesis in the liver. Should blood glucose exceed the renal threshold then it will be excreted in the urine (see section 5.3).

19. The gastric secretions are as follows: (a) **Hydrochloric acid** helps to kill bacteria and provides an acidic environment for the functioning of digestive enzymes; (b) **Pepsinogen** is converted into the active enzyme pepsin that starts the breakdown of proteins; (c) **Rennin** is produced in the stomach of unweaned animals. It facilitates the clotting of milk; (d) **Lipase** is produced in the stomach of unweaned animals to start the digestion of fats.

20. The Crypts of Lieberkhun produce new cells that replace those that are shed in the small intestine. As they are shed they secrete brush border enzymes such as Enterokinase. The Crypts also secrete the hormones Cholecystokinin and Secretin that control the activity and secretory activity of the digestive tract.

21. b. The larger plasma proteins are unable to pass through the capillary membrane of the glomerulus.

22. d.

23. a.

24. d. Remember that diabetes insipidus is related to the inability to secrete sufficient effective ADH.

25. c. The PCT reabsorbs some water, salts and glucose from the filtrate.

26. a.

27. c

28. c. The DCT can secrete bicarbonate and hydrogen ions to assist with maintenance of the acid/base balance.

29. d. 85–99% of the glomerular filtrate is reabsorbed in the healthy animal.

30. a.

31. Diabetes insipidus occurs when the animal is unable to produce sufficient effective ADH. It is therefore unable to regulate the loss of water via the kidneys and is unable to produce concentrated urine. As a result, animals show polydipsia and polyuria, producing copious quantities of dilute urine.

32. The distal convoluted tubule can selectively reabsorb some substances and actively secrete others to finally adjust the composition of the tubular fluid. It can reabsorb sodium and chloride ions into the peritubular fluid under the influence of the hormone aldosterone, thereby reducing their excretion. It can also reabsorb calcium ions, under the influence of calcitriol and PTH, secrete potassium, bicarbonate and hydrogen ions should their levels in the peritubular fluid become too high, and aid regulation of the acid/base balance.

33. ADH is secreted in response to dehydration. It causes the walls of the nephron, in particular the walls of the collecting duct, to become more permeable to water. In this way, water can be reabsorbed into the peritubular fluid and retained within the body rather than being lost in urine.

34. The JGA secretes the hormones erythropoietin and renin (see Chapter 4).

35. The JGA is stimulated by Angiotensin II to produce renin (see Chapter 4).

36. See Figure 5.11.

37. The urethra connects the bladder to the external urinary opening, whereas the ureter connect the kidney to the bladder.

38. The PCT is associated with a network of capillaries and it is here that glucose, some water and salts are reabsorbed back into the peritubular fluid to return to the circulation.

39. As the transport is against a concentration gradient, energy is required and this is described as active transport.

40. b. During inspiration the muscles of the diaphragm contract and the diaphragm becomes flattened and lowered, increasing the volume of the thoracic cavity.

41. a.

42. c. Remember that 16% is expired air and 20% is inspired air.

43. a.

44. c.

45. c.

46. d.

47. d. Chemorecoptors are located centrally in the medulla of the brain and peripherally in the aortic arch and carotid bodies.

48. a.

49. b.

50. d. Bronchodilation is under involuntary control and occurs when the animal is frightened, stressed or prepares to defend itself.
51. See Figure 5.14a.
52. The nasal chamber is highly vascular so the blood within the capillaries can warm the inspired air. The mucous helps to moisten the air and to trap any particles/foreign bodies that are moved towards the back of the throat by the cilia. It is then swallowed. By warming, moistening and filtering the inspired air the lower respiratory tract is protected from damage.
53. The soft palate moves upwards and forwards during swallowing preventing any food entering the respiratory tract. In cases of a cleft palate food may escape into the respiratory tract; this can be seen in young puppies when milk dribbles down the nose when suckling.
54. Surfactant lines the surfaces of the alveoli and reduces surface tension thereby preventing their collapse, helping to keep them open.
55. See Figure 5.17.
56. Tidal volume describes the amount of air breathed in and out at rest.
57. Four conditions that may reduce lung function include pneumothorax, pyothorax, a ruptured diaphragm or pulmonary congestion/oedema.
58. Chemoreceptors are located centrally, within the medulla of the brain and peripherally, in the aortic arch and carotid bodies. They are stimulated by a fall in pH due to increased levels of CO_2 of the CSF and blood. When stimulated they trigger an increase in the rate and depth of respiration to eliminate any excess CO_2.
59. During inspiration the muscles of the diaphragm contract, pulling it from its domed shape to a more flattened position. During expiration, the muscles of the diaphragm relax and the diaphragm becomes dome shaped again.
60. The two areas of the brain associated with the control of respiration are the medulla and the pons.

Chapter 6

1. d. 4 digital pads, 1 metacarpal pad, 1 carpal pad. The dew claw normally has a pad, although in some individuals it may not.
2. a. The stratum corneum is the outermost layer and the inner most is the stratum germinativum.
3. d. Sweat glands are located in the dermis.
4. c. Sebum does not promote the further growth of hair.
5. d. Vitamin D_3 is produced by skin in response to UV light.
6. d. Lymphocytes are associated with the immune response.
7. a. Anti-histamines are given in some cases to combat the production of histamine during an allergic response.
8. d. Mast cells are activated during anaphylaxis.
9. c. Active immunity best describes the process of vaccination.
10. a. Another term for macrophage is histiocyte.
11. Sunlight is necessary for the formation of Vitamin D_3 by the skin. This is then converted by the liver into an intermediate compound that is then used to synthesize the hormone calcitriol. Calcitriol is necessary for the absorption of calcium and phosphorus from the digestive tract. Consequently, if the animal is deficient in vitamin D_3 through lack of exposure to sunlight, it will be unable to absorb dietary calcium.
12. There are two types of sweat glands. Apocrine sweat glands produce a secretion that contains pheremones and is thought to be associated with individual recognition and territory marking. Eccrine sweat glands produce sweat that is composed of water, sodium chloride, urea, lactic acid and potassium ions. This type of sweat is associated with the regulation of heat loss.
13. Interferons are small proteins that bind to membranes of healthy cells triggering the production of antiviral proteins in neighbouring cells. If the cells are invaded by a virus then antiviral proteins prevent viral replication within the cells.
14. Subcutaneous fat acts as an energy reserve in addition to providing some degree of mechanical and thermal protection.
15. The testes have to be maintained at lower than normal body temperature for the production of viable sperm. Consequently, there is little subcutaneous fat in order that the area can remain as cool as possible.
16. A cat's claws are sharp and retractable when compared to the dog's and are less pigmented. They are more brittle and easily shed, being laterally flattened rather than tubular.
17. During inflammation histamine is released by mast cells, basophils and platelets. Heparin

and prostaglandins are also released in the area. The chemicals all act to increase the permeability of the capillaries in the injured area resulting in an increased supply of blood, in particular white blood cells that help to protect against infection and remove damaged cells from the injured site. Vasodilation also raises the temperature locally. This is thought to help prevent infection by increased activity of the antimicrobial enzymes.

18. Certain pathogens cause the release of pyrogens. These small proteins reset the temperature control centre in the hypothalamus of the brain, and body temperature can increase (i.e. fever might occur). Fever may help by inhibiting the replication of some viruses and bacteria; it will also increase the body's cellular metabolism in order that cellular reactions occur at a faster rate, helping to combat the effects of disease.

19. Colostrum confers passive (or maternal) immunity to the neonate.

20. During anaphylaxis a very rapid allergic reaction occurs due to activation of mast cells. Symptoms can include swelling and oedema in the dermis of the skin and contraction of the smooth muscle of the respiratory system (hence difficulty breathing). A severe response can cause sudden peripheral vasodilation leading to circulatory collapse.

21. a. Fats are transported in the lymphatic system before entering the circulatory system.

22. c. Lymphocytes are produced by the lymphatic tissue of the lymph nodes.

23. b.

24. a.

25. a.

26. b.

27. d. Progesterone is secreted by the corpus luteum whereas oestrogen is secreted by the developing follicle.

28. b. The vas deferens is part of the male reproductive tract.

29. a. Luteinizing hormone is released by the anterior pituitary gland and has its effects on the ovary.

30. a. Oxytocin is responsible for milk let down. Prolactin is responsible for stimulating the synthesis of milk.

31. Lymph is formed as fluid from blood arriving at the capillary bed leaks through the capillary walls into the interstitial tissue spaces, due to a difference in hydrostatic pressure between the blood and tissue fluid. Some of this fluid returns to the circulation at the venous end of the capillary bed; however, not all can return due to the difference in hydrostatic pressure. The remaining fluid is collected and returned to the circulation by the lymphatic system, the fluid within the system being called lymph.

32. Dietary fats are converted into chylomicrons via the addition of a protein coat. The chylomicrons enter the lacteals of the lymphatic system within the villus of the digestive epithelium. From here they pass within the lymphatic system and eventually enter the circulatory system via the subclavian vein. Only at this stage are they available for metabolism.

33. The three different types of cell in the seminiferous tubule are the Interstitial cells of Leydig, Spermatogenic cells and Sertoli cells. Interstitial cells secrete testosterone, spermatogenic cells produce spermatozoa, and Sertoli cells provide support and nourishment for the developing spermatozoa. They also have some regulatory effects upon the rate of spermatogenesis and the release of spermatozoa into the seminiferous tubule.

34. Refer to Figure 6.10.

35. Refer to Table 6.2.

36. A bitch should be mated as close a possible to the time of ovulation to ensure conception. Detection of the optimal time for mating is most commonly achieved either through the use of vaginal smears (mating when the percentage of anuclear cells is maximal) or through a simple blood test detecting the increased levels of plasma progesterone that occur immediately post-ovulation as the corpus luteum is formed. Another method includes the use of clinical observation, mating on days 12–14 following the first signs of bleeding. This coincides with the estimated time of ovulation; however, it may not be accurate for some bitches.

37. Prolactin is now thought to be a major contributor in cases of pseudopregnancy in the bitch.

38. The stages of parturition of the bitch are: (a) **Stage of preparation**. pre-partum hypothermia may be observed indication parturition will commence within the following 24–26 hours. Other than this there are few obvious signs; (b) **First stage parturition**: uterine contractions begin. Milk may appear within the mammary glands and the dam may show some signs of discomfort, restlessness, panting

and nesting behaviour. She may try to seek seclusion. Allantoic fluid may be seen at the vulva as the allantochorion ruptures; (c) **Second stage parturition**: uterine contractions are stronger as the foetus is propelled through the cervix into the vagina. Strong abdominal straining is seen as the foetus is presented and delivered. Considered as a separate stage in some species, the third stage, passage of the placenta occurs during this stage for the bitch. (d) **Pueperium**: the period during which the reproductive tract returns to its normal state. This takes approximately 4–6 weeks during which a mucoid vaginal discharge may be seen.

39. Placental lactogen, progesterone and oestrogens are all involved in the development and growth of the mammary gland during pregnancy.

40. Suckling causes the release of prolactin and oxytocin which stimulate milk secretion and let down during lactation.

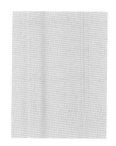

Glossary of terms

ABSOLUTE REFRACTORY PERIOD. The first period during which the neurone cannot respond to a second stimulus.

ACCOMMODATION. The ability to change the shape of the lens to allow focusing on both near and distant objects.

ACETYLCHOLINE. A neurotransmitter of the peripheral nervous system, released at neuromuscular junctions and parasympathetic synapses.

ACID. A molecule with a tendency to release protons or hydrogen ions (H^+) in solution.

ACINAR CELLS. Cells of the pancreas that secrete an alkaline juice containing digestive enzymes.

ACTIN. One of the two proteins involved in muscle contraction forming the myofibrils of muscle.

ACTION POTENTIAL. A change in the transmembrane potential of a cell (usually a neurone) due to a change in permeability of the cell to sodium ions.

ACTIVE TRANSPORT. The movement of ions or molecules across the cell membrane against a concentration gradient requiring the use of energy obtained from ATP.

ADAPTATION. Response seen by some receptors that are exposed to a constant stimulus in that the stimulus fails to trigger the receptor if the stimulus remains.

ADDISON'S DISEASE. *See* hypoadrenocorticism.

ADENOHYPOPHYSIS. *See* anterior pituitary gland.

ADENOSINE TRIPHOSPHATE (ATP). A molecule that acts as an energy store via the chemical bonds between its adenosine and phosphate molecules. When ATP is converted into ADP (adenosine diphosphate) and a chemical bond is broken, energy is released that can be used to drive many biochemical processes, e.g. active transport. The re-synthesis of ATP from ADP and phosphate requires the formation of a chemical bond and hence the input of energy.

ADRENAL GLAND. An endocrine gland that is located on the superior portion of each kidney. They consist of a cortex and medulla and secrete steroid hormones and catecholamines, e.g. adrenaline (epinephrine) and noradrenaline (norepinephrine).

ADRENERGIC SYNAPSE. A synapse that is associated with the release of epinephrine (adrenaline).

ADRENOCORTICOTROPIC HORMONE. Secreted by the anterior pituitary gland under regulation of a corticotropin-releasing hormone from the hypothalamus. Adrenocorticotropic hormone regulates the production of glucocorticoids from the cortex of the adrenal gland.

AEROBIC RESPIRATION. Respiration that occurs with freely available oxygen, producing energy (in the form of ATP), water and carbon dioxide.

AFFERENT. Conducting towards, incoming. An afferent nerve fibre carries impulses towards the CNS.

AGONIST. A muscle responsible for producing a specific movement.

AGRANULOCYTE. A division of white blood cells that includes lymphocytes and monocytes. The cytoplasm appears agranular on staining.

ALBINO. An animal that lacks pigmentation due to the inability to produce melanin.

ALDOSTERONE. Corticosteroid produced by the cortex of the adrenal gland that stimulates the retention of sodium ions and water by the kidney.

ALKALI. A molecule that accepts protons or hydrogen ions (H^+) in solution. Alkalis react with acids, neutralizing them.

ALL-OR-NONE LAW. States that neurones respond only to a stimulus above a specific threshold when they respond maximally, the magnitude and duration of the response being the same. A graded response does not exist.

ALPHA CELLS. One of the four endocrine cells of the Islets of Langerhans. Alpha cells secrete a hormone called glucagon that causes an increase in blood glucose levels through the breakdown of glycogen.

ALVEOLUS. Pleural=alveoli. A pocket within the lungs, at the termination of the bronchioles, where gaseous exchange occurs. Also the bony socket that holds the tooth.

AMACRINE CELLS. Neurons within the retina of the eye that are adapted to facilitate or inhibit transmission between the bipolar cells and the ganglion cells.

AMINO ACID. An organic compound containing nitrogen that forms the building blocks of proteins.

AMPHI-ARTHROSIS. Also known as a cartilaginous joint, formed either by hyaline cartilage, fibrocartilage or a combination of the two. A joint that permits limited movement.

AMPULLA. The expanded end of the semi-circular canal of the inner ear.

ANABOLIC REACTION. A chemical reaction that results in the formation of chemical bonds and the use of energy.

ANAEROBIC RESPIRATION. Respiration that occurs when oxygen is not available, producing energy (in the form of ATP), water, carbon dioxide and lactic acid.

ANAL SAC. Also known as anal glands. A pair of glands between the internal and external anal sphincters. The secretion from the glands aids with defecation and territory marking.

ANAPHYLAXIS. An unusual or extreme allergic response.

ANASTAMOSIS. A connection between two vessels without an intervening capillary bed.

ANDROGEN. A hormone that stimulates male characteristics, e.g. testosterone.

ANGIOTENSIN. Angiotensin I is converted from Angiotensinogen by renin into Angiotensin II by Angiotensin-converting enzymes.

ANGIOTENSIN CONVERTING ENZYME. An enzyme produced in the lungs that converts Angiotensin I into Angiotensin II.

ANGIOTENSINOGEN. An inactive plasma protein that is produced by the liver. It is converted into Angiotensin I in the presence of renin.

ANION. A negatively charged ion, e.g. chloride ion Cl^-.

ANTAGONIST. A muscle that opposes the movement of an agonist.

ANTERIOR PITUITARY GLAND. Also known as the adenohypophysis. The anterior pituitary gland secretes a total of seven hormones all under the control of regulatory hormones from the hypothalamus.

ANTIBODY. Also called immunoglobulin or gamma globulin. A protein produced by B-lymphocytes when exposed to an antigen.

ANTIDIURETIC HORMONE. Also known as vasopressin. A hormone synthesized in the hypothalamus but stored and secreted from the posterior pituitary gland. It stimulates the retention of water by the body through effects on the kidney.

ANTIGEN. A substance that triggers an immune response, e.g. a toxin or bacterium.

ANUS. The terminal opening of the digestive tract.

AORTIC STENOSIS. A narrowing of the aorta on leaving the heart.

APOCRINE SWEAT GLAND. Coiled sweat glands that secrete a component of sweat containing pheremones.

APONEUROSIS. A broadsheet of connective tissue/tendon that connects skeletal to bone.

APPENDICULAR SKELETON. Part of the skeleton including the bones of the forelimb and hindlimb, including the scapula and pelvic bones.

AQUEOUS HUMOUR. The watery fluid contained within the anterior chamber of the eye, secreted by the glandular tissue of the ciliary body.

ARACHNOID LAYER. The middle layer of the meninges.

ARTERIOLE. A small branch of an artery that delivers blood to the capillary bed.

ARTERY. A large blood vessel that carries blood away from the heart.

ARTICULAR. Associated with a joint.

ATOM. The smallest part or 'building blocks' of an element.

ATOMIC NUMBER. The number of protons OR electrons of an atom.

ATRIAL NATRUIRETIC PEPTIDE. A hormone produced by cells of the atrium of the heart in response to abnormal stretching. It stimulates fluid loss and a consequent reduction in circulating blood volume.

ATRIO-VENTRICULAR NODE. Specialized area within the septum of the heart that relays the wave of cardiac contraction to the Bundle of His and Purkinje fibres.

ATRIO-VENTRICULAR VALVE. Also known as the bicuspid (mitral) and tricuspid valves.

ATRIUM. Pleural=atria. The upper, thin walled chambers of the heart that receive blood from the pulmonary and systemic circuits.

ATROPHY. The wasting away of tissue, usually muscle due to lack of use.

AUDITION. The sensation of hearing.

AUDITORY CANAL. Also known as the ear canal or external acoustic meatus. The tube (both vertical and horizontal) leading from the pinna to the tympanic membrane.

AUDITORY NERVE. Cranial nerve VIII. Transmits impulses associated with audition and balance from the inner ear to the brain.

AUDITORY OSSICLES. *See* ear ossicles.

AUSCULTATION. Listening for sounds produced within the body, usually used with particular reference to the heart.

AUTOLYSIS. The breakdown of cells by their own digestive enzymes contained within lysosomes.

AUTONOMIC NERVOUS SYSTEM. Part of the nervous system associated with the involuntary control of the viscera (organs).

AVASCULAR. Without a blood supply.

AXIAL SKELETON. Part of the skeleton including the skull, vertebral column, ribs and sternum.

AXOLEMMA. The cell membrane of the axon.

AXON. The process that conducts impulses away from the cell body in the form of an action potential.

BAND CELLS. The immature form of a leucocyte.

BARORECEPTORS. A sensory receptor that is stimulated by a change in pressure, usually that of blood.

BASOPHIL. The least numerous granulocyte that manufactures histamine and heparin that are released at the site of inflammation.

BETA CELLS. One of the four endocrine cells of the Islets of Langerhans. Beta cells secrete a hormone called insulin that causes a fall in blood glucose levels by promoting its conversion into glycogen.

BICUSPID VALVE. The left atrioventricular valve, also known as the Mitral valve. The valve that separates the left atrium from the left ventricle.

BILE PIGMENTS. The pigments that give bile its colour including bilirubin and biliverdin.

BILE SALTS. The part of bile that is responsible for the emulsification of lipid.

BILIRUBIN. One of the bile pigments produced by the breakdown of haemoglobin.

BILIVERDIN. One of the bile pigments produced by the breakdown of haemoglobin. Converted to bilirubin in the liver.

BIOCHEMISTRY. The study of the chemical reactions and process that occur in biological (living) systems such as plants and animals.

BODY. Largest region of the stomach.

BONY LABYRINTH. A series of canals within the temporal bone that contain the component parts of the inner ear.

BOWMAN'S CAPSULE. A capsule or cup that encloses the glomerulus of the nephron.

BRADYCARDIA. An abnormal, slow heart rate.

BRONCHIOLE. A small division of a bronchus.

BRONCHOCONSTRICTION. Constriction of the bronchi.

BRONCHODILATION. Dilation of the bronchi, usually caused by activity in the sympathetic nervous system.

BRONCHUS. Pleural=bronchi. One of two airways supplying air to the lungs between the trachea and bronchioles.

BUFFER. A substance or molecule that can cause a change in pH by releasing or accepting hydrogen ions (protons). Buffers help to maintain the pH of biological systems within normal ranges and are part of the homeostatic mechanisms of the system.

BULBO-URETHRAL GLAND. An accessory gland found in the cat that contributes towards the seminal fluid.

BUNDLE OF HIS. Specialized cells within the interventricular septum that conduct the wave of cardiac contraction from the atrioventricular node to the Purkinje fibres.

BURSA. A small, synovial fluid filled sac that reduces friction and cushions adjacent structures.

CAECOTROPHS. Also known as 'night faeces'. Soft pellets that are produces by rabbits (and some other herbivorous species) and are ingested to pass through the digestive tract a second time.

CAECUM. Proximal part of the large intestine. It is well developed in herbivorous species such as the rabbit.

CALCITONIN. A hormone secreted by the thyroid gland that assists with the regulation of calcium in the circulation. It is secreted in response to an elevated level of calcium in the blood having opposite effects to parathyroid hormone, causing a decrease in the levels of circulatory calcium ions.

CALCITRIOL. Another name for cholecalciferol that is secreted by the kidney in response to the parathyroid hormone due to falling levels of circulating calcium ions. Calcitriol acts to increase the efficiency of calcium absorption from the digestive tract.

CALLUS. A network of bone that forms around the site of a fracture. The first stage of bone repair that is remodelled and replaced gradually as the fracture site heals.

CANAL OF SCHLEMM. The tract that allows the passage of the aqueous humour from the anterior chamber of the eye to the venous circulation.

CANAL OF VOLKMANN. Canals within the bone structure that contain the blood supply that runs from the periosteum to the osteons.

CANCELLOUS BONE. Also known as spongy bone due to the loose network of trabeculae that branch out in a less rigid structure. Cancellous bone contains spaces that may be filled with red bone marrow. It is located in the vertebrae, in flat bones and in the end of long bones of the skeleton (the epiphysis).

CANTHUS. Both medial and lateral. The area between the upper and lower eyelids at the corners of the eyes.

CAPILLARY. A very small blood vessel that runs between an arteriole and a venule within body tissues with a thin wall that permits the exchange of nutrients and waste products between the interstitial fluid and plasma.

CARBOHYDRATE. An organic compound that can be classified as a monosaccharide, disaccharide or polysaccharide.

CARDIA. Region of the stomach at the entrance to the oesophagus.

CARDIAC CENTRE. The area within the medulla oblongata of the brain that regulates heart rate via the sympathetic and parasympathetic nervous systems.

CARDIAC MUSCLE. Muscle of the heart that is under involuntary control.

CARDIAC SPHINCTER. A circular ring of smooth muscle that lies at the entrance to the stomach.

CARDIOVASCULAR CENTRE. The area of the medulla oblongata of the brain comprising the cardiac and vasomotor centres that together regulate heart rate and vasodilation/constriction, thereby controlling blood pressure.

CARINA. A ridge between the openings of the left and right bronchi.

CARNASSIAL TOOTH. A tooth adapted for shearing meat from bones. In dogs it is the upper fourth premolar and lower first molar and in cats it is the upper third premolar and lower first molar.

CARNIVORE. An animal that primarily eats meat.

CARTILAGE. A type of connective tissue.

CASTRATION. Surgical removal of the testes.

CATABOLIC REACTION. A chemical reaction that results in the breaking of chemical bonds and the release of energy.

CATALASE. The enzyme contained within microbodies or peroxisomes that converts toxic hydrogen peroxide produced by many cellular reactions into oxygen and water.

CATION. A positively charged ion, e.g. sodium ion Na^+.

CAUDA EQUINA. Caudal aspect of the spinal cord ending in a group of nerves whose structure resembles that of a mare's tail.

CELLULOSE. An undigestible polysaccharide that forms plant cells walls. Herbivorous species have bacteria and protozoa in the rumen or caecum that can digest the cellulose, making its products available to the animal.

CENTRAL NERVOUS SYSTEM (CNS). A division of the nervous system that includes the brain and spinal cord.

CENTRE OF OSSIFICATION. A point where ossification (the formation of bone) starts and spreads throughout as a bone is formed.

CEREBELLUM. Part of the hindbrain controlling motor co-ordination.

CEREBROSPINAL FLUID. Fluid contained within the central nervous system secreted by the choroid plexus in the ventricles of the brain.

CEREBRUM. Largest part of the brain (forebrain) composed of two cerebral hemispheres. Thought to control learning, emotions and behaviour.

CERUMEN. Also known as ear wax. A waxy secretion from glands in the wall of the external auditory meatus.

CERUMINOUS GLANDS. Modified sweat glands in the external ear that secrete cerumen.

CHEMORECEPTORS. A sensory receptor that is stimulated by a change in the chemical composition of a fluid, usually blood, e.g. changes in pH.

CHIEF CELLS. Also known as zymogen cells. Cells of the stomach that secrete pepsinogen. *See* parathyroid gland.

CHOLECALCIFEROL. Vitamin D_3. *See* calcitriol.

CHOLECYSTOKININ. A hormone secreted by endocrine cells of the crypts of Lieberkuhn. It regulates the secretory activity of the acinar cells of the pancreas and the secretion of bile from the gall bladder.

CHOLINERGENIC SYNAPSE. A synapse that is associated with the release of acetylcholine.

CHONDROCYTE. A cartilage cell.

CHORDA TENDINA. Pleural=chordae tendinae. One of the many chords that attach the atrioventicular valves of the heart to the papillary muscle, preventing backflow of blood into the atria during ventricular systole.

CHOROID PLEUXUS. A vascular region within the ventricles of the brain that secretes cerebrospinal fluid.

CHROMOSOMES. Structures within the nucleus of the cell containing fine threads of chromatin, containing DNA.

CHYLOMICRON. A large molecule that contains triglyceride (fatty acids) and proteins that are synthesized within the wall of the intestine and transported via the lacteal into the lymphatic system.

CHYME. The semi-fluid mixture of digested food and gastric secretions that leaves the stomach.

CHYMOSIN. An enzyme found in the stomach of unweaned animals that coagulates milk protein.

CILIA. Small projections on the surface of a cell formed from microtubules. They beat to move fluid or mucus over the surface of the cell and are particularly important in the movement of mucus in the upper respiratory tract.

CILIARY BODY. An area of the choroid that includes both ciliary muscle and glandular tissue. It supports the suspensory ligaments of the lens.

CIRCADIAN RHYTHM. The regular occurrence of certain physiological events that occur at about the same time, irrespective of daylength, e.g. sleep cycles. Implies an inbuilt 'body clock'.

CISTERNA MAGNA. An enlarged subarachnoid space between the cerebellum and the medulla oblongata. Can be used for the collection of cerebrospinal fluid or for the injection of contrast media for radiography.

COCHLEA. The coil shaped part of the bony labyrinth that contains the organ of hearing, located in the inner ear.

COLLAGEN. A structural protein found in connective tissue.

COLLECTING DUCT. Part of the nephron that runs from the distal convoluted tubule to the renal pelvis.

COLLOID. A solution that contains molecules that are unable to pass through a semi-permeable membrane. Used in practice to treat severe haemorrhage due to their plasma expanding effects, they have a high osmotic pressure and thereby pull fluid from the interstitial spaces acting as a short-term solution to counteract the effects of hypovolaemia.

COLON. Located between the caecum and the rectum, the colon compacts the remains of the digestive process and also contains bacteria that produce vitamins that are absorbed.

COLOSTRUM. The first milk following parturition that is rich in maternal antibodies.

COMPACT BONE. A type of bone that is compact in structure with the osteons or haversian systems located close together. It is located on the outer surfaces of bones.

COMPOUND. A substance composed of two or more elements combined together in a chemical reaction. Examples include sodium chloride, potassium permanganate and nitrous oxide.

CONCENTRATION GRADIENT. Local differences that exist in the concentration of a substance.

CONES. Light sensitive cells (photoreceptors) that are stimulated in bright light and are responsible for the perception of colour.

CONJUNCTIVA. A covering of the inner surface of the eyelids and anterior surface of the eye formed from stratified squamous epithelium.

CONNECTIVE TISSUE. One of the four types of tissue. Can be loose or areolar connective tissue, dense connective tissue, bone, blood or cartilage.

COPROPHAGIA. The ingestion of faeces. Also known as caecotrophy in rabbits and other herbivorous species.

CORNEA. The transparent rostral surface of the outer layer of the eye.

CORONARY BAND. Area of the epidermis where growth of the claw occurs.

CORPUS CALLOSUM. The body that connects the left and right cerebral hemispheres.

CORPUS LUTEUM. Part of the ovary that remains after ovulation. Produces the female hormone progesterone that maintains the uterus in a state fit for pregnancy.

CORPUSCLE. A small mass or body usually use with reference to blood corpuscle or blood cell.

CORTEX. The outer region of an organ or bone.

CORTICOSTERONE. *See* glucocorticoids.

CORTICOTROPIN-RELEASING HORMONE. Produced by the hypothalamus and regulates the production of adrenocorticotropic hormones by the anterior pituitary gland.

CORTISOL. *See* glucocorticoids.

COVALENT BONDING. The sharing of electrons between atoms in the formation of a molecule during a chemical reaction, e.g. water or H_2O.

CREMASTER MUSCLE. A small strip of muscle that attaches to the spermatic cord and can draw the testes close to the abdomen.

CRENATION. The shrinking of a red blood cell (erythrocyte) due to being placed in a hypertonic solution.

CRYPTORCHIDISM. A condition where both testes fail to descend into the scrotum and are retained in the abdominal or pelvic cavities.

CRYPTS OF LIEBERKUHN. Glandular tissue at the base of the villi of the small intestine.

CRYSTALLIOD. An isotonic electrolyte solution that is capable of passing through a semi-permeable membrane. Used in practice to treat dehydration or fluid loss.

CUPULA. A mass that sits in the ampullae of the semi-circular canals (of the inner ear). Sensory hair cells of the crista are stimulated by movement of the endolymph within the canals.

CUSHING'S DISEASE. *See* hyperadrenocorticism.

CYTOPLASM. The semi-fluid content of the cell that contains the nucleus and organelles.

DECIDUOUS TEETH. Also known as 'milk teeth'. Teeth that are shed in puppies and kittens and are replaced by the permanent adult dentition.

DELTA CELLS. On of the four endocrine cells of the Islets of Langerhans. Delta cells secrete a hormone called Somatostatin that prevents dramatic swings in blood glucose and also reduces the movement of food along the digestive tract.

DENATURED. The destruction of proteins within the body due to changes in pH or temperature that are outside normal ranges. Denaturing a protein changes its shape and structure and hence its biological activity is reduced or prevented.

DENDRITE. Short processes that extend out of the cell body where nervous impulses enter the neurone.

DENTINE. The layer of tooth inside the outer layer of enamel.

DEOXYRIBONUCLEIC ACID (DNA). A double stranded structure formed from sequences of bases (adenine, guanine, cytosine and thiamine) that codes for the synthesis of all proteins and polypeptides made by the cell, i.e. the genetic code.

DEPOLARIZATION. A change in the transmembrane potential from the resting potential of $-70\,mV$ towards a slight positive charge.

DERMIS. The layer of connective tissue below the epidermis of the skin.

DIABETES INSIPIDUS. An inability to produce sufficient amounts of effective anti-diuretic hormone causing retention of water within the body. The animal is polydipsic and polyuric producing copious quantities of dilute urine.

DIAPHRAGM. A musculotendinous structure that separates the thorax from the abdomen.

DIAPHYSIS. The shaft of a long bone formed by a primary centre of ossification.

DIARTHROSIS. Also known as a synovial joint. A joint that is freely movable with bone surfaces separated by synovial fluid.

DIASTOLE. The period of relaxation of cardiac muscle.

DIABETES MELLITUS. An inability to produce sufficient amounts of effective insulin or a decrease in the sensitivity of the animal to the insulin produced. The animal is unable to regulate its blood glucose levels and consequently exceeds the renal threshold and glucose appears in the urine. Fat may be used for cellular metabolism as glucose is unavailable.

DIFFUSION. The movement of molecules from high concentration to low concentration until their concentration is equal in all areas.

DIPLOID. Describes a cell that contains two sets of chromosomes, a paternal set and a maternal set. Sometimes termed $2n$ (where n is the number of chromosomes).

DISTAL CONVOLUTED TUBULE. Part of the nephron that runs between the loop of Henle and the collecting duct. A site of active secretion.

DISTICHIASIS. A condition cause by having an additional row of eyelashes which are turned in towards the eyeball.

DUODENUM. The proximal part of the small intestine.

DURA MATER. The tough, outer protective layer of the meninges.

DYSPNOEA. Difficulty or laboured breathing.

DYSRHYTHMIA. A disturbance of heart rate.

DYSTOCIA. Difficulty giving birth.

EAR OSSICLES. Also known as auditory ossicles. Three small bones in the middle ear that transmit the vibration of the ear drum across the middle ear. Known as the malleus (hammer), incus (anvil) and stapes (stirrup).

ECCRINE SWEAT GLAND. Also known as merocrine sweat glands. Sweat glands that produce the main component of sweat comprising water, sodium chloride, urea, lactic acid and potassium ions.

ECTROPION. Turning outwards of the eyelid margins.

EFFERENT. Conducting away from, outgoing. An efferent nerve fibre carries information away from the CNS to the periphery.

EICOSANOID. A compound derived from arachidonic acid.

ELASTIN. A protein that is found in elastic connective tissue.

ELECTROCHEMICAL GRADIENT. The combination of electrical gradients and chemical gradients that exist across a membrane.

ELECTROLYTE. A compound that dissolves in water to form a solution of ions, e.g. sodium chloride, an important component of fluid therapy in treating dehydration.

ELECTROMAGNETIC RECEPTORS. Those receptors that are triggered by changes in electromagnetic stimuli.

ELECTRON. Negatively charged sub-atomic particles that orbit the nucleus of the atom in orbits. They are involved in chemical bonding.

ELECTRON TRANSPORTER/CARRIER. A molecule that carries/transfers electrons across the cell membrane.

ELEMENT. A simple substance that cannot be broken down or divided by any chemical means. Examples of elements include sodium, potassium and magnesium.

EMESIS. Vomiting.

EMULSIFICATION. The breakdown of large lipid droplets into smaller droplets that are more accessible to digestive enzymes.

ENAMEL. The very hard, outer layer of the tooth.

ENDOCARDIUM. The layer of simple squamous epithelia tissue that lines the inner surface of the heart.

ENDOCHONDRIAL OSSIFICATION. The formation of bone based upon a cartilage model.

ENDOCRINE GLANDS. 'Ductless glands' that secrete their products (usually hormones) directly into the blood stream, e.g. the thyroid gland.

ENDOCYTOSIS. The uptake of material into a cell from the environment (outside), including both pinocytosis and phagocytosis.

ENDOLYMPH. Fluid contained within the membranous labyrinth of the inner ear (the utricle, saccule, semi-circular canals and cochlear duct).

ENDOMETRIUM. The mucous membrane lining the uterus.

ENDOMYSIUM. A delicate membrane of connective tissue that surrounds each muscle cell.

ENDONEURIUM. Connective tissue surrounding the axon.

ENDOPLASMIC RETICULUM. Both smooth and rough form fine tubules that run throughout the cytoplasm of the cell. Smooth endoplasmic reticulum synthesizes and stores lipid and some carbohydrates, whereas rough endoplasmic reticulum is associated with the synthesis and storage of proteins.

ENDOSTEUM. Tissue lining the medullary cavity of bone.

ENTEROKINASE. A brush border enzyme that activates the pancreatic pro-enzyme trypsinogen.

ENTROPION. Turning inwards of the margins of the eyelids.

ENZYME. A protein that acts as a catalyst during a chemical reaction in that it speeds up the chemical reaction but is not directly involved in the reaction itself.

EOSINOPHIL. A type of granulocyte that increases in number during allergic reactions and nematode infections. They are phagocytic.

EPAXIAL. Above the vertebral column.

EPICARDIUM. The outer membrane covering the heart. Also known as the visceral pericardium.

EPIDERMIS. The outer layer of the skin.

EPIDIDYMIS. Coiled tubules where sperm maturation occurs.

EPIGLOTTIS. A flap of tissue that contains cartilage that covers the entrance to the larynx during swallowing.

EPIMYSIUM. The dense outer layer of skeletal muscle that is continuous with tendons and the perimysium.

EPINEURIUM. An outer fibrous sheath holding together groups of bundles in addition to enclosing a blood supply and fatty deposits.

EPIPHYSEAL PLATE. *See* growth plate.

EPIPHYSIS. The end of a long bone formed by a secondary centre of ossification.

EPITHELIUM. One of the four types of tissue. Can be simple squamous, simple cuboidal or simple columnar. May also be stratified (compound) epithelium consisting of several layers of cells or glandular eplithelium producing secretions.

ERYTHROCYTE. A red blood cell that transports oxygen in the form of oxyhaemoglobin.

ERYTHROPOIESIS. Formation of red blood cells (erythrocytes). This is under the regulation of the hormone erythropoietin.

ERYTHRPOIETIN. A hormone secreted by the kidneys in response to low oxygen content of the blood. It stimulates erythropoiesis in bone marrow.

EUSTACIAN TUBE. A channel that connects the middle ear with the nasopharynx which permits pressure to be equalized on either side of the tympanic membrane.

EXOCRINE GLANDS. Glands that secrete onto the surfaces of a cavity (or skin). Formed from epithelial tissue pockets with ducts to the surface, e.g. sweat glands.

EXOCYTOSIS. The opposite of endocytosis. The discharge of materials from within a cell that are too large to pass out via diffusion or osmosis.

EXTERNAL NARES. Also known as nostrils.

EXTERNAL RESPIRATION. Diffusion of air between the air in the alveoli and the blood.

EXTRACELLULAR FLUID. Fluid located outside cells. Includes interstitial fluid, plasma and transcellular fluid.

F CELLS. On of the four endocrine cells of the Islets of Langerhans. F cells produce a hormone called pancreatic peptide that is thought to affect the production of some pancreatic digestive enzymes.

FACIAL NERVE. Cranial nerve VII. Innervates the muscles of the face and tongue.

FACILITATED DIFFUSION. The use of a protein carrier molecule to carry a substance across a cell membrane in the direction of the concentration gradient. This is a passive process, i.e. requires no energy expenditure.

FASCIA. A sheet of connective tissue that separates muscles and other internal organs.

FASICLE. A small bundle or cluster of muscle fibres.

FAT. Also known as lipid. An organic compound called a triglyceride composed of fatty acids and glycerol.

FIBRIN. Insoluble fibres of protein that form a mesh like structure as the sits of the wound.

FIBRINOGEN. A plasma protein that forms fibrin when exposed to the enzyme thrombin.

FIBRINOLYSIS. The process where a blood clot gradually dissolves as the wound heals.

FIBROBLAST. A cell of connective tissue that produces collagen fibres.

FOLLICLE. The ovum and surrounding cells during its development in the ovary.

FOLLICLE STIMULATING HORMONE. A hormone secreted by the anterior pituitary gland that stimulates development of the gametes in both the male and female animal.

FORAMEN. Pleural=foramina. A hole or passageway, usually through bone.

FOSSA OVALIS. A depression in the wall of the right atrium representing the location of the foramen ovale in the foetus, a hole in the septum between the left and right atrium that normally closes at birth.

FOVEA. Part of the retina that provides the sharpest vision due to the high density of cones. Also known as the Macula Lutea.

FUNDUS. Region of the stomach lying to the left and dorsal to the cardia.

G CELLS. Cells within the pyloric region of the stomach that secrete the hormone gastrin.

GAMETE. The male of female reproductive cell that contains a haploid number of chromosomes. The spermatozoon or ovum.

GAMMA-AMINOBUTYRIC ACID. An amino acid that acts as an inhibitory neurotransmitter of the CNS.

GANGLION. A group of cell bodies of neurones outside the CNS.

GASTRIC JUICE. The collective term used to describe the secretory contents of the stomach including hydrochloric acid, intrinsic factor and pepsinogen.

GASTRIC LIPASE. An enzyme found in the stomach of unweaned animals that starts the digestion of fat in milk.

GASTRIN. A hormone secretes by G cells of the stomach in response to the presence of food in the stomach. Gastrin stimulates the production of gastric juice and contractions of the stomach wall.

GLIAL CELL. *See* neuroglia.

GLOMERULAR FILTRATE. The fluid that is produced due to filtration at the glomerulus, that passes along the nephron.

GLOMERULUS. A knot of capillaries in the kidney that sits in the Bowman's capsule. The site of filtration.

GLOSSOPHARYNGEAL NERVE. Cranial nerve IX. Innervates the pharynx, tongue and salivary glands.

GLUCAGON. A hormone produced by the alpha cells of the pancreatic islets of Langerhans that stimulates the breakdown of glucagon into glucose.

GLUCOCORTIOCOIDS. Hormones such as cortisol, corticosterone and cortisone secreted by the cortex of the adrenal gland. Also known as steroid hormones.

GLUCOGENESIS. *See* glycogenolysis.

GLYCOGEN. A carbohydrate that is the principal storage material in animals, primarily in the liver and muscles.

GLYCOGENESIS. The creation of glycogen from glucose.

GLYCOGENOLYSIS. The breakdown of glycogen into glucose. Also known as glucogenesis.

GLYCOPROTEIN. A protein molecule combined with a carbohydrate group.

GOBLET CELL. A specialized mucus secreting cell.

GOLGI APPARATUS. Membrane bound sacs that modify, synthesize and transport cellular materials, e.g. glycoproteins and lysosomal enzymes.

GOMPHOSIS. A classification of joint also known as a type of fibrous joint, e.g. the joint between the tooth and the alveolar socket of the mandible.

GONADOTROPIN-RELEASING HORMONE. A hormone secreted by the hypothalamus that regulates the secretion of follicle stimulating hormone by the anterior pituitary gland.

GONADS. The reproductive organs of the male and female animal that produce the gametes (spermatozoa and ova, respectively).

GRANULOCYTE. *See* polymorphonuclear leucocyte.

GREY MATTER. Area of the brain and spinal cord containing the cell bodies of the neurones.

GROWTH HORMONE. Also known as somatotropin. A hormone released by the anterior pituitary gland that stimulates the growth of tissues and the longterm regulation of energy stores.

GROWTH HORMONE-INHIBITING HORMONE. A hormone secreted by the hypothalamus that inhibits the release of growth hormone.

GROWTH HORMONE-RELEASING HORMONE. A hormone secreted by the hypothalamus that stimulates the release of growth hormone.

GROWTH PLATE. Also known as the epiphyseal plate. The cartillaginous region in developing bone between the epiphysis and diaphysis.

GUSTATION. The sensation of taste.

GUT ASSOCIATED LYMPHOID TISSUE. Lymphoid tissue within the digestive system.

GYRUS (pl=GYRI). A fold or ridge on the surface of the cerebrum.

HAEMOGLOBIN. A protein that is contained in red blood cells that has a high affinity for oxygen.

HAEMOLYSIS. The rupture of red blood cells (erythrocytes).

HAEMOPOIESIS. Also known as haematopoiesis. Refers to the production of blood cells.

HAEMOSTASIS. Also known as blood clotting/coagulation. The stopping of bleeding.

HAPLOID. Describes a cell that contains only one set of chromosomes (n), half the number of the original parent cell. These form the gametes of the organism.

HAUSTRA. Pouches within the colon that permit considerable expansion.

HAVERSIAN CANAL. The central canal to an osteon carrying the blood vessels that supply the bone tissue.

HAVERSIAN SYSTEM. *See* osteons.

HERBIVORE. A species of animal that eats only plant/vegetable matter.

HERING BREUER REFLEX. A reflex that triggers the regulation of breathing by preventing over-inflation of the lungs.

HISTIOCYTE. Also referred to as a macrophage. A large phagocytic cell of the reticulo-endothelial system, usually located within connective tissue.

HISTOLOGY. The study of tissue structure and function.

HOMEOSTASIS. The ability of a biological system to maintain a relatively constant internal environment, e.g. pH and body temperature, whilst adapting to cope with a fluctuating external environment.

HORMONE. A chemical messenger that is released by an endocrine gland or tissue which is carried in the circulation to reach target cells in other tissues around the body.

HYDROGEN BONDING. Weak bonds that exist between water molecules (intermolecular bonds).

HYDROPHILIC. Describes a substance that reacts readily with water.

HYDROPHOBIC. Describes a substance that does not react with water.

HYOID APPARATUS. A structure of small bones that forms a suspensory mechanism for the tongue and larynx.

HYPAXIAL. Below the vertebral column.

HYPERADRENOCORTICISM. Also known as Cushing's disease. The adrenal cortex produces excessive amounts of glucocorticoids especially cortisol. This is either due to neoplasia of the gland or the excessive production of adrenocorticotrophic hormone.

HYPERPARATHYROIDISM. Overproduction of parathyroid hormone due to neoplasia of the parathyroid gland, chronic renal failure or a diet low in calcium. It causes excess calcium to be reabsorbed from the bones leading to brittle/soft bones affecting the growth of young animals.

HYPERPOLARIZATION. Movement of the transmembrane potential below $-70\,mV$ for a brief period as the resting potential returns.

HYPERTENSION. High blood pressure.

HYPERTHERMIA. An abnormally high body temperature.

HYPERTHYROIDISM. Overproduction of T_4 and T_3 usually as a consequence of enlargement of the thyroid gland.

HYPERTONIC/HYPEROSMOTIC. Describes a solution that has an osmotic pressure greater than the one to which it is being compared. In biological systems the comparable solution is usually plasma.

HYPERTROPHY. Enlargement, usually of muscle, due to repeated use or exercise.

HYPOADRENOCORTICISM. Also known as Addison's disease. The adrenal cortex is unable to produce sufficient aldosterone and potassium is retained within the body.

HYPODERMIS. Also known as the subcutaneous layer. The layer of loose connective tissue below the dermis of the skin.

HYPOPHYSIS. *See* pituitary gland.

HYPOTENSION. Low blood pressure.

HYPOTHALAMUS. Part of the brain closely linked with the pituitary gland. Responsible for the co-ordination of neural and endocrine functions.

HYPOTHERMIA. An abnormally low body temperature.

HYPOTHYROIDISM. Underactivity of the thyroid gland produces lower than normal levels of T_4 and T_3. In some cases production may stop completely.

HYPOTONIC/HYPO-OSMOTIC. Describes a solution that has an osmotic pressure less that the one to which it is compared. In biological systems the comparable solution is usually plasma.

HYPOVOLAEMIA. Abnormally low circulatory blood volume.

ILEUM. The terminal part of the small intestine.

IMMUNOGLOBULIN. *See* antibody.

INCUS. The second ear ossicles (also known as the anvil) articulating with the malleus and the stapes.

INHIBIN. The hormone produced by the testis or the ovary that has a negative feedback upon the production of follicle stimulating hormone.

INSERTION. The point of attachment of a muscle to bone that is most movable during muscle contraction.

INSULIN. A hormone produced by the beta cells of the pancreatic islets of Langerhans that stimulates a fall in blood glucose by promoting its conversion into glycogen.

INTEGUMENT. The skin.

INTERFERON. A glycoprotein released by cells invaded by a virus. It stimulates uninfected cells to produce an antiviral agent preventing viral replication if the cells which have been invaded by the virus.

INTERNAL RESPIRATION. Also known as tissue respiration. The diffusion of gases between the interstitial fluid and the blood.

INTERSTITIAL CELLS OF LEYDIG. Cells of the testis that secrete the male hormone testosterone.

INTERSTITIAL CELL STIMULATING HORMONE. *See* luteinizing hormone.

INTERSTITIAL FLUID. Fluid located in the spaces between cells, part of the extracellular fluid compartment. Also known as tissue fluid.

INTRACELLULAR FLUID. Fluid located within the cell.

INTRAMEMBRANOUS OSSIFICATION. The formation of bone within connective tissue, without the prior development of cartilage.

INTRINSIC FACTOR. A glycoproteins secreted by the parietal cells of the stomach that is necessary for the absorption of vitamin B_{12}.

INVOLUNTARY MUSCLE. *See* smooth muscle.

ION. A charged particle formed when an atom gains or loses and electron(s), e.g. sodium ion Na^+ or a chloride ion Cl^-.

IONIC BONDING. The transfer of electrons from one atom to another in the formation of a molecule during a chemical reaction, e.g. sodium chloride NaCl.

IRIS. A structure composed of circular and radial smooth muscle fibres that forms the coloured part of the eye. It determines the size of the pupil thereby controlling the amount of light entering the eye.

ISLETS OF LANGERHANS. Also known as pancreatic islets. Endocrine cells of the pancreas that consist of four different cell types: alpha, beta, delta and F cells.

ISOMETRIC CONTRACTION. Contraction of skeletal muscle that increases tone within the muscle, length of the muscle remaining constant.

ISOTONIC CONTRACTION. Contraction of skeletal muscle that produces muscle shortening, tone within the muscle remaining constant.

ISOTONIC/ISO-OSMOTIC. Describes a solution that has an osmotic pressure equal to the one to which it is compared. In biological systems an isotonic fluid is usually taken to have the same osmotic pressure to plasma, e.g. normal saline (0.9% NaCl).

ISOTOTOPE. An element that has the same atomic number but different mass number, i.e. with the same number of protons but with a different number of neutrons. Some isotopes are radioactive and give off radioactive particles as they decay into a more stable form.

JACOBSON'S ORGAN. Also known as the vomeronasal organ. Thought to act as a supplement to the olfactory system being stimulated by pheremones. In snakes it is particularly well developed and is involved with the detection of prey.

JEJUNUM. Part of the small intestine between the duodenum and ileum.

JUXTAGLOMERULAR APPARATUS. A collection of specialized smooth muscle fibres and cells of the distal convoluted tubule that release the hormones renin and erythropoietin.

KERATIN. A structural scleroprotein that has waterproof properties. The principle constituent of the epidermis, hair and claws.

KININ. A peptide that increases the permeability of blood vessels.

KUPFFER CELLS. Phagocytic cells of the liver.

LACRIMAL CANALICULI. A term used to describe the lacrimal ducts within the eyelid itself.

LACRIMAL GLAND. Also known as the tear gland located on the dorsolateral surface of the eye. It produces watery tears.

LACRIMAL SAC. Located at the proximal end of the nasolacrimal duct. The lacrimal ducts empty into them.

LACTEAL. Terminal part of the lymphatic system that is located within the small intestine.

LACUNA. A small cavity within the bone matrix that contains and osteocyte.

LARYNX. Contains the vocal folds that are responsible for the production of sound. Also called the voice box it is composed of cartilage and muscle.

LENS. The transparent biconvex body lying behind the iris and pupil that can change shape to allow the focusing of light from both near and distant objects.

LEUCOCYTE. A white blood cell. White blood cells can be further divided into granulocytes and agranulocytes depending upon their structure and function.

LEUCOPOIESIS. The production of leucocytes.

LIGAMENT. A band of connective tissue that connects one bone to another.

LIMBIC SYSTEM. An area of the brain that is associated with the emotional aspect of behaviour.

LIMBUS. The junction between the cornea and the sclera.

LIPASE. An enzyme that breaks down lipids. Produced predominantly by the pancreas.

LIPID. *See* fat.

LONGITUDINAL SULCUS. The divide fissure between the two cerebral hemispheres.

LOOP OF HENLE. Part of the nephron that runs between the proximal and distal convoluted tubules. It creates a concentration gradient in the renal medulla.

LORDOSIS. Arching of the spine. Seen in bitches and queens that are sexually receptive.

LUMEN. A central space within a tube or duct.

LUTEINIZING HORMONE. A hormone secreted by the anterior pituitary gland that promotes the secretion of FSH and ovulation in the female and promotes spermatogenesis in the male where it is also known as interstitial cell stimulating hormone.

LYMPHADENOPATHY. Swollen, inflamed lymph nodes.

LYMPHOCYTE. A type of agranulocyte that can be classified as a B-lymphocyte or T-lymphocyte. Both are involved with defence of the animal against invading cells, B-lymphocytes produce antibodies and T-lymphocytes attack invading cells directly.

LYSOSOME. A vesicle within the cytoplasm that contains digestive enzymes.

LYSOZYMES. An enzyme that destroys baceteria.

MACROPHAGE. *See* histiocyte.

MACULA. Plural=maculae. Endings of the auditory nerve located in the utricle and saccule.

MACULA LUTEA. *See* fovea.

MALLEUS. The first of the ear ossicles (also known as the hammer) articulating with the tympanic membrane and the second ear ossicles, the incus.

MASS NUMBER. The mass of the nucleus of an atom. Equal to the number of protons PLUS neutrons.

MAST CELL. A cell within connective tissue that releases serotonin, histamine and heparin when triggered by tissue damage.

MASTICATION. The action of chewing.

MECHANORECEPTORS. Those receptors that are triggered by mechanical pressures or distortions, e.g. those responding to touch.

MEDIASTINUM. The tissues and organs that separate the two lungs (including the heart and vessels, trachea, oesophagus, thymus and other associated tissues).

MEDULLA. The inner region of an organ or bone.

MEDULLA OBLONGATA. Part of the hindbrain controlling basic functions such as respiratory rate and heart rate.

MEGAKARYOCYTE. Large cells in bone marrow that produce thrombocytes.

MEIBOMIAN GLAND. Also known as the tarsal gland, meibomian glands are found between the cartilage and conjunctiva of the eyelids. They secrete a fatty material that forms part of the tear film.

MEIOSIS. The process of cell replication that occur in gametes, producing cells that are haploid with genetic material different in structure from the parent cell.

MELAENA. Black, tar like faeces.

MELANOCYTES. A specialized cell in the skin that produces the pigment melanin.

MELANOCYTE-STIMULATING HORMONE. A hormone released by the anterior pituitary gland that stimulates the production of skin pigments based on melanin by melanocytes.

MELATONIN. Produced by the pineal gland during periods of darkness, melatonin is a precursor of serotonin and it is thought linked to timing of oestrus, sexual maturation and maintenance of circadian rhythms.

MENINGES. The three layers of tissue that surround the central nervous system.

MENISCUS. A piece of fibrocartilage between opposing surfaces in a joint, e.g. the stifle.

MEROCRINE SWEAT GLAND. *See* eccrine sweat gland.

MESENTERY. A layer of serous membranes that supports organs in the abdominal and pelvic cavities, holding them in place and providing a route for the blood and nervous supply.

MESOVARIUM. A fold of mesentery that encloses the ovary.

METAPHYSIS. The area between the epiphysis and diaphysis of a long bone, usually the location of the epiphyseal plate (growth plate) of developing bone.

MICROBODIES or PEROXISOMES. Small membrane bound structures found particularly in liver cells containing catalase and other oxidases.

MICROTUBULES and MICROFILAMENTS. Small filaments found in the cytoplasm that are associated with the maintenance of the shape of the cell. They may form cilia and are also involved in the formation of the spindle during cell division.

MICROVILLUS. Pleural=microvilli. Small finger-like projections on the surface of an epithelial cell.

MICTURITION. Meaning urination.

MINERALOCORTICOIDS. Corticosteroids, e.g. aldosterone, produced by the cortex of the adrenal gland that effect the regulation of electrolytes (sodium and potassium).

MISALLIANCE. Also called mismating. When the female animal is mated to the wrong male or is mated when unplanned.

MITOCHONDRION. The organelle that generates ATP for cellular use.

MITOSIS. The process of cell replication whereby identical, diploid daughter cells are produced.

MITRAL VALVE. *See* bicuspid valve.

MOLE. A minute quantity of a substance where 1 mole is the weight of 1 molecule of that substance, i.e. its molecular weight. A mole is always equal to 6.023×10^{23} molecules, sometimes referred to as the Avogadro's Number.

MOLECULE. The smallest amount of a compound.

MONOCYTE. A type of agranulocyte that is phagocytic, engulfing foreign bodies at the site of injury/infection.

MONOESTRUS. An animal that has one period of oestrus during a breeding season.

MONOGASTRIC. A species of animal having a single stomach, e.g. the dog and cat.

MONORCHIDISM. A condition where one of the two testicles has failed to descend into the scrotum and is retained in the abdominal or pelvic cavities.

MONOSACCHARIDE. A simple sugar or carbohydrate that cannot be broken down any further, e.g. glucose, fructose and galactose.

MOTOR. Associated with movement. A motor nerve fibre carries impulses from the CNS to skeletal muscle (somatic) or to organs (visceral).

MULTIPAROUS. Describing a species that gives birth to many offspring.

MUSCARININC RECEPTORS. Receptors sensitive to acetylcholine found at all parasympathetic effector junctions and a few sympathetic effector junctions.

MYELIN. A phospholipid/protein-type substance that forms a sheath around certain axons (known as myelinated nerve fibres).

MYOCARDIUM. The muscular tissue layer of the heart.

MYOEPITHELIAL CELLS. Epithelial cells that are contractile in nature found in glandular epithelium. Contraction assists with the secretory ability of the cell.

MYOFIBRIL. One of the threads of a muscle fibre composed of myofilaments.

MYOFILAMENT. Protein filaments from myofibrils, composed of actin and myosin.

MYOSIN. One of the two proteins involved in muscle contraction forming the myofibrils of muscle.

NASOLACRIMAL DUCT. The duct that carries tears from the nasolacrimal sac to the nasal cavity.

NASOPHARYNX. Part of the pharynx above the soft palate.

NATURAL KILLER CELL. A cell that recognizes and destroys abnormal cells/antigens without themselves being sensitized against the target.

NEOPLASIA. Any new abnormal growth. Usually referring to a tumour that may be benign or malignant.

NEPHRON. The functional unit of the kidney.

NEURILEMMA. The outer membrane of a glial cell that surrounds an axon.

NEUROGLIA. Cells that provide support and protection for the neurone (also known as satellite or glial cells). These include astrocytes, oligodendrocytes, microglia, ependymal cells, satellite cells and Schwann cells.

NEUROHYPOPHYSIS. *See* posterior pituitary gland.

NEUROMUSCULAR JUNCTION. The junction between a neurone and a muscle fibre.

NEURONE. A cell within the nervous system specialized for the transmission of nervous impulses. They can be bipolar, unipolar or multipolar.

NEUROTRANSMITTER. A chemical compound synthesized by a neurone that, when released, affects the transmembrane potential of another neurone.

NEUTRON. An uncharged (neutral) subatomic particle that exists in the nucleus of all atoms, except the hydrogen atom that consists only of one proton and one electron.

NEUTROPHIL. The most numerous granulocytes that ingest bacteria and cellular debris (phagocytosis) particularly in areas of infection.

NICOTINIC RECEPTORS. Receptors of the autonomic ganglion cells and motor-end plates of skeletal muscle sensitive to acethylcholine.

NICTITANS GLAND. Located at the medial canthus producing a secretion that contributes to the tear film. The gland can become prolapsed causing a condition known as 'Cherry eye' appearing as a large pink swelling at the medial canthus.

NICTITATING MEMBRANE. Also known as the membrana nictitans or third eyelid. A fold of conjunctiva with cartilage that is attached at the medial canthus.

NISSL BODY. A region of cell body of a neurone that stains darkly due to the density of endoplasmic reticulum and ribosomes.

NOCICEPTORS. Those receptors that are triggered by pain or injury.

NODE OF RANVIER. Region between glial cells where there is a gap in the myelin sheath.

NORADRENALINE. Also known as norepinephrine. A neurotransmitter of most of the sympathetic postganglionic neurones in addition to being a hormone released from the adrenal medulla in response to stimulation of the sympathetic nervous system.

NUCLEASE. *See* nucleotidase.

NUCLEOLUS. A dense region in the nucleus that is the site of RNA synthesis.

NUCLEOTIDASE. Also called nuclease. An enzyme produced by the acinar cells of the pancreas that breaks down nucleotides.

NUCLEUS. Part of the cell that contains genetic material (DNA) in the form of chromatin, RNA and protein. It controls the cells' activities.

OEDEMA. An abnormal accumulation of fluid usually within tissue or a body cavity.

OESOPHAGUS. A muscular tube connecting the pharynx to the stomach.

OESTROGEN. Female sex steroid hormone produced by the developing oocyte.

OESTRUS. The period of sexual receptivity during which the female will accept the male for mating.

OLFACTION. The sensation of smell.

OLFACTORY BULB. End of the olfactory tract that synapses with the CNS below the lobes of the cerebrum.

OMNIVORE. An animal that eats both plant and animal material.

OOGENESIS. The production of ova.

OPTIC DISC. The region where the optic nerve enters the eye. Also known as the blind spot due to an absence of photoreceptors in this area.

OPTIC NERVE. Cranial nerve II, carrying impulses from the retina of the eye to the brain.

ORGAN OF CORTI. Part of the cochlea that contains the sensory hair cells that provide the sensation of hearing.

ORGANELLE. One of the many specialized structures within the cell (not including the nucleus).

ORIGIN. The point of attachment of a muscle to bone that is least moveable during muscle contraction.

OSMOSIS. The movement of a solvent, usually water, across a semi-permeable membrane from low solute concentration (weak or dilute solution) to high solute concentration (strong or concentrated solution) until the concentrations of both solutions on either side of the membrane are equal.

OSMOTIC PRESSURE. The pressure that is required to prevent osmosis, i.e. to prevent the movement of solvent molecules.

OSTEOBLASTS. Cells that produce bone matrix.

OSTEOCLASTS. Cells that break down bone matrix.

OSTEOCYTE. A bone cell that is unable to divide but which recycles the minerals within the bone matrix. Found within the osteons in layers around the Haversian canal.

OSTEON. The structural unit of compact bone, consisting of concentric layers of osteocytes around a central canal (the Haversian canal) containing the blood vessels that supply the bone tissue. Osteons are also known as Haverisan systems.

OSTEOPROGENITOR CELL. Cells that divide to produce cells that become osteoblasts within the bone matrix.

OTODECTES CYANOTIS. The ear mite commonly seen in cats and dogs.

OTOLITH. A fragment of calcium carbonate that is located within the maculae of the utricle and saccule of the inner ear.

OVAL WINDOW. An opening in the bony labyrinth where the stapes conducts its vibrations into the fluid filled inner ear.

OVARIOHYSTERECTOMY. Surgical removal of the ovaries and uterus of the female animal to prevent breeding.

OVARY. The female gonad.

OVIDUCT. Also called the fallopian or uterine tube. The tube that carries the ova from the ovary to the uterine horns.

OVUM. Pleural=ova. The female gamete.

OXYGEN DEBT. That build up during the process of anaerobic respiration and 'repaid' after exercise by panting.

OXYHAEMOGLOBIN. Haemoglobin that is carrying/combined with oxygen.

OXYNTIC CELLS. Also known as parietal cells. Cells of the stomach that secrete hydrochloric acid and intrinsic factor.

OXYTOCIN. A hormone synthesized in the hypothalamus but stored and secreted from the posterior pituitary gland. It causes the contraction of smooth muscle of the uterus during labour and milk let down during lactation.

PALPEBRAE. Meaning eyelids.

PANCREATIC AMYLASE. An enzyme produced by the acinar cells of the pancreas that breaks down carbohydrates.

PANCREATIC AMYLASE. The enzyme produced by the acinar cells of the pancreas that breaks down polysaccharides.

PANCREATIC PEPTIDE. A hormone produced by the F cells of the pancreatic islets of Langerhans that is thought to affect the production of some pancreatic digestive enzymes.

PARASYMPATHETIC NERVOUS SYSTEM. That part of the autonomic nervous system that is responsible for stimulating activities that conserve energy and lower metabolic rate. Predominates when the animal is in a relaxed state.

PARATHYROID GLAND. Endocrine glands (two) that lie close to the thyroid glands. Chief cell secrete the hormone parathyroid hormone that stimulates an increase in the circulating levels of calcium ions in the blood.

PARATHYROID HORMONE. Also known as parathormone. It is secreted by the chief cells of the parathyroid glands causing an increase in the circulating levels of calcium ions. Works in conjunction with calcitonin to maintain homeostatic levels of blood calcium ions.

PARENCHYMA. The functional cells of an organ (compared to those associated with structure/framework).

PARIETAL CELLS. *See* oxyntic cells.

PARTURITION. The act of giving birth.

PATHOGEN. A disease causing organism.

PEPSIN. A proteolytic enzyme that breaks down proteins in the stomach.

PEPSINOGEN. An inactive pro-enzyme that is converted into its active form, pepsin when exposed to hydrochloric acid.

PEPTIDASE. An enzyme that breaks the bonds within a peptide releasing amino acids.

PEPTIDE. Formed from amino acids. Several peptides from a polypeptide and several polypeptides from a protein.

PERICARDIUM. Fibrous sac surrounding the heart. The visceral (serous) pericardium lies adjacent to the heart whereas the parietal (fibrous) pericardium lines the pericardial cavity.

PERICHONDRIUM. A layer of fibrous connective tissue surrounding cartilage.

PERILYMPH. Fluid found between the membranous labyrinth and bony labyrinth of the inner ear.

PERIMYSIUM. Connective tissue that surrounds individual muscle fascicles.

PERINEUM. The region between the tail and genitalia.

PERINEURIUM. Connective tissue holding bundles of axons together.

PERIODONTAL LIGAMENT. The ligament that connects the tooth to the alveolar socket.

PERIOSTEUM. The layer of connective tissue that surrounds bone consisting of a tough, protective outer layer and an inner layer of osteogenic cells.

PERIPHERAL NERVOUS SYSTEM (PNS). The remaining neural tissue outside the CNS.

PERISTALSIS. Waves of contraction of the smooth muscle that propel contents along the intestine.

PERITONEUM. Parietal peritoneum and visceral peritoneum.

PEYER'S PATCHES. A type of gut associated lymphoid tissue associated with the small intestine.

pH. The relative strength of an acid or alkali expressed in relation to water with a pH of 7 (neutral). Strong acids have a pH of 1 or 2 and strong alkalis have a pH of 13 or 14. Weak alkalis are sometimes called bases.

PHAGOCYTOSIS. The engulfing of extracellular materials by a cell into membrane bound vacuoles within the cytoplasm. The cell is known as a phagocyte.

PHARYNX. A muscular passageway common to both the respiratory and digestive tracts. It can be subdivided into the nasopharynx, the oropharynx and the laryngopharynx.

PHOSPHOLIPID BILAYER. A double-layered membrane formed from phosphate and lipid molecules with hydrophilic and hydrophobic properties.

PIA MATER. The inner layer of the meninges covering the brain and spinal cord.

PILOERECTION. The erection of hair.

PINEAL GLAND. Also known as the 'third eye'. The pineal gland is located in the brain and is thought to be sensitive to light, stimulating the production of melatonin.

PINEALOCYTES. Specialized secretory cells of the pineal gland that secrete melatonin.

PINNA. The expanded part of the external ear that in most species, acts as a funnel for sound.

PINOCYTOSIS. The ingestion of extracellular fluid and it contents by a cell into membrane bound vesicles within the cytoplasm.

PITUITARY GLAND. Often referred to as the 'master gland' of the body or hypophysis, an endocrine gland located at the base of the brain that is connected to the hypothalamus. It is comprised of the posterior and anterior parts.

PLACENTA. An organ that joins the mother and foetus during pregnancy.

PLASMA. A clear, straw-coloured fluid that forms approximately half the volume of whole blood. The fluid part of blood in which the blood cells are suspended. Part of the extracellular fluid compartment.

PLASMA MEMBRANE. Sometimes used to mean cell membrane.

PLEURA. The membranes surrounding the pleural cavities containing the lungs. Visceral (pulmonary) pleura lining the lungs and parietal pleura lining the pleural cavities.

PLEURAL FLUID. Lubricating fluid that reduces friction between the pleural membranes as the lungs inflate and deflate.

PLEXUS. A network, usually in relation to nerves.

PNEUMOTHORAX. Air in the pleural cavity.

POLARIZED. Cells that have a transmembrane potential can be described as polarized.

POLYDIPSIA. Excessive drinking.

POLYMORPHONUCLEAR LEUCOCYTE. A type of white blood cell also known as a granulocyte. They include neutrophils, eosinophils and basophils. Their cytoplasm appears granular on staining.

POLYOESTRUS. An animal that has two or more oestrus cycles in a breeding season.

POLYPHAGIA. Excessive eating.

POLYUREA. Excessive urination.

PONS. Part of the hindbrain connecting the medulla oblongata to the midbrain.

POSTERIOR PITUITARY GLAND. Also known as the neurohypophysis. The posterior pituitary gland acts as a storage site for two hormones synthesized by the hypothalamus, oxytocin and antidiuretic hormone.

POSTGANGLIONIC NEURONE. These refer to neurones that exists distal to a ganglion.

PREGANGLIONIC NEURONE. These usually form part of the autonomic nervous system and are located proximal to a ganglion.

PROENYZME. An inactive enzyme, e.g. trypsinogen, pepsinogen.

PROGESTERONE. The hormone that is produced by the corpus luteum of the ovary following ovulation. Responsible for the maintenance of pregnancy.

PROLACTIN. A hormone secreted by the anterior pituitary gland that promotes the development of mammary tissue and plays and active role in lactation.

PROLACTIN-INHIBITING HORMONE. A hormone secreted by the hypothalamus that inhibits the release of prolactin.

PROLACTIN-RELEASING FACTOR. A hormone secreted by the hypothalamus that stimulates the release of prolactin.

PROPRIOCEPTORS. Those receptors that relay information regarding the position and movements of the body.

PROSTATE GLAND. An accessory gland of the dog and cat that produces the bulk of the seminal fluid.

PROTEIN. A large organic compound formed from chains of polypeptides that are themselves formed from chains of amino acids.

PROTEOLYTIC. The breaking of peptide bonds that form proteins.

PROTHROMBINASE. *See* thrombokinase.

PROTON. A small sub-atomic particle that forms the nucleus of the atom. It has a mass of 1 with a positive charge.

PROXIMAL CONVOLUTED TUBULE. The proximal part of the nephron that is situated between the Bowman's capsule and the loop of Henle. The major site of active reabsorption of glucose.

PSEUDOCYESIS. *See* pseudopregnancy.

PSEUDOPREGNANCY. Also known as pseudocyesis, false pregnancy or phantom pregnancy. Development of the signs of pregnancy without the presence of an embryo.

PTYALIN. *See* salivary amylase.

PULMONARY CIRCULATION. The circulation that runs from the right ventricle of the heart to the lungs and back into the left atrium.

PULMONIC STENOSIS. The most common cardiac defect in the dog. A narrowing of the pulmonary artery leaving the heart.

PUNCTUM. Pleural=punctae. A small hole on each eyelid, close to the medial canthus that drains tears into the lacrimal duct.

PURKINJE FIBRES. Specialized conducting cells that spread across the left and right ventricles causing ventricular contraction when stimulated.

PYLORIC GLANDS. Glands in the pyloric regions of the stomach that secrete mucus to line the stomach mucosa.

PYLORIC SPINCTER. A circular ring of smooth muscle that lies at the exit of the stomach.

PYLORUS. The distal third of the stomach close to the pyloric sphincter.

PYOMETRA. Pus within the uterus.

PYOTHORAX. Pus in the thorax causing the accumulation of large amounts of pleural fluid.

PYROGEN. An agent that causes fever.

RECEPTOR MOLECULE. A molecule either within the cell membrane or in the cell itself that recognises and binds with specific molecules, such a binding triggering a change within the cell.

RECEPTORS. A sensory nerve ending that responds to a specific stimulus and triggers a nervous impulse.

RECTUM. The terminal part of the large intestine that acts as an expandable, temporary store for faecal material.

REFLEX OVULATOR. An animal in which the act of mating stimulates ovulation.

REFRACTION. The bending of light rays as they move between media of differing density.

REFRACTORY STAGE. The period of depolarization and repolarization of a neurone existing in two phases, the absolute refractory period and the relative refractory period.

RELATIVE REFRACTORY PERIOD. The latter period of the refractory stage during which the neurone can be stimulated but only be a stronger than normal stimulus.

RELAXIN. A hormone produced during pregnancy by the corpus luteum, placenta and uterus that helps to prepare the female for birth.

RENIN. A hormone produced by the kidney in response to a fall in blood pressure.

RENNIN. *See* chymosin.

REPOLARIZATION. Return from the positive charge of depolarization towards the resting potential.

RESPIRATORY CENTRE. An area within the medulla oblongata and pons that co-ordinate respiration.

RETICULO-ENDOTHELIAL SYSTEM. A population of macrophages that are distributed throughout the body.

RETINA. The inner layer of the eye that contains the light sensitive cells or photoreceptors called rods and cones.

RHINARIUM. Skin of the nose.

RHODOPSIN. The visual pigment found in the photoreceptor cells.

RIBONUCLEIC ACID (RNA). Molecules that are contained within the nucleolus of the cell and within the ribosomes that copy and translate the genetic code of the DNA into proteins and polypeptides.

RIBOSOME. An organelle that contains ribosomal RNA that is associated with the manufacture of proteins.

RODS. Light sensitive cells (photoreceptors) that are stimulated in dim light conditions.

ROUND WINDOW. An opening in the bony labyrinth that exposes the membrane of the tympanic duct within the cochlea to the middle ear.

RUGAE. Folds of the mucosa of the stomach when empty that stretch with gastric distension.

RUMINANT. A species of animal that has a rumen. The rumen is the largest of the stomachs that acts as a fermentation vat.

SACCULE. Part of the membranous labyrinth of the inner ear. Contains maculae which are important in the sense of balance.

SALIVARY AMYLASE. The enzyme that is secreted by the parotid and submandibular salivary glands that starts the digestion of carbohydrate.

SALT. Any compound that is formed from ions, e.g. sodium chloride, magnesium sulphate, potassium chloride although more specifically used to describe sodium chloride or common table salt.

SARCOLEMMA. The cell membrane of a muscle cell.

SARCOMERE. The smallest contractile unit of skeletal muscle. SCLERA. The outer layer of the eye forming the white of the eye on the anterior surface.

SEASONALLY POLYOESTRUS. An animal that has oestrus cycles during a particular time of year.

SEBACEOUS GLAND. Gland in the skin that secretes sebum.

SEBUM. The secretion produced from sebaceous glands to lubricate the hair and skin.

SECRETIN. A hormone secreted by endocrine cells of the crypts of Lieberkuhn. It regulates the secretory activity of the duct cells of the pancreas.

SEMICIRCULAR CANALS. Three canals in each ear, located perpendicular to each other that are associated with the detection of movement.

SEMI-LUNAR VALVE. The valves that prevent the back flow of blood back into the ventricles on ventricular dystole. The pulmonary semi-lunar valve prevents the flow of blood back into the right ventricle whereas the aortic semi-lunar valve prevents blood flowing back into the left ventricle.

SEMINIFEROUS TUBULES. Small tubules within the testis where spermatogenesis occurs.

SENSORY. Associated with sensation. A sensory nerve fibre carries information from the periphery towards the CNS.

SEPTAL CELLS. Also known as type II cells. Cells within the alveoli that secrete surfactant.

SEPTUM. The wall that divides the left and right chambers of the heart.

SEROTONIN. A neurotransmitter produced from melatonin secreted by the pineal gland.

SERTOLI CELLS. Cells of the testis that secrete small quantities of oestrogen.

SINO-ATRIAL NODE. Also referred to as the pacemaker of the heart. An area within the right atrium where the rhythm of cardiac contraction arises spontaneously.

SINUS ARRHYTHMIA. The normal cyclic variation in heart rate.

SMOOTH MUSCLE. Also known as involuntary muscle. Muscle found in the walls of visceral organs and the digestive, respiratory, urinary and reproductive tracts.

SOLUTE. A solid that dissolves in a liquid to form a solution.

SOLUTION. The liquid that is formed by dissolving a solute in a solvent.

SOLVENT. The liquid that dissolves a solid to form a solution. In biological systems the solvent is water.

SOMA. The cell body of neurone, containing the nucleus.

SOMATIC. Relating to the body.

SOMATOSTATIN. A hormone produced by the delta cells of the pancreatic islets of Langerhans that prevents dramatic swings in blood glucose and also reduces the movement of food along the digestive tract.

SOMATOTROPIN. *See* growth hormone.

SPERMATOGENIC CELLS. Cells of the testis that produce spermatozoa by meiosis.

SPERMATOZOON. Pleural=spermatozoa. The male gamete.

SPLANCHNIC SKELETON. Bones that develop in tissue that are unattached to any other bone. In the dog, this is the os penis. The cat does not have an os penis.

SPONGY BONE. *See* cancellous bone.

SPONTANEOUS OVULATOR. An animal that ovulates whether or not mating occurs.

STAPES. The last ear ossicles (also known as the stirrup) articulating with the incus and the oval window at the entrance to the inner ear.

STRATUM BASALE. *See* stratum germinativum.

STRATUM CORNEUM. The outer layer of the epidermis above the stratum lucidum.

STRATUM GERMINATIVUM. Also called the stratum basale. The lower layer within the epidermis of the skin that contains cells that divide rapidly by mitosis.

STRATUM GRANULOSUM. The layer within the epidermis above the stratum germinativum.

STRATUM LUCIDUM. The layer within the epidermis above the stratum granulosum.

STRIATED MUSCLE. Also known as skeletal or voluntary muscle. Muscle of the skeletal system that is under voluntary control.

SUBARACHNOID SPACE. A space within the meninges that contains cerebrospinal fluid.

SULCUS (pl=SULCI). A groove.

SURFACTANT. A phospholipid that reduces surface tension within the alveoli of the lungs.

SUSPENSORY LIGAMENTS. A delicate ligament that suspends the lens from the ciliary body of the eye.

SUTURE. A classification of joint also known as a type of fibrous joint, e.g. joints between the bones of the skull.

SYMBIOSIS. An association between two organisms where the existence of one benefits the other or both.

SYMPATHETIC NERVOUS SYSTEM. Part of the autonomic nervous system that is responsible for the 'fight or flight' response, i.e. those responses that lead to an increase in use of energy and metabolic rate.

SYNAPSE. The junction between one neurone and another or between a neurone and an organ.

SYNAPTIC CLEFT. The gap between the two neurones at the synapse.

SYNARTHROSIS. Also known as a fibrous joint. A joint that does not permit relative movement between two surfaces.

SYNDESMOSIS. A classification of joint also known as a type of fibrous joint, e.g. attachment of the hyoid apparatus to the temporal bone of the skull.

SYNOTOSIS. A classification of joint also known as a type of fibrous joint, e.g. any normal or abnormal union of two bones by osseous material.

SYSTEMIC CIRCULATION. The circulation that runs from the left ventricle of the heart around the body and back into the right atrium.

SYSTOLE. The period of contraction of cardiac muscle.

TACHYCARDIA. An abnormal, fast heart rate.

TAIL GLAND. Areas of specialized cells that are located at the base of the tail in dogs and extend along the dorsal surface of the tail in cats. They secrete a scent thought to be important in individual recognition.

TAPETUM. A layer of reflective cells on the surface of the choroid, characteristic of animals that have good night vision. It reflects light back into the eye giving it a second opportunity to stimulate the retinal receptors.

TARSAL GLAND. *See* meibomian gland.

TARSAL PLATE. Fibrous tissue within the eyelids.

TENDON. A band of connective tissue that connects skeletal muscle to bone.

TESTIS. Pleural=testes. Also known as testicle. The male gonad.

TESTOSTERONE. The primary male reproductive hormone produced by the interstitial cells of the testis.

THALAMUS. Part of the mammalian brain that acts as a relay between the spinal cord/brainstem and the cerebral hemispheres.

THERMORECEPTORS. Those receptors that are triggered by changes in temperature.

THRESHOLD. The level of depolarization that is required before an action potential can be generated.

THROMBIN. The enzyme that converts fibrinogen to fibrin during coagulation.

THROMBOCYTE. Also known as a platelet. The smallest of the blood cells, appearing as non-nucleated fragments. They assist with haemostasis (blood clotting).

THROMBOKINASE. Also known as prothrombinase. The enzyme that triggers the conversion of prothrombin to thrombin during coagulation.

THROMBOPLASTIN. Formed by the combination of clotting factors and calcium ions through both the extrinsic and intrinsic pathways, during haemostasis. Thromboplastin triggers the formation of the enzyme prothominase (or thrombokinase).

THROMBOPOIESIS. Also known as thrombocytopoeisis. The formation of thrombocytes (platelets).

THROMBOPOIETIN. The hormone controlling the rate of thrombopoiesis.

THYMUS. An endocrine gland located in the mediastinum that is large in young animals decreasing in size with age. It secretes a hormone called thymosin that promotes the development and maturation of lymphocytes.

THYROID GLAND. An endocrine gland situated below the larynx. It secretes three hormones, thyroxine (T_4), tri-iodothyrodine (T_3) and calcitonin.

THYROID STIMULATING HORMONE. Also known as Thyrotropin. It is secreted by the anterior pituitary and stimulates the thyroid gland to produce thyroid hormones under the regulation of thyrotropin releasing hormone secreted by the hypothalamus.

THYROXINE. Also known as T_4. Hormone secreted by the thyroid gland that increases cellular metabolism.

TISSUE RESPIRATION. *See* internal respiration.

TONICITY. The equivalent osmotic pressure of a solution.

TRABECULAE. Bony spindles in cancellous bone that form a framework whose spaces are usually filled with bone marrow. Also layers of connective tissue within the lymph node.

TRACHEA. The windpipe, connecting the larynx to the bronchi.

TRANSCELLULAR FLUID. Part of the extracellular fluid compartment. Secreted by specialized cells.

TRANSMEMBRANE POTENTIAL. The potential difference that exists across a cell membrane due to the difference in concentration of ions on either side. Also known as the resting potential.

TRICUSPID VALVE. The right atrio-ventricular valve separating the right atrium from the right ventricle.

TRI-IODOTHYRODINE. Also known as T_3. Hormone secreted by the thyroid gland that has similar effects to T_4.

TRYPSINOGEN. An inactive pro-enzyme secreted by the acinar cells of the pancreas that is converted into trypsin by the enzyme enterokinase.

TUNICA ADVENTITIA. The outer protective layer of blood vessels.

TUNICA INTIMA. The inner most layer of blood vessels, consisting of endothelial cells.

TUNICA MEDIA. The middle layer of arteries and veins containing smooth muscle and elastic fibres in varying proportions.

TUNICA MUCOSA. The inner mucosal layer of the intestine.

TUNICA MUSCULARIS. The middle muscular layer of the intestine containing smooth muscle.

TUNICA SEROSA. The protective outer layer of the intestine.

TURBINATES. Bones within the nasal cavity that are covered with vascular, mucous epithelium.

TYMPANIC MEMBRANE. Also known as the ear drum. A thin membrane that separates the outer ear from the middle ear.

TYPE II CELLS. *See* septal cells.

UREA. The end product of protein metabolism formed in the liver from amino acids and other compounds containing nitrogen. Secreted in urine.

URETER. The tube that carries urine from the kidney to the bladder.

URETHRA. The tube that carries urine from the bladder to the exterior during urination.

UTERUS. A hollow muscular organ in female animals where the fertilized ovum implants and develops through pregnancy. In dogs and cats the uterus consists of a short body and a pair of elongated uterine horns.

UTRICLE. Part of the membranous labyrinth of the inner ear. Contains maculae which are important in the sense of balance.

UVEA. A term used to describe the middle, vascular layer of the eye consisting of the choroid, ciliary body and iris.

VACUOLE. A small cavity inside a cell, usually taken to contain a solid material, distinguishing it from a vesicle although sometimes the terms are used ambiguously.

VAGINA. The tract in the female animal that runs from the cervix of the uterus to the vestibule.

VAGUS NERVE. The tenth cranial nerve that supplies parasympathetic and sensory fibres to most of the thoracic and abdominal viscera.

VALENCY. The ability of an atom to combine with another through the exchange or sharing of electrons. An atom with a valency of 1 can share, donate or receive one electron during formation of a molecule.

VAS DEFERENS. Plural=vasa deferentia. The duct that carries spermatozoa from the epididymis to the urethra on ejaculation.

VASCULAR. Having a rich supply of blood vessels.

VASECTOMY. Surgical excision of the vas deferens to cause sterility.

VASOMOTOR CENTRE. The area within the medulla oblongata of the brain that regulates vasoconstriction and vasodilation.

VASOPRESSIN. *See* antidiuretic hormone.

VEIN. A large blood vessel that carries blood towards the heart.

VENTRICLE. One of the four fluid-filled chambers of the brain or one of the two lower, muscular chambers of the heart that pump blood into the pulmonary and systemic circulations.

VENULE. A small blood vessel that carries blood from the capillary bed to a vein.

VESICLE. A small sac containing liquid.

VESTIBULE. A cavity at the entrance to another structure. In the case of the ear, the entrance to the middle ear. Also, entrance to the vagina.

VIBRISSAE. Whiskers, large tactile hairs.

VILLUS. Pleural=villi. A finger-like projection of the intestinal mucosa into the lumen of the intestine for absorption.

VISCERAL. Relating to an organ (usually within the abdomen).

VITREOUS HUMOUR. The 'jelly'-like fluid in the posterior chamber of the eye.

VOLUNTARY MUSCLE. *See* striated muscle.

VULVA. The external genitalia of the female animal.

ZYMOGEN CELLS. *See* chief cells.

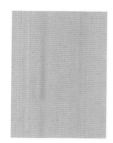

Index

acid base *see* pH balance
acids 6–7
action potential, muscle 84
active transport 11, 12–13, 40
adaptation 53
Addison's disease 71
adenosine triphosphate 85–6
adrenal
    glands 70–1
    medulla 54, 71
adrenaline 65
alimentary canal *see* oesophagus
alkalis 6–7
alpha receptors 54
amino acids 65, 122
anaemia 97
anaerobic respiration, muscles 85
anaphylaxis 143
anatomical terms 24
angiotensin 109–10
anions 4
ANS 45, 53
    heart 102
antibodies 145–6
antidiuretic hormone (ADH) 126–7
anus 144
aorta 105
arteries 104, 105
atomic number 2
atoms 2
    bonding 3
ATP *see* adenosine triphosphate
audition *see* ear, the
autonomic nervous system *see*
    ANS
avieolar ducts 132
axon 35

balance 63–4
beta receptors 54
bile 120
biochemistry basics 1–10

blood 93–9
    chemical content 109
    clotting 97
    and the liver 123
    pressure 108–10
        hormones 109
    vessels, bone 80
        see also vascular system

blood–brain barrier 36, 47
body
    cavities 24–8
    fluids 29–30
bonding *see* chemical bonding
bone 77–82
    anatomical features 82
    blood vessels 80
    cancellous 79
    development 79–80
    fractures 81
    ossification 80–1
    terminology 82
Bowman's capsule, liver 124–5
brain 46–8
    and cardovascular system 109
breathing *see* respiratory system
breeding 154–60
bronchi 132

caecum 113–14, 118
calcitriol 141
capillaries 104, 106–8
    kidney 124
    small intestine 117–18
carbon dioxide 135
cardiac muscle 86, 100
cardiovascular system 99–101
cartilage 21–2
cartilaginous joints 88
castration 160
cations 4

cavities in the body 24–8
cells 12–23
    blood 94–6
    bone 78
    communication between 64–5
    division 14, 15
    membrane 10–13
    see also neurones; Schwann
    cells
cellular exchange 28
central nervous system *see* CNS
cerebral hemispheres 46
cerebrospinal fluid 46–7
chemical bonding 3–5
chemoreceptors 109, 135
circulation
    of the lymphatic system 147–9
    see also cardiovascular system
circulatory shock 110–11
citric acid cycle 129
claws 142–3
clots, blood 97
CNS 34, 45–55
    blood pressure 109
cochlea 62
collateral gangia 54
complement proteins 144–5
compounds 1, 3
concentrations of substances 9
cones, the eye 57, 58, 59
contraception *see* reproduction,
    controlling
converting units 8–9
coronary band 142
coughing 132
covalent bonding 3–4
crenation 5–6

DCT *see* distel convoluted tubule
defecation 122
dendrites 35
dentine 115
depolarization 40
dermis 139
diabetes
    insipidus 72, 127
    mellitus 72, 128
diffusion 5, 11–12
digestion 113–23
    absorption of products 120–2
    herbivores 114
    secretions 118–19
distel convoluted tubule (DCT)
    128–9
DNA 13
duodenum 117

ear, the 60–1
    sweat glands 141
ECG *see* electrocardiogram
efferent nerves 48, 49
electrocardiogram 103
electrolytes 4, 5
electrovalent bond 4

elements 1
endocrine system 64
endo/exocytosis 13
endoplasmic reliculum 13
energy 146
enzymes 115–20
epidermis 139, 142
epididymis 151–2
erythrocytes 94–5
Eustacian tube, ear 62, 130
eye, the 56–60
eyelids 60

fallopian tubes 154
false pregnancy 161
feet 141
female reproductive system 152–4
fever 145
fibrinolysis 99
fluids *see* body fluids
foot pads 142
forebrain 46
fractures, bone 81

gall bladder 120
gametes 149–50
gastric secretions 119
glucocorticoids 71
glycoproteins 11
Golgi apparatus 13, 14
gonads *see* ovaries; testes
growth hormone 68
gustation 64

haemolysis 5–6
haemopoiesis 96–7
haemorrhage 110–11
hair 143–4
Haversian systems 79
hearing 61
heart 70
    anatomy 99–100
    beat 102
    capillaries 108
    rate 108
    valves 100–2
herbivores, digestion 114
Hering-Breuer reflex 135
hindbrain 48
histiocytes *see* microphages
homeostasis 30–1
hormones 65–74
    blood pressure 109
    and control of reproduction 160
    lactation 163–4
    liver 123
    secretions 66
hydrogen bonding 4–5
hypo-adrenocorticism 79
hypophysis *see* pituitary gland
hypothalamus 47, 66, 68
hypothyroidism 70

ilium 117
immunity 145–7
immunological
    competence 146
    surveillance 144
imperial to metric 8
inflammation 145
inner layer, the eye 57
innervation, bones 80–1
integument *see* skin
interferons 144
intermolecular bonding 4–5
intestines 117–18
ionic bonding 4
isotopes 3

joints 88–91
jujunum 117
juxtaglomerular apparatus 127

kidneys 70, 109, 123–9
Krebs cycle 129
Kupffere cells 123

lactation 163–4
large intestine 118
larynx 116, 130
lens, eye 58–9
leucocytes 95–6, 97
ligaments 90–1
limbic system 48
lipids 65
liver, the 122–3
loop of Henle 125–6
lungs 132
    capacity 133
    factors affecting 134
lymph nodes 148
lymphatic system 147–9
lymphocytes 96, 145, 149
lysosomes 14

male reproductive system 150–2
mass number 2
mathematical notation 7–8
mating 154, 158–9
medulla oblongata 55
meiosis 15
melanocytes 141
melatonin 69
metabolism 23
metric from imperial 8
microbodies 14
microphages 144
midbrain 42
milk, producing *see* lactation
mitochondria 14
mitosis 14–15
molecule 3
monoestrus species 154
motor neurones 38
mouth 114–15

muscles
    action potential 84
    anaerobic respiration 85
    atrophy and hypertrophy 86
    classification 87
    contraction 83–5
    opposing groups 87
    relaxants 45
    skeletal 86–7
    types 83
myofilaments 83
myelin sheath 36

natural killer (NK) cells 144
nerve fibres 38
nerves, SNS 49–50
    efferent 48, 49
nervous
    impulse, the 41
        transmission of 45
    system *see* CNS
neural control of respiration 135
neuromuscular junction 43–4
neurones 34
    classification 36–8
neurophysiology 39
neurotransmitters 42–3
    muscle 84
    PNS 55
    SNS 54
neutrons 2–3
noradrenaline 54, 65
nose 130
    skin of 142
NSSI bodies 35
nucleus of a cell 13

oesophagus 116, 132
oestrogen 72
oestrus
    cycle 155–7
    suppressing after mating 160
olfaction 64
optic chambers 58
oral cavity *see* mouth
organs 23
    PNS and SNS 55
osmosis 5–6, 11, 12
ossification 80–1
osteocytes *see* bone
ovaries 72, 152
oviducts *see* fallopian tubes
ovulation 152–4
    see also mating
oxygen 129, 130

pain receptors 53
pancreas 119–20
parathyroid glands 69
parietal pleura 132
parturition 162
penis 152
peripheral nervous system *see* PNS

pH balance 127
phagocytic cells 144
phagocytosis 149
pharynx 116, 130
photoreceptors 57
pigmentation 141
pineal gland 69
pituitary gland 67–9
plasma 93–4
    membrane 10–13
platelets *see* thrombocytes
postganglionic neurone 53
potassium 39
PNS 45, 48–9, 53–5
    heart 102
    neurotransmitters 55
    and SNS integration 55
polyoestrus species 154
postsynaptic receptors 44–5
preganglionic neurone 53, 55
pregnancy 156, 157, 161–4
    false 161
pressure, units 10
progesterone 72
prostate gland 152, 160
protons 2–3, 6
pseudopregnancy 161
pulate, the 115–16
pulmonary
    circulation 100
    pleura 132
pulse 108

radioactive isotopes 3
radiography, diagnosing
    pregnancy 161
receptors
    alpha, beta 54
    in the ear 63
    pain 53
    postsynaptic 44–5
    sense of smell 64
    sensory 52–3
    see also photoreceptors
reflexes 50–2
reproduction 149–64
    controlling 159–60
respiratory system 127–35
    mechanism of 132–4
resting potential 39–41
retina 56, 57
ribosomes 13
rickets 141
RNA 134
rods, the eye 57, 58, 59

salivary glands 116, 118
sarcolemma 83
Schwann cells 35–6
scrotum 142, 150–1
sebaceous glands 140–1, 143, 144
sensation, skin 141
senses, special 55–64

sensory receptors 52–3
septicaemia 148
seratonin 69
shock 110–11
SI units 7
skeletal muscles 86–7
skeleton, the 77
skin
    functions 140
    specialization 141–14
    structure 139
small intestine 117–18
    secretions 119
smell, sense of 64
SNS 45–6, 49–50, 53
sodium 39–40
solutes 5
solvents 5
somatic nervous system *see* SNS
spaying 159
spermatozoa 150, 151–2
spinal
    cord 48
    nerves 49
    see also myelin sheath
spleen 149
stomach 116–17
subcutaneous layer 139
sweat glands 141, 142
sympathetic chain ganglia 54
synapse 41–2
synovial joints 88–90
systemic circulation 100

T-cells 146
T-lymphocytes 145
taste 64
teeth 114–15
temperature, converting 9
tendons 87, 91
terminology, anatomy 24
testes 72, 150–1
testosterone 72
thrombocytes 95, 97, 98
thoracic duct 148
thymus 70, 149
thyroid gland 69
tissue 17–22
    connective 20–2
    epithelium 18–20
    fluid, circulation 147–8
tongue 114–15
tonicity 5
trachea 132
transmembrane potential 39
tubular fluid *see* kidneys

ultrasound 161
units, converting 8–9
urethra 128, 152
urinary system 123–8
urine 128
uterus 154

valency of an atom 3
valves
    see heart valves; veins
vas deferens 152
vascular
    layer of the eye 57
    system 104–8
vasectomy 160
veins 105
visceral reflexes 55
vision 56

vitamin D 141
vitamins, absorption 121–2
vocal cords 132
vomiting 122
vagina 154

water, absorption 122
weight, converting 8
white blood cells *see* leucocytes